Recent Results in Cancer Research

Volume 212

Series editors

Alwin Krämer, German Cancer Research Center (DKFZ) and University of Heidelberg, Heidelberg, Germany

Jiade J. Lu, Shanghai Proton and Heavy Ion Center, Shanghai, China

More information about this series at http://www.springer.com/series/392

Uwe M. Martens

Editor

Small Molecules in Hematology

Third Edition

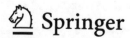

Editor
Uwe M. Martens
MOLIT Institute
Cancer Center Heilbronn-Franken,
  SLK-Clinics
Heilbronn, Baden-Württemberg
Germany

ISSN 0080-0015   ISSN 2197-6767   (electronic)
Recent Results in Cancer Research
ISBN 978-3-030-08256-7   ISBN 978-3-319-91439-8   (eBook)
https://doi.org/10.1007/978-3-319-91439-8

Preface

Over the past two decades, hematologic malignancies have been extensively evaluated by powerful technologies, evolving from conventional karyotyping and FISH analysis to high-throughput next-generation sequencing (NGS). These analyses have allowed to refine our understanding of the underlying disease mechanisms in leukemia and lymphomas, elucidating the roles of different pathways involved in carcinogenesis and enabling the development of molecularly targeted drugs.

One of the early pioneers has been imatinib mesylate (Glivec®), a first-generation small-molecule tyrosine kinase inhibitor (TKI), that showed remarkable efficacy for the treatment of patients with Philadelphia chromosome-positive CML, changing the course of this formerly deadly disease profoundly. Nowadays, second- and third-generation TKIs for the treatment of CML are already in clinical use. Also, the portfolio of targeted anticancer drugs has been further expanded by agents such as ibrutinib, idelalisib, and venetoclax that all target B-cell cancers by blocking the action of the BCL2 molecule—and even more agents are currently investigated in clinical trials.

With the third edition of "Small Molecules in Oncology series", we aim to give you a comprehensive survey of both, already established drugs as well as promising new substances. Therefore, all chapters of this book have been contributed by renowned scientists and clinicians, offering first-hand insight into the exciting and rapidly evolving field of targeted cancer therapies. Due to the tremendous amount of available agents, the book has been divided into two volumes, while "Small Molecules in Oncology" covers the treatment options in solid tumors and "Small Molecules in Hematology" focuses mainly on molecularly targeted drugs in hematologic malignancies.

Heilbronn, Germany   Uwe M. Martens

Contents

Imatinib Mesylate

Cornelius F. Waller

Contents

C. F. Waller (✉)
Department of Haematology, Oncology and Stem Cell Transplantation, Faculty of Medicine,
University Medical Centre Freiburg, University of Freiburg,
Hugstetter Str. 55, 79106 Freiburg, Germany
e-mail: cornelius.waller@uniklinik-freiburg.de

© Springer International Publishing AG, part of Springer Nature 2018
U. M. Martens (ed.), *Small Molecules in Hematology*, Recent Results
in Cancer Research 211, https://doi.org/10.1007/978-3-319-91439-8_1

Abstract

Imatinib mesylate (Gleevec, Glivec [Novartis, Basel, Switzerland], formerly referred to as STI571 or CGP57148B) represents the paradigm of a new class of anticancer agents, so-called small molecules. They have a high selectivity against a specific molecular target known to be the cause for the establishment and maintenance of the malignant phenotype. Imatinib is a rationally designed oral signal transduction inhibitor that specifically targets several protein tyrosine kinases, Abl, Arg (*Abl*-related gene), the stem cell factor receptor (c-KIT), platelet-derived growth factor receptor (PDGF-R), and their oncogenic forms, most notably BCR-ABL. Imatinib has been shown to have remarkable clinical activity in patients with chronic myeloid leukemia (CML) and malignant gastrointestinal stroma tumors (GIST) leading to its approval for treatment of these diseases. Treatment with imatinib is generally well tolerated with a low incidence of severe side effects. The most common adverse events include mild to moderate edema, muscle cramps, diarrhea, nausea, skin rashes, and myelosuppression. Several mechanisms of resistance have been identified. Clonal evolution, amplification, or overexpression of BCR-ABL as well as mutations in the catalytic domain, P-loop, and other mutations have been demonstrated to play a role in primary and secondary resistance to imatinib, respectively. Understanding of the underlying mechanisms of resistance has led to the development of new second- and third-generation tyrosine kinase inhibitors (see chapters on dasatinib, nilotinib, bosutinib, and ponatinib).

Keywords

CML · Tyrosine kinase inhibitor · Imatinib

1 Introduction

Chronic myeloid leukemia (CML) is a clonal disorder of the hematopoietic stem cell. The clinical presentation often includes granulocytosis, a hypercellular bone marrow, and splenomegaly. The natural course of the disease involves three sequential phases—chronic phase (CP), progressing often through an accelerated phase (AP) into the terminal blast crisis (BC). The duration of CP is several years, while AP and BC usually last only for months. In the past, prior to the introduction of TKIs into the treatment of CML, median survival was in the range of 4–5 years (Hehlmann et al. 2007b; Sawyers 1999).

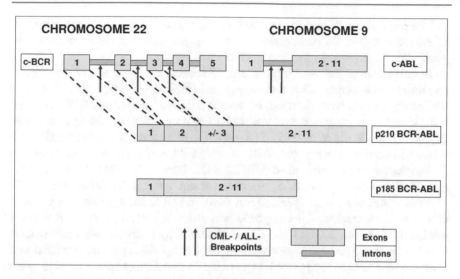

Fig. 1 Common breakpoints in CML and Ph⁺ ALL: In CML, *BCR* breakpoints occur after the second or third exon, whereas in Ph⁺ ALL, breaks can occur after the first exon. In *c-ABL*, a break occurs between the first and second exon (CML and Ph⁺ ALL)

CML is characterized by the presence of the Philadelphia chromosome (Ph), a unique reciprocal translocation between the long arms of chromosomes 9 and 22, t(9:22), which is present in >90% of patients with CML and approximately 15–30% of ALL (Nowell and Hungerford 1960; Rowley 1973). On the molecular level, t(9:22) results in the generation of an oncogene, the BCR-ABL fusion gene, encoding the BCR-ABL protein which has constitutive tyrosine kinase activity (Konopka et al. 1984; Fig. 1).

Its causal role in the development of CML has been demonstrated in vitro as well as in several animal models (Daley et al. 1990; Heisterkamp et al. 1990; Lugo et al. 1990; Voncken et al. 1995).

The pathological effects of BCR-ABL include increased proliferation, protection from programmed cell death, altered stem cell adhesion, and possibly genetic instability that leads to disease progression (Deininger and Goldman 1998; Deininger et al. 2000).

Before the introduction of imatinib, standard therapy of CML was interferon-α alone or in combination with cytarabine (ara-C) leading to hematologic remissions in the majority of patients, but major cytogenetic responses—i.e., <35% Ph⁺ metaphases—were only seen in 6–25% of patients (Hehlmann et al. 2007b). The only curative treatment of CML is allogeneic stem cell transplantation from an HLA-compatible donor. However, it is only an option for a part of the patients and still associated with considerable morbidity and mortality (Gratwohl et al. 1998; Hehlmann et al. 2007a).

The presence of BCR-ABL in >90% of CML patients and the identification of its essential role in the pathogenesis of the disease provided the rationale of targeting this fusion protein for treatment of CML.

In the nineties of the twentieth century, first data of compounds with an effect on tyrosine kinases were published (Levitzky and Gazit 1995). Tyrphostins and other similar compounds were shown to inhibit the ABL—as well as the BCR-ABL tyrosine kinase at micromolar concentrations but had only limited specificity (Anafi et al. 1993a, b; Carlo-Stella et al. 1999). This led to the rational design of further TKI with selective activity against the ABL tyrosine kinase, one of which was a 2-phenylaminopyrimidine called CGP57148B, later called STI571 or imatinib mesylate (Buchdunger et al. 1995, 1996; Druker and Lydon 2000; Druker et al. 1996).

After demonstration of specificity in vitro, in cell-based systems as well as in different animal models, this compound was tested in several phase I and phase II studies (Druker et al. 2001a; Kantarjian et al. 2002a, b). Imatinib was shown to have very high rates of hematologic remissions in CP-CML patients previously treated with interferon-α as well as in advanced stages of the disease. Cytogenetic remissions were achieved in a considerable portion of patients. Based on these good results, imatinib was approved for treatment of CML patients in CP after treatment failure with interferon-α and the advanced stages, i.e., AP and BC (Cohen et al. 2002b).

The phase III (IRIS-) trial led to establishment of imatinib as standard for first-line therapy of CP-CML (Cohen et al. 2009; Dagher et al. 2002; Hochhaus et al. 2017). The very good clinical results for imatinib of the IRIS trial were reproduced by several large phase III studies, including the German CML IV trial (Hehlmann et al. 2017). Patients who optimally respond to imatinib or next-generation TKIs have a near-normal life expectancy and, in this population, the impact of comorbidities on survival outcomes is considered as greater than that of CML itself. However, lifelong treatment is still recommended (Saußele et al. 2015, 2016; Rea and Mahon 2018).

Currently, several trials investigate the effect of stopping imatinib or second-generation TKIs in patients reaching a very good long-lasting remission based upon the results of the so-called STIM trial where it could be shown that approximately half of patients stayed in a very good molecular remission after the end of the therapy (Mahon et al. 2010; Etienne et al. 2017; Mahon et al. 2016; Rea et al. 2017). This has prompted the development of a new concept in the evaluation of CML patients known as "treatment-free remission" (Saußele et al. 2016).

Other molecular targets of imatinib are the stem cell factor receptor (c-KIT) and platelet-derived growth factor receptor (PDGF-R) (Buchdunger et al. 1995, 1996, 2000; Heinrich et al. 2002a, b).

c-KIT is expressed in a variety of human cancers, including germ cell tumors, neuroblastoma, melanoma, small cell lung cancer, breast and ovarian cancers, acute myeloid leukemia, mast cell disorders as well as malignant gastrointestinal stroma tumors (GIST). While in most of these diseases, the exact role of c-KIT expression is not defined, in mastocytosis and GISTs activating mutations of c-KIT have been identified.

Based upon data of a single open-label phase II trial and two large phase III trials by the EORTC and SWOG, imatinib received approval for treatment of metastatic/unresectable GIST (Cohen et al. 2009; Dagher et al. 2002). In addition, the role of neoadjuvant therapy and adjuvant treatment with imatinib after successful resection of primary GIST has been clearly demonstrated and led to its approval (Joensuu et al. 2012; von Mehren and Joensuu 2018). The duration of adjuvant imatinib therapy in patients with a substantial risk of recurrence should be at least 3 years. However, the optimal duration is unknown. As in CML, several resistance mutations in c-kit as well as in the PDGFRA have been identified in patients with GIST (von Mehren and Joensuu 2018).

Furthermore, imatinib has been successfully used in diseases with aberrant PDGF receptors. They have been shown to deregulate the growth of a variety of cancers, such as GIST; myeloproliferative disorders (Pardanani and Tefferi 2004), e.g., in hypereosinophilic syndrome (FIP1L1/PDGFRα-rearrangement), chronic myelomonocytic leukemia (CMML), harboring the activating translocations involving the PDGF receptor beta locus on chromosome 5q33 (FIP1/PDGFR-translocation); carcinomas; melanoma; gliomas; and sarcomas, including dermatofibrosarcoma protuberans (Barnhill et al. 1996; Greco et al. 2001).

In addition, in several non-malignant diseases, e.g., pulmonary veno-occlusive disease and pulmonary capillary hemangiomatosis imatinib, has a positive effect on the disease (Ogawa et al. 2017). Its role in the treatment of autoimmune disease has been investigated (Hoeper et al. 2013; Moinzadeh et al. 2013).

2 Structure and Mechanisms of Action

Imatinib mesylate is designated chemically as 4-[(4-methyl-1-piperazinyl)methyl]-N-[4-methyl-3-[[4-(3-pyridinyl)-2-pyrimidinyl] aminophenyl] benzamide methanesulfonate. Its molecular formula is $C_{29}H_{31}N_7O.CH_4SO_3$, and its relative molecular mass is 589.7 (Fig. 2).

Fig. 2 Structure of imatinib mesylate (formerly STI 571 bzw. CGP57148)

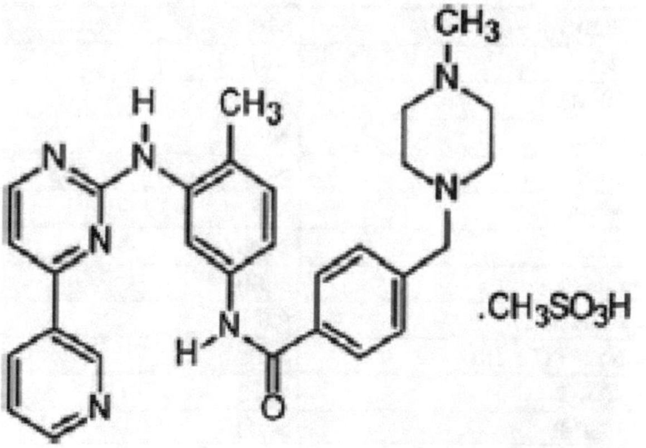

Imatinib functions as a specific competitive inhibitor of ATP. It binds with high affinity at the ATP binding site in the inactive form of the kinase domain, blocks ATP binding, and thereby inhibits kinase activity by interrupting the transfer of phosphate from ATP to tyrosine residues on substrate proteins (Cohen et al. 2002a, b, 2005; Lyseng-Williamson and Jarvis 2001; Mauro et al. 2002).

Imatinib selectively inhibits all the ABL tyrosine kinases, including BCR-ABL, cellular homolog of the Abelson murine leukemia viral oncogene product (c-ABL), v-ABL, TEL-ABL, and Abelson-related gene (ARG). In addition, it was found to potently inhibit the tyrosine kinase activity of the α- and β-platelet-derived growth factor receptors (PDGF-R) and the receptor for stem cell factor (c-KIT; CD117). The concentrations required for a 50% kinase inhibition were in the range of 0.025 μM in in vitro kinase assays and approximately 0.25 μM in intact cells. Extensive screening did not show activity against other tyrosine kinases or serine/threonine kinases (Buchdunger et al. 1995, 1996, 2000, 2001; Deininger et al. 2005; Druker and Lydon 2000; Druker et al. 1996; Heinrich et al. 2002a; Okuda et al. 2001; Table 1).

Table 1 Inhibition of protein kinases by imatinib mesylate (formerly STI 571 bzw. CGP57148) (adapted from Deininger et al. 2005)

Protein kinase	Substrate phosphorylation IC50[a] (μM)	Cellular tyrosine phosphorylation IC50[a] (μM)
c-abl	0.2; 0.025	ND
v-abl	0.038	0.1–0.3
p210[BCR→ABL]	0.025	0.25
p185[BCR→ABL]	0.025	0.25
TEL-ABL	ND	0.35
PDGF-Rα and β	0.38 (PDGF-Rβ)	0.1
Tel-PDGF-R	ND	0.15
c-KIT	0.41	0.1
FLT-3	>10	>10
Btk	>10	ND
c-FMS	ND	>10
v-FMS	ND	>10
c-SRC	>100	ND
v-SRC	ND	>10
c-LYN	>100	ND
c-FGR	>100	ND
LCK	9.0	ND
SYK (TPK-IIB)	>100	ND
JAK-2	>100	>100
EGF-R	>100	>100

(continued)

Table 1 (continued)

Protein kinase	Substrate phosphorylation IC50[a] (μM)	Cellular tyrosine phosphorylation IC50[a] (μM)
Insulin receptor	>10	>100
IGF-IR	>10	>100
FGF-R1	31.2	ND
VEGF-R1 (FLT-1)	19.5	ND
VEGF-R2 (KDR)	10.7	ND
VEGF-R3 (FLT-4)	5.7	ND
TIE-2 (TEK)	>50	ND
c-MET	>100	ND
PKA	>500	ND
PPK	>500	ND
PKC α, $\beta1$, γ, δ, ε, ξ, η	>100	ND
Protein kinase CK-1, CK-2	>100	ND
PKB	>10	ND
P39	>10	ND
PDK1	>10	ND
c-RAF-1	0.97	ND
CDC2/cyclin B	>100	ND

ND not done, PDGF-R platelet-derived growth factor receptor, Btk Bruton tyrosine kinase, TPK tyrosine-protein kinase, EGF-R epidermal growth factor receptor, IGF-IR insulin-like growth factor receptor I, FGF-R1 fibroblast growth factor receptor 1, VEGF-R vascular endothelial growth factor receptor, PKA cAMP-dependent protein kinase, PPK phosphorylase kinase; PKC protein kinase C, CK casein kinase, PKB protein kinase B (also known as Akt), PKD1 3-phosphoinoside-dependent protein kinase 1
[a]IC50 was determined in immunocomplex assays

Imatinib concentrations causing a 50% reduction in kinase activity (IC50) are given.

3 Preclinical Data

In vitro studies demonstrated specific inhibition of myeloid cell lines expressing BCR-ABL without killing the parental cell lines from which they were derived (Deininger et al. 1997; Druker et al. 1996; Gambacorti-Passerini et al. 1997). Continuous treatment with imatinib inhibited tumor formation in syngeneic mice as well as in a nude mouse model after inoculation of BCR-ABL-expressing cells in a dose-dependent manner, treated intraperitoneally or with oral administration of STI571, respectively (Druker et al. 1996; le Coutre et al. 1999). Activity on primary CML cells could be demonstrated, and a >90% reduction of BCR-ABL-expressing colonies in colony-forming assays from peripheral blood or bone marrow from CML patients was achieved at a concentration of imatinib of 1 μM while normal colonies did not show growth inhibition (Deininger et al. 1997; Druker et al. 1996; Gambacorti-Passerini et al. 1997).

4   Clinical Data in CML

4.1   Phase I Trials

In 1998, a phase I clinical trial with imatinib was initiated. This study was a dose escalation trial designed to determine the maximally tolerated dose, with clinical benefit as a secondary endpoint. 83 patients with CP-CML who had failed standard therapy with interferon-α (IFN-α) or were intolerant to it were enrolled. One-third of patients had signs of early progression to AP. They received escalating oral doses of imatinib, ranging from 25 to 1000 mg/day. Clinical features of patients were typical of the disease. Dose-limiting toxicity was not reached, although a higher frequency of severe toxicities was encountered at imatinib doses >750 mg/day. The most common adverse events were nausea (43%), myalgia (41%), edema (39%), and diarrhea (25%). After 29 patients were enrolled, therapeutic doses of 300 mg or more per day were reached. 53 of 54 patients achieved a complete hematologic response, reaching normal blood counts typically within four weeks of treatment. 51 of these 53 patients maintained normal blood counts after one year of therapy. Furthermore, these patients had a 31% rate of major cytogenetic responses (MCyR; <35% Ph$^+$ metaphases) and a 13% rate of complete cytogenetic responses (CCyR; eradication of Ph$^+$ bone marrow cells) (Druker 2008; Druker et al. 2001b).

In another phase I trial, patients with myeloid and lymphoid blast crisis and patients with relapsed or refractory Ph$^+$ lymphoblastic leukemia (ALL) were treated with daily doses of 300–1000 mg of imatinib. 55% of patients with myeloid blast crisis responded to therapy (45% of patients with <5% blasts in the bone marrow, and 11% reached a complete remission with full recovery of peripheral blood counts, respectively) but only in 18% response was maintained longer than one year.

Of 20 patients with Ph$^+$ ALL or lymphoid blast crisis, 70% responded, 20% reached a complete hematologic remission. Nevertheless, all but one relapsed between days 45 and 117 (Druker et al. 2001a).

Based on the results of the phase I trials, the use of imatinib was expanded to large phase II and phase III clinical trials.

4.2   Phase II Studies

Three open-label, single-arm phase II studies using imatinib as a single agent were conducted in patients with Ph$^+$ CML in three clinical settings: CML-CP after IFN-α failure or with intolerance to the drug, CML-AP, and CML-BC. Imatinib was administered orally once daily. Initially, all patients received 400 mg/day. Early in the study, however, the imatinib dose was increased to 600 mg daily for CML-AP and CML-BC trials. Patients with resistant or progressive disease receiving a dose of 400 or 600 mg/day could receive doses of 600 or 800 mg daily (administered as 400 mg twice daily).

In 532 patients with CP-CML who had failed IFN-α therapy, 95% of patients reached a complete hematologic response, with CCR rates of 41% and major cytogenetic remission (MCR) of 60%. The estimated rates of freedom from progression to accelerated or blastic phase and overall survival at 6 years were 61 and 76%, respectively (Druker 2008; Hochhaus et al. 2008; Kantarjian et al. 2002a).

For patients in BC and with Ph+ ALL, the studies confirmed the results of the phase I trial. Response rates were also high; however, relapses were seen frequently. The majority of patients in BC relapsed during the first year of treatment. Hematologic responses were observed in 52% of patients (n = 260) with myeloid BC, with a median response duration of 10 months. Interestingly, 48% of patients in this trial developed new cytogenetic abnormalities during treatment, demonstrating clonal evolution (Druker et al. 2001a; Ottmann et al. 2002; Sawyers et al. 2002).

The efficacy in patients with AP CML was intermediate between CP and BC. Of 181 patients with AP, 82% showed a hematologic response, 53% reached a CHR which was sustained in 69%. Major cytogenetic remissions were seen in 24% of patients with a CCR rate of 17% (Talpaz et al. 2002).

The treatment results in advanced phase CML and Ph+ ALL underline the necessity of combination therapies with conventional chemotherapy as well as the use of second-generation tyrosine kinase inhibitors.

The results of the phase I and phase II trials led to the approval by the Food and Drug Administration (FDA) of imatinib for the treatment of CML in advanced phase and after failure of IFN therapy in CP CML (Cohen et al. 2002b; Deininger et al. 2005; Druker 2008).

4.3 Phase III Study (IRIS Trial)

In a landmark phase III study, the International Randomized Study of Interferon and STI571 (IRIS) trial, imatinib and the combination of IFN plus cytarabine were compared in newly diagnosed CP-CML patients. More than 1000 patients were accrued in less than 7 months. 553 patients were randomized to each of the two treatments, imatinib at 400 mg per day or interferon-α plus Ara-C. There were no significant differences in prognostic or clinical features between the two treatment arms. After a median follow-up of 19 months, patients randomized to imatinib had significantly better results for CHR, MCR, and CCR, as well as progression-free survival than patients treated with interferon-α plus Ara-C (O'Brien et al. 2003a, b).

The remarkable superiority of imatinib led to early disclosure of study results. Thereafter, most patients were crossed over from interferon-α plus Ara-C to the imatinib arm.

The IRIS trial is now a long-term follow-up study of patients who received imatinib as initial therapy. After a follow-up of 5 years, the overall survival for newly diagnosed CP patients treated with imatinib was 89%. An estimated 93% of imatinib-treated patients remained free from disease progression to the AP or BC. The estimated annual rate of treatment failure was 3.3% in the first year, 7.5% in

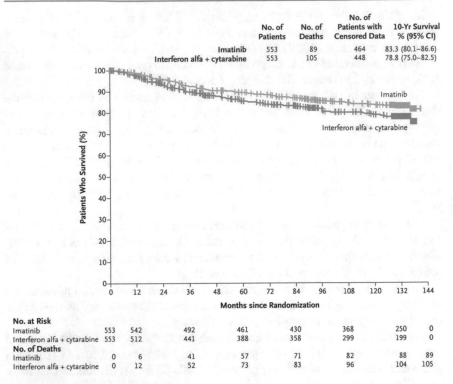

	No. of Patients	No. of Deaths	No. of Patients with Censored Data	10-Yr Survival % (95% CI)
Imatinib	553	89	464	83.3 (80.1–86.6)
Interferon alfa + cytarabine	553	105	448	78.8 (75.0–82.5)

No. at Risk

Imatinib	553	542	492	461	430	368	250	0
Interferon alfa + cytarabine	553	512	441	388	358	299	199	0

No. of Deaths

Imatinib	0	6	41	57	71	82	88	89
Interferon alfa + cytarabine	0	12	52	73	83	96	104	105

Fig. 3 Kaplan–Meier Estimated Overall Survival Rates at 10 Years in the Intention-to-Treat Population. Shown is the overall survival over time among patients assigned to each trial group. For the curve for the group of patients who had been randomly assigned to receive interferon alfa plus cytarabine, data include survival among the 363 patients who crossed over to imatinib (65.6%). These patients crossed over to imatinib after a median of 0.8 years of receiving interferon alfa plus cytarabine. In patients with no reported death (whether because they were known to be alive or because their survival status was unknown), survival was censored (tick marks) at the date of last contact. (Adapted from Hochhaus et al. NEJM 2017)

year two, 4.8% in year three, 1.5% in year four, and 0.9% in year five. The progression rate did not increase over time (Druker et al. 2006; Hochhaus et al. 2017; Fig. 3). Survival rates in the IRIS trial were especially high in patients who had a major molecular response at 12 months or 18 months and those with low Sokal scores. These results are consistent with previous reports from IRIS and other studies as, e.g., the CML IV trial showing that early response to TKI therapy is a valuable prognostic marker for long-term outcome (Hochhaus et al. 2017; Hehlmann et al. 2017).

Most of the side effects of imatinib were mild to moderate, with the most common being edema, muscle cramps, diarrhea, nausea, skin rashes, and myelosuppression (Druker et al. 2006; Hochhaus et al. 2017). Serious adverse cardiac events were reported in 7.1%. No new safety signals were observed after the 5-year analysis. Quality of life was far better in patients treated with imatinib (Hahn et al. 2003).

Table 2 Results from the IRIS trial (Druker et al. 2006; O'Brien et al. 2003a, b)

Timepoint of follow-up	First-line treatment	Estimated cumulative rate of CHR (%)	Estimated cumulative rate of MCR (%)	Estimated cumulative rate of CCR (%)	Progression-free survival (PFS) (%)	Freedom from progression to AP or BC (%)	OAS (%)	References
18 months	IFN + Ara-C n = 553	55.5	22.1	8.5	73.5	91.5		O'Brien et al. (2003a, b)
	Imatinib n = 553	95.3*	85.2*	73.8*	92.1	96.7		O'Brien et al. (2003a, b)
60 months	Imatinib	98	92	87	83	95.0	89.4	Druker et al. (2006)
10.9 years	Imatinib	98.6	89	82.8		92.4	83.3	Hochhaus et al. (2017)

*Statistically significant difference to treatment with IFN + Ara-C (p = 0.001)

Rates of hematologic and cytogenetic responses are shown in Table 2. A recent update at 10.9 years showed an estimated overall survival of 83.3% which is similar to the rate of 84% reported among patients who were treated with imatinib-based regimens in the German CML IV study, which was initiated shortly after IRIS to investigate alternative dosing strategies and drug combinations in patients with newly diagnosed CML in first chronic phase (Hehlmann et al. 2017). The estimated EFS at 10.9 years was 79.6%.

The estimated rate without progression to AP or BC is 93%. A CCR was achieved by 456 of 553 (82%) of patients on first-line imatinib (O'Brien et al. 2008).

Monitoring of residual disease by quantitative RT-PCR in complete cytogenetic responders showed that the risk of disease progression was inversely correlated with the reduction of BCR-ABL mRNA compared with pre-therapeutic levels (Hughes et al. 2003). The rates of major molecular remissions as well as the depth of molecular responses increase over time with a downward trend of relapse (O'Brien et al. 2008).

Investigation of pharmacokinetics in the imatinib-treated patients showed a correlation between imatinib trough plasma concentrations with clinical responses, EFS, and adverse events. Patients with high imatinib exposure had better rates of CCR, major molecular responses, and event-free survival (Larsen et al. 2008).

The results of the IRIS trial have led to FDA approval of imatinib for first-line treatment of patients with CP-CML in 2002 (Cohen et al. 2002b, 2005; Druker et al. 2001b).

5 Treatment Recommendations for the Use of Imatinib in Chronic Phase CML

Based upon the results achieved in the phase I, II, and III trials with imatinib, expert panels of the European Leukemia Net and the NCCN have developed guidelines for monitoring and treatment of CP-CML with imatinib (http://www.nccn.org/professionals/physician_gls/PDF/cml.pdf; Baccarani et al. 2013; http://www.nccn.org/professionals/physician_gls/PDF/cml.pdf; Table 3).

While the IRIS trial was performed, new guidelines for CML treatment were published and new BCR-ABL1 inhibitors dasatinib, nilotinib, bosutinib were developed. Nilotinib, dasatinib and bosutinib have been approved as first-line therapies in patients with CML in chronic phase based on results from phase III trials showing higher response rates than the comparator imatinib.

In case of suboptimal response to imatinib, a mutation analysis should be performed and treatment with a 2nd generation TKI such as dasatinib, nilotinib, bosutinib or third-generation TKI as ponatinib should be discussed as they are approved in this setting (see according chapters). Furthermore, the option of allogeneic stem cell transplantation should be considered. New third-generation TKI are currently under investigation.

Table 3 Response definitions to first-line treatment with TKIs (any TKI) (adapted from Baccarani et al. 2013)

Timepoint	Optimal response	Warning	Treatment failure
Baseline	NA	High risk or CCA/Ph$^+$ Major Route	NA
3 months	BCR-ABL1 $\leq$ 10% and/or Ph$^+$ $\leq$ 35%	BCR-ABL1 > 10% and/or Ph$^+$ 36–95%	Non-CHR and/or Ph$^+$ > 95%
6 months	BCR-ABL1 < 1% and/or Ph$^+$ 0	BCR-ABL1 1–10% and/or Ph$^+$ 1–35%	BCR-ABL1 > 10% and/or Ph$^+$ > 35%
12 months	BCR-ABL1 $\leq$ 0.1%	BCR-ABL1 > 0.1–1%	BCR-ABL1 > 1% and/or Ph$^+$ > 0
Any time point	BCR-ABL1 $\leq$ 0.1%	CCA/Ph$^-$ (−7, or 7q−)	Loss of CHR/CCgR
			Confirmed loss of MMR[a]
			Mutation
			CCA/Ph$^+$

CHR complete hematologic response
CCgR complete cytogenetic response (absence of Ph$^+$)
MMR major molecular response (ratio BCR-ABL/ABL > 0,10)
CCA/Ph$^+$ clonal chromosome abnormalities in Ph $^+$ cells
CCA/Ph$^-$ clonal chromosome abnormalities in Ph$^-$ cells
[a]In 2 consecutive tests, of which one with a BCR-ABL1 transcripts level $\geq$ 1%

6 Imatinib in Combination with Other Drugs

In order to further optimize the efficacy of imatinib in CML, a number of approaches have been investigated in phase II trials. Increase in the dose of imatinib monotherapy to 800 mg/d in CP-CML has shown earlier complete cytogenetic responses but is associated with more side effects (Cortes et al. 2003; Hehlmann et al. 2011; Hehlmann et al. 2017). In addition, imatinib in combination with other agents, such as interferon-α, cytarabine, and homoharringtonine, has been examined. Patients treated with combination therapy reached faster cytogenetic remission, but also experienced higher rates of toxicity, in particular myelotoxicity (Baccarani et al. 2003, 2004; Gardembas et al. 2003). Several major phase III trials compared standard dose imatinib with increased doses and combinations with cytarabine or interferon. In these trials, the induction of faster cytogenetic as well as molecular remissions could be shown in patients receiving higher dosages of imatinib. However, the increased dosage if imatinib as well as when used in combination with cytarabine was more toxic than standard dose (Hehlmann et al. 2017; Preudhomme et al. 2010).

7 Imatinib: Other Targets

Other molecular targets of imatinib are the platelet-derived growth factor receptor (PDGF-R) and the stem cell factor receptor (c-KIT) (Buchdunger et al. 1995, 2000; Heinrich et al. 2002a).

Aberrant PDGF receptors have been shown to deregulate the growth of a variety of cancers, such as myeloproliferative disorders (Pardanani and Tefferi 2004), e.g., in hypereosinophilic syndrome (FIP1L1/PDGFR-rearrangement) (Jovanovic et al. 2007), CMML involving the 5q33 translocations (Jovanovic et al. 2007), carcinomas, melanoma, gliomas, and sarcomas, including dermatofibrosarcoma protuberans (Barnhill et al. 1996; Greco et al. 2001).

c-KIT is expressed in a variety of human malignancies, including germ cell tumors, neuroblastoma, melanoma, small cell lung cancer, breast and ovarian cancer, acute myeloid leukemia, mast cell disorders, and malignant GIST.

In most of these diseases, the exact role of c-KIT expression is not defined in mastocytosis and GISTs, activating mutations of c-KIT have been identified (Heinrich et al. 2003a, b).

In approximately 60% of cases of GIST, there are mutations in c-kit[105] in the juxtamembrane domain. In most of the remaining cases, mutations in exon 13 and exon 9 have been found. The mutations lead to constitutive activation of the receptor without its ligand (Lux et al. 2000). Imatinib at a dosage of 400 mg once or twice daily was investigated in the EORTC 62,005 and S0033 trials. Both studies confirmed the benefit of imatinib 400 mg once daily, which was first reported in the B2222 study, (CR rates 3–6%, PR rates 45–48%, and SD rates 26–32%) (Verweij et al. 2004; Casali et al. 2015; Demetri 2002). No OS difference (47–55 months) was demonstrated between the 400 and 800 mg doses, establishing 400 mg once daily as the standard dose. Pooled analysis of the two EORTC trials showed that patients with exon 9 mutations treated with the higher imatinib dose had a longer PFS. These patients should therefore receive 2 mg × 400 mg, if tolerated. In the BFR14 trial patients were randomly assigned to stop therapy after 1, 3, or 5 years. Patients who stopped therapy had a shorter PFS compared with those who remained on treatment. These data support uninterrupted treatment with imatinib (von Mehren and Joentsuu 2018).

After approval of imatinib in metastatic GIST, the role of adjuvant treatment after successful resection was investigated.

In two of three randomized trials, adjuvant imatinib administered for 1 or 2 years improved recurrence-free survival compared with observation or placebo. However, an overall survival benefit was not demonstrated in either study. In the third trial, GIST patients with a high risk for relapse were randomized to receive adjuvant imatinib for 1 or 3 years after surgery, respectively. After a median follow-up of 7.5 years, patients who received 3 years of imatinib had longer recurrence-free survival while OS was comparable between both arms. In all three studies, patients with KIT exon 11 deletion mutations had the most benefit from adjuvant imatinib (Corless et al. 2014; Joensuu et al. 2012). Two further phase III trials are ongoing.

Table 4 Randomized trials that led to approval of imatinib (FDA) for advanced GIST (modified from von Mehren and Joentsuu 2018)

Trial/reference	Line of therapy	Allocation group	Median PFS	Median OS
B2222 van Oosterom et al. (2001), Blanke et al. (2008)	Imatinib, first line	Imatinib 400 versus 600 mg	20 versus 26 months ($p = 0.371$)	57 versus 57 months; HR, 0.87 ($p = 0.551$).
S0033 Demetri et al. (2002), Verweij et al. (2004)	Imatinib, first line	Imatinib 400 mg daily versus 400 mg twice daily	18 versus 20 months ($p = 0.13$)	55 versus 51 months; HR, 0.98; (95% CI, 0.79 to 1.21) ($p = 0.83$).
EORTC Casali et al. (2015)	Imatinib, first line	Imatinib 400 mg daily versus 400 mg twice daily	1.7 versus 2.0 years; HR, 0.91; (95% CI, 0.79–1.04) ($p = 0.18$)	3.9 years in both arms; HR, 0.93; (95% CI, 0.80–1.07) ($p = 0.31$)

Patients with a substantial risk for relapse should be treated for at least 3 years with imatinib. However, the optimal duration remains unknown. Mutation analysis of kit and PDGFRA is mandatory prior to initiation of adjuvant therapy because GISTs with PDGFRA D842 V mutation or lacking a mutation in KIT or PDGFRA are unlikely to benefit from adjuvant imatinib (see for review von Mehren and Joensuu 2018) (Table 4).

8 Side Effects/Toxicity

Hematologic side effects of imatinib are shown in Tables 5 and 6. Grade 3 or 4 neutropenia, thrombocytopenia, or anemia was seen in all phase II trials and the phase III study. While grade 3/4 neutropenia occurred in first-line treatment of CP-CML in about 17%, in accelerated and blastic phase, it could be detected in approximately 60% of patients. In addition, in advanced phase, CML thrombocytopenia and anemia are more frequently than in CP-CML (first or second line).

Typical non-hematologic side effects in phase II trials of imatinib in CML are shown in Table 5 (Cohen et al. 2002b, 2005; Guilhot 2004). In the IRIS trial, most of the side effects of imatinib were mild to moderate, with the most common being edema, muscle cramps, diarrhea, nausea, skin rashes, and myelosuppression as shown in Table 5 (Druker et al. 2006; O'Brien et al. 2003b).

Recently, it has been suggested that imatinib may cause cardiotoxicity (Kerkela et al. 2006). However, a preexisting condition predisposing to congestive heart failure (CHF) could not be excluded in these patients. Furthermore, a follow-up

Table 5 Adverse events >10% in the phase II CML trials (Guilhot 2004; Cohen et al. 2002a, b)

Reported or specified term	CML-CP[a] after IFN-failure/ intolerance		CML-AP[b]		CML-myeloid BC[b]	
	$N = 532$		$N = 235$		$N = 260$	
	Dosage: 400 mg		Dosage 600 mg: $n = 158$		Dosage 600 mg: $n = 223$	
			Dosage 400 mg: $n = 77$		Dosage 400 mg: $n = 37$	
	All grades (%)	Grades 3/4%	All grades (%)	Grades 3/4%	All grades (%)	Grades 3/4%
Hematologic adverse events						
Anemia		4		36		50
Neutropenia		33		58		62
Thrombocythemia		16		42		58
Non-hematologic AEs						
Nausea	60	2	71	5	70	4
Fluid retention	66	3	73	6	71	12
Superficial edema	64	2	71	4	67	5
Other fluid retention	7	2	7	2	22	8
Muscle cramps	55	1	42	0.4	27	0.8
Diarrhea	43	2	55	4	42	2
Vomiting	32	1	56	3	54	4
Hemorrhage	22	2	44	9	52	19
GI hemorrhage	2	0.4	5	3	8	3
CNS hemorrhage	1	1	2	0.9	7	5
Musculoskeletal pain	35	2	46	9	43	9
Skin rash	42	3	44	4	35	5
Headache	34	0.2	30	2	27	5
Fatigue	40	1	41	4	29	3
Arthralgia/joint pain	36	1	31	6	25	4
Dyspepsia	24	0	21	0	11	0
Myalgia	25	0.2	22	2	8	0
Weight gain	30	5	14	3	5	0.8
Pyrexia	17	1	39	8	41	7
Abdominal pain	29	0.6	33	3	31	6
Cough	17	0	26	0.9	14	0.8
Dyspnea	9	0.6	20	7	14	4
Anorexia	6	0	17	2	14	2
Constipation	6	0.2	15	0.9	15	2
Nasopharyngitis	18	0.2	16	0	8	0
Night sweats	10	0.2	14	1	12	0.8
Pruritus	12	0.8	13	0.9	8	1
Epistaxis	5	0.2	13	0	13	3

(continued)

Table 5 (continued)

Reported or specified term	CML-CP[a] after IFN-failure/ intolerance		CML-AP[b]		CML-myeloid BC[b]	
	N = 532		N = 235		N = 260	
	Dosage: 400 mg		Dosage 600 mg: n = 158		Dosage 600 mg: n = 223	
			Dosage 400 mg: n = 77		Dosage 400 mg: n = 37	
	All grades (%)	Grades 3/4%	All grades (%)	Grades 3/4%	All grades (%)	Grades 3/4%
Hypokalemia	5	0.2	8	2	13	4
Petechiae	1	0	5	0.9	10	2
Pneumonia	3	0.8	8	6	12	6
Weakness	7	0.2	9	3	12	3
Upper respiratory tract infection	15	0	9	0.4	3	0
Dizziness	13.0	0.2	12	0	11	0.4
Insomnia	13	0.2	13	0	10	0
Sore throat	11	0	11	0	8	0
Ecchymosis	2	0	6	0.9	11	0.4
Rigors	8	0	11	0.4	10	0
Asthenia	6	0	11	2	5	2
Influenza	10	0.2	6	0	0.8	0.4

CP chronic phase, *AP* accelerated phase; *BC* blast crisis, *AE* adverse event
[a]Adverse events considered possibly related to treatment
[b]All adverse events regardless of relationship to treatment

Table 6 Most frequently reported AEs: first-line imatinib at 7-year follow-up: (Druker et al. 2006; O'Brien et al. 2008)

Most common adverse events (by 5 years)	All grade AEs patients (%)	Grade 3/4 AEs patients (%)
Superficial edema	60	2
Nausea	50	1
Muscle cramps	49	2
Musculoskeletal pain	47	5
Diarrhea	45	3
Rash/skin problems	40	3
Fatigue	39	2
Headache	37	<1
Abdominal pain	37	4
Joint pain	31	3
Elevated liver enzymes	5	5
Hematologic toxicity		
Neutropenia	60.8	17
Thrombocytopenia	56.6	9
Anemia	44.6	4

Only serious adverse events (SAEs) were collected after 2005. Grade 3/4 adverse events decreased in incidence after years 1–2

examination of the Novartis database of imatinib clinical trials includ- '
ing >5600 years of exposure to imatinib found an incidence of CHF in imatinib
recipients of 0.2% cases per year with a possible or probable relationship to the
drug. In the IRIS trial, the incidence of cardiac failure and left ventricular dysfunction was estimated at 0.04% per year in the imatinib arm compared to 0.75% in
interferon-a- and ara-C-treated patients (Hatfield et al. 2007). The final analysis
after a median follow-up of 10.9 years showed cardiac SAEs, regardless of study
drug relationship in 7.1% of patients treated with frontline imatinib. Serious events
of a second neoplasm could be seen in 11.3%. No new safety signals were observed
since the 5-year analysis (Hochhaus et al. 2017).

In an early trial in GIST, adverse events were similar to CML patients and
included edema, fluid retention, nausea, vomiting, diarrhea, myalgia, skin rash,
bone marrow suppression, bleeding, and elevations in aspartate aminotransferase,
alanine aminotransferase, or bilirubin. Gastrointestinal bleeding or intratumoral
hemorrhage occurred in seven patients (5%) and was not correlated with thrombocytopenia or tumor bulk. Other non-hematologic side effects included fatigue and
gastrointestinal complaints which were usually mild to moderate. The most common laboratory abnormality was anemia. Fluid retention and skin rash were
reported more often in patients treated with 800 mg/day. Based upon these data,
escalation of imatinib dosing up to 800 mg/day for patients with progressive disease was approved (Blanke et al. 2008; Heinrich et al. 2008). However, 26% of
patients receiving imatinib for 3 years in the adjuvant setting discontinued treatment for causes other than relapse (Joensuu et al. 2012).

9 Clinical Pharmacology and Drug Interactions

Imatinib AUC is dose proportional at the recommended daily dose range of 400 and
600 mg. Within 7 days, approximately 81% of the dose is eliminated, 68% in feces,
and 13% in urine.

Cytochrome P450 (CYP3A4) is the major enzyme responsible for imatinib
metabolism, and both imatinib and CGP74588 appear to be potent in vitro CYP2D6
inhibitors. Imatinib plasma concentrations may be altered when the drug is administered with inhibitors or inducers of CYP3A4. When CYP3A4 inhibitors, e.g.,
itroconazole, ketoconazole, erythromycin, or clarithromycin, are co-administered
with imatinib, its metabolization may be decreased. CYP3A4 inducers, such as
dexamethasone, phenytoin, rifampicin, carbamazepine, phenobarbital, may increase
imatinib metabolism. Furthermore, increased plasma concentrations of drugs which
are substrates of CYP3A4, e.g., simvastatin, cyclosporine, and others, may be the
result of imatinib use (Cohen et al. 2002b, 2005; Lyseng-Williamson and Jarvis
2001; Mauro et al. 2002).

In a small number of children with Ph$^+$ ALL imatinib plasma levels as well as of
its metabolite CGP74588 were measured. Imatinib plasma levels were similar to
those in adult patients. However, AUC of CGP74588 was only 5–24% of the parent

drug's AUC, and it was eliminated much faster than in adults indicating a lesser role of the metabolite in antileukemic activity (Marangon et al. 2009).

In the phase III (IRIS) trial, the correlation of imatinib pharmacokinetics and the response to treatment as well as to side effects could be shown (Larsen et al. 2008).

10 Biomarkers

10.1 CML

10.1.1 Disease Progression and Imatinib Resistance

Resistance to imatinib includes de novo resistance and relapse after an initial response. The frequent and durable responses in CP-CML are caused by the selective inhibition of BCR-ABL by imatinib. In accelerated and blastic phase CML as well as in Ph$^+$ ALL, the combination of high numbers of proliferating tumor cells and genomic instability may lead to secondary genetic alterations, independent of BCR-ABL (von Bubnoff et al. 2003). In the majority of patients who respond to imatinib and then relapse, reactivation of the BCR-ABL tyrosine kinase could be shown. This indicates that BCR-ABL-dependent mechanisms either prevent imatinib from reaching its target or render the target insensitive to BCR-ABL. In the former category are mechanisms such as increased drug efflux through the multidrug resistance gene or protein binding of imatinib while the latter include mutations in the catalytic domain, the P-loop, and other mutations (Druker 2008; Gorre et al. 2001). Over 70 point mutations have been demonstrated to play a role in primary and secondary resistance to imatinib, respectively (Hochhaus et al. 2011; Fig. 4).

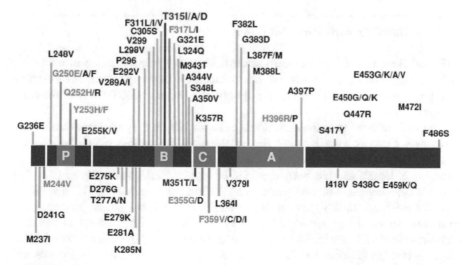

Fig. 4 Map of BCR-ABL kinase domain mutations associated with clinical resistance to imatinib (adapted from Branford and Hughes 2006). *P* P-loop, *B* imatinib binding site, *C* catalytic domain, *A* activation loop. Amino acid substitutions in *green indicate* mutations detected in 2–10% and in *red* in >10% of patients with mutations.

Gene amplification or overexpression of BCR-ABL as reason for resistance is seen occasionally (Shah et al. 2008; Shah and Sawyers 2003).

Understanding the underlying mechanisms of resistance has led to the development and investigation of new second- and third-generation tyrosine kinase inhibitors (Mueller 2009; Schiffer 2007) (see chapters bosutinib, dasatinib, nilotinib, and ponatinib).

10.2 GIST

Other molecular targets of imatinib are the platelet-derived growth factor receptor (PDGF-R) and the stem cell factor receptor (c-KIT) (Buchdunger et al. 1995, 2000; Heinrich et al. 2002a).

In GISTs, activating mutations of c-KIT and PDGF-R have been identified (Heinrich et al. 2003a, b).

In approximately 60% of cases of GIST, there are mutations in c-kit[105] in the juxtamembrane domain. In most of the remaining cases, mutations in exon 13 and exon 9 have been found. The mutations lead to constitutive activation of the receptor without its ligand (Lux et al. 2000). The mutational status is being used for the choice and duration of adjuvant therapy. In case of a PDGFRA D842V mutation, no adjuvant therapy is indicated. In the presence of wild-type kit, the situation has to be discussed on an individual base. In exon-11 and all mutations except exon-9 mutations, adjuvant therapy should be performed with 400 mg imatinib while in the presence of exon-9-mutations, 800 mg/d should be used (Joensuu et al. 2012; von Mehren and Joentsuu 2018).

11 Summary and Perspectives

The development of imatinib mesylate resembles the progress made in molecular biology over the past 30 years and has changed the landscape of cancer treatment leading toward causative treatment not only of CML and GIST but also for other malignancies.

After identification of the critical role of BCR-ABL in the pathogenesis of CML, less than 15 years went by until the development of imatinib which became the standard of care for patients in CP-CML. It has specific activity against a limited number of targets and has been shown to be highly effective not only in CML but also in other hematologic malignancies and solid tumors such as GIST. Side effects of treatment are mild to moderate. In addition to the originator product, after running out of the patent rights there are several generic versions of imatinib available in the EU and in the USA. The understanding of mechanisms of resistance and disease progression has furthermore lead to the development of second- and third-generation tyrosine kinase inhibitors which are even more effective in first-line therapy of CP-CML and have each a distinct profile of side effects.

References

Anafi M, Gazit A, Gilon C, Neriah YB, Levitzki A (1993a) Tyrphostin-induced differentiation of mouse erythroleukemia cells. FEBS Lett 330:260–264

Anafi M, Gazit A, Zehavi A, Ben-Neriah Y, Levitzki A (1993b) Tyrphostin-induced inhibition of p210bcr-abl tyrosine kinase activity induces K562 to differentiate. Blood 82:3524–3529

Baccarani M, Russo D, Rosti G, Martinelli G (2003) Interferon-alfa for chronic myeloid leukemia. Semin Hematol 40:22–33

Baccarani M, Martinelli G, Rosti G, Trabacchi E, Testoni N, Bassi S, Amabile M, Soverini S, Castagnetti F, Cilloni D et al (2004) Imatinib and pegylated human recombinant interferon-alpha2b in early chronic-phase chronic myeloid leukemia. Blood 104:4245–4251

Baccarani M, Deininger MW, Rosti G, Hochhaus A, Soverini S, Apperley JF, Cervantes F, Clark RE, Cortes JE, Guilhot F et al (2013) European LeukemiaNet recommendations for the management of chronic myeloid leukemia: 2013. Blood 122:872–884

Barnhill RL, Xiao M, Graves D, Antoniades HN (1996) Expression of platelet-derived growth factor (PDGF)-A, PDGF-B and the PDGF-alpha receptor, but not the PDGF-beta receptor, in human malignant melanoma in vivo. Br J Dermatol 135:898–904

Blanke CD, Rankin C, Demetri GD, Ryan CW, von Mehren M, Benjamin RS, Raymond AK, Bramwell VH, Baker LH, Maki RG et al (2008) Phase III randomized, intergroup trial assessing imatinib mesylate at two dose levels in patients with unresectable or metastatic gastrointestinal stromal tumors expressing the kit receptor tyrosine kinase: S0033. J Clin Oncol 26:626–632

Branford S, Hughes T (2006) Detection of BCR-ABL mutations and resistance to imatinib mesylate. Methods Mol Med 125:93–106

Buchdunger E, Zimmermann J, Mett H, Meyer T, Muller M, Regenass U, Lydon NB (1995) Selective inhibition of the platelet-derived growth factor signal transduction pathway by a protein-tyrosine kinase inhibitor of the 2-phenylaminopyrimidine class. Proc Natl Acad Sci U S A 92:2558–2562

Buchdunger E, Zimmermann J, Mett H, Meyer T, Muller M, Druker BJ, Lydon NB (1996) Inhibition of the Abl protein-tyrosine kinase in vitro and in vivo by a 2-phenylaminopyrimidine derivative. Cancer Res 56:100–104

Buchdunger E, Cioffi CL, Law N, Stover D, Ohno-Jones S, Druker BJ, Lydon NB (2000) Abl protein-tyrosine kinase inhibitor STI571 inhibits in vitro signal transduction mediated by c-kit and platelet-derived growth factor receptors. J Pharmacol Exp Ther 295:139–145

Buchdunger E, Matter A, Druker BJ (2001) Bcr-Abl inhibition as a modality of CML therapeutics. Biochim Biophys Acta 1551:M11–M18

Carlo-Stella C, Regazzi E, Sammarelli G, Colla S, Garau D, Gazit A, Savoldo B, Cilloni D, Tabilio A, Levitzki A, Rizzoli V (1999) Effects of the tyrosine kinase inhibitor AG957 and an Anti-Fas receptor antibody on CD34(+) chronic myelogenous leukemia progenitor cells. Blood 93:3973–3982

Casali PG, Le Cesne A, Poveda Velasco A, et al (2015) Time to definitive failure to the first tyrosine kinase inhibitor in localized GI stromal tumors treated with imatinib as an adjuvant: A European Organisation for Research and Treatment of Cancer Soft Tissue and Bone Sarcoma Group Intergroup randomized trial in collaboration with the Australasian Gastro-Intestinal Trials Group, UNICANCER, French Sarcoma Group, Italian Sarcoma Group, and Spanish Group for Research on Sarcomas. J Clin Oncol 33:4276–4283

Cohen MH, Dagher R, Griebel DJ, Ibrahim A, Martin A, Scher NS, Sokol GH, Williams GA, Pazdur R (2002a) US Food and Drug Administration drug approval summaries: imatinib mesylate, mesna tablets, and zoledronic acid. Oncologist 7:393–400

Cohen MH, Williams G, Johnson JR, Duan J, Gobburu J, Rahman A, Benson K, Leighton J, Kim SK, Wood R et al (2002b) Approval summary for imatinib mesylate capsules in the treatment of chronic myelogenous leukemia. Clin Cancer Res 8:935–942

Cohen MH, Johnson JR, Pazdur R (2005) U.S. Food and Drug Administration drug approval summary: conversion of imatinib mesylate (STI571; Gleevec) tablets from accelerated approval to full approval. Clin Cancer Res 11:12–19

Cohen MH, Farrell A, Justice R, Pazdur R (2009) Approval summary: imatinib mesylate in the treatment of metastatic and/or unresectable malignant gastrointestinal stromal tumors. Oncologist

Corless CL, Ballman KV, Antonescu CR et al (2014) Pathologic and molecular features correlate with long-term outcome after adjuvant therapy of resected primary GI stromal tumor: the ACOSOG Z900 trial. J Clin Oncol 32:1563–1570

Cortes J, Giles F, O'Brien S, Thomas D, Garcia-Manero G, Rios MB, Faderl S, Verstovsek S, Ferrajoli A, Freireich EJ et al (2003) Result of high-dose imatinib mesylate in patients with Philadelphia chromosome-positive chronic myeloid leukemia after failure of interferon-alpha. Blood 102:83–86

Dagher R, Cohen M, Williams G, Rothmann M, Gobburu J, Robbie G, Rahman A, Chen G, Staten A, Griebel D, Pazdur R (2002) Approval summary: imatinib mesylate in the treatment of metastatic and/or unresectable malignant gastrointestinal stromal tumors. Clin Cancer Res 8:3034–3038

Daley GQ, Van Etten RA, Baltimore D (1990) Induction of chronic myelogenous leukemia in mice by the P210bcr/abl gene of the Philadelphia chromosome. Science 247:824–830

Deininger MW, Goldman JM (1998) Chronic myeloid leukemia. Curr Opin Hematol 5:302–308

Deininger MW, Goldman JM, Lydon N, Melo JV (1997) The tyrosine kinase inhibitor CGP57148B selectively inhibits the growth of BCR-ABL-positive cells. Blood 90:3691–3698

Deininger MW, Goldman JM, Melo JV (2000) The molecular biology of chronic myeloid leukemia. Blood 96:3343–3356

Deininger M, Buchdunger E, Druker BJ (2005) The development of imatinib as a therapeutic agent for chronic myeloid leukemia. Blood 105:2640–2653

Demetri GD (2002) Identification and treatment of chemoresistant inoperable or metastatic GIST: experience with the selective tyrosine kinase inhibitor imatinib mesylate (STI571). Eur J Cancer 38(Suppl 5):S52–S59

Demetri GD, von Mehren M, Blanke CD, Van den Abbeele AD, Eisenberg B, Roberts PJ, Heinrich MC, Tuveson DA, Singer S, Janicek M et al (2002) Efficacy and safety of imatinib mesylate in advanced gastrointestinal stromal tumors. N Engl J Med 347:472–480

Druker BJ (2008) Translation of the Philadelphia chromosome into therapy for CML. Blood 112:4808–4817

Druker BJ, Lydon NB (2000) Lessons learned from the development of an abl tyrosine kinase inhibitor for chronic myelogenous leukemia. J Clin Invest 105:3–7

Druker BJ, Tamura S, Buchdunger E, Ohno S, Segal GM, Fanning S, Zimmermann J, Lydon NB (1996) Effects of a selective inhibitor of the Abl tyrosine kinase on the growth of BCR-ABL positive cells. Nat Med 2:561–566

Druker BJ, Sawyers CL, Kantarjian H, Resta DJ, Reese SF, Ford JM, Capdeville R, Talpaz M (2001a) Activity of a specific inhibitor of the BCR-ABL tyrosine kinase in the blast crisis of chronic myeloid leukemia and acute lymphoblastic leukemia with the Philadelphia chromosome. N Engl J Med 344:1038–1042

Druker BJ, Talpaz M, Resta DJ, Peng B, Buchdunger E, Ford JM, Lydon NB, Kantarjian H, Capdeville R, Ohno-Jones S, Sawyers CL (2001b) Efficacy and safety of a specific inhibitor of the BCR-ABL tyrosine kinase in chronic myeloid leukemia. N Engl J Med 344:1031–1037

Druker BJ, Guilhot F, O'Brien SG, Gathmann I, Kantarjian H, Gattermann N, Deininger MW, Silver RT, Goldman JM, Stone RM et al (2006) Five-year follow-up of patients receiving imatinib for chronic myeloid leukemia. N Engl J Med 355:2408–2417

Etienne G, Guilhot J, Rea D, Rigal-Huguet F, Nicolini F, Charbonnier A, Guerci-Bresler A, Legros L, Varet B, Gardembas M, Dubruille V, Tulliez M, Noel MP, Ianotto JC, Villemagne B, Carré M, Guilhot F, Rousselot P, Mahon FX (2017) Long-term follow-up of the french stop imatinib (STIM1) study in patients with chronic myeloid leukemia. J Clin Oncol 35(3):298–305. https://doi.org/10.1200/JCO.2016.68.2914 Epub 2016 Oct 31

Gambacorti-Passerini C, Le Coutre P, Mologni L, Fanelli M, Bertazolli C, Marchesi E, Di Nicola M, Biondi A, Corneo GM, Belotti D et al (1997) Inhibition of the ABL kinase activity blocks the proliferation of BCR/ABL + leukemic cells and induces apoptosis. Blood Cells Mol Dis 23:380–394

Gardembas M, Rousselot P, Tulliez M, Vigier M, Buzyn A, Rigal-Huguet F, Legros L, Michallet M, Berthou C, Cheron N et al (2003) Results of a prospective phase 2 study combining imatinib mesylate and cytarabine for the treatment of Philadelphia-positive patients with chronic myelogenous leukemia in chronic phase. Blood 102:4298–4305

Gorre ME, Mohammed M, Ellwood K, Hsu N, Paquette R, Rao PN, Sawyers CL (2001) Clinical resistance to STI-571 cancer therapy caused by BCR-ABL gene mutation or amplification. Science 293:876–880

Gratwohl A, Hermans J, Goldman JM, Arcese W, Carreras E, Devergie A, Frassoni F, Gahrton G, Kolb HJ, Niederwieser D et al (1998) Risk assessment for patients with chronic myeloid leukaemia before allogeneic blood or marrow transplantation. Chronic leukemia working party of the European group for blood and marrow transplantation. Lancet 352:1087–1092

Greco A, Roccato E, Miranda C, Cleris L, Formelli F, Pierotti MA (2001) Growth-inhibitory effect of STI571 on cells transformed by the COL1A1/PDGFB rearrangement. Int J Cancer 92:354–360

Guilhot F (2004) Indications for imatinib mesylate therapy and clinical management. Oncologist 9:271–281

Hahn EA, Glendenning GA, Sorensen MV, Hudgens SA, Druker BJ, Guilhot F, Larson RA, O'Brien SG, Dobrez DG, Hensley ML, Cella D (2003) Quality of life in patients with newly diagnosed chronic phase chronic myeloid leukemia on imatinib versus interferon alfa plus low-dose cytarabine: results from the IRIS Study. J Clin Oncol 21:2138–2146

Hatfield A, Owen S, Pilot PR (2007) In reply to 'Cardiotoxicity of the cancer therapeutic agent imatinib mesylate'. Nat Med 13, 13: author reply 15–16

Hehlmann R, Berger U, Pfirrmann M, Heimpel H, Hochhaus A, Hasford J, Kolb HJ, Lahaye T, Maywald O, Reiter A et al (2007a) Drug treatment is superior to allografting as first-line therapy in chronic myeloid leukemia. Blood 109:4686–4692

Hehlmann R, Hochhaus A, Baccarani M (2007b) Chronic myeloid leukaemia. Lancet 370:342–350

Hehlmann R, Lauseker M, Jung-Munkwitz S, Leitner A, Muller MC, Pletsch N, Proetel U, Haferlach C, Schlegelberger B, Balleisen L et al (2011) Tolerability-adapted imatinib 800 mg/d versus 400 mg/d versus 400 mg/d plus interferon-alpha in newly diagnosed chronic myeloid leukemia. J Clin Oncol 29:1634–1642

Hehlmann R, Lauseker M, Saußele S, Pfirrmann M, Krause S, Kolb HJ, Neubauer A, Hossfeld DK, Nerl C, Gratwohl A, Baerlocher GM, Heim D, Brümmendorf TH, Fabarius A, Haferlach C, Schlegelberger B, Müller MC, Jeromin S, Proetel U, Kohlbrenner K, Voskanyan A, Rinaldetti S, Seifarth W, Spieß B, Balleisen L, Goebeler MC, Hänel M, Ho A, Dengler J, Falge C, Kanz L, Kremers S, Burchert A, Kneba M, Stegelmann F, Köhne CA, Lindemann HW, Waller CF, Pfreundschuh M, Spiekermann K, Berdel WE, Müller L, Edinger M, Mayer J, Beelen DW, Bentz M, Link H, Hertenstein B, Fuchs R, Wernli M, Schlegel F, Schlag R, de Wit M, Trümper L, Hebart H, Hahn M, Thomalla J, Scheid C, Schafhausen P, Verbeek W, Eckart MJ, Gassmann W, Pezzutto A, Schenk M, Brossart P, Geer T, Bildat S, Schäfer E, Hochhaus A, Hasford J (2017) Assessment of imatinib as first-line treatment of chronic myeloid leukemia: 10-year survival results of the randomized CML study IV and impact of non-CML determinants. Leukemia 31(11):2398–2406. https://doi.org/10.1038/leu.2017.253 Epub 2017 Aug 14

Heinrich MC, Blanke CD, Druker BJ, Corless CL (2002a) Inhibition of KIT tyrosine kinase activity: a novel molecular approach to the treatment of KIT-positive malignancies. J Clin Oncol 20:1692–1703

Heinrich MC, Rubin BP, Longley BJ, Fletcher JA (2002b) Biology and genetic aspects of gastrointestinal stromal tumors: KIT activation and cytogenetic alterations. Hum Pathol 33:484–495

Heinrich MC, Corless CL, Demetri GD, Blanke CD, von Mehren M, Joensuu H, McGreevey LS, Chen CJ, Van den Abbeele AD, Druker BJ et al (2003a) Kinase mutations and imatinib response in patients with metastatic gastrointestinal stromal tumor. J Clin Oncol 21:4342–4349

Heinrich MC, Corless CL, Duensing A, McGreevey L, Chen CJ, Joseph N, Singer S, Griffith DJ, Haley A, Town A et al (2003b) PDGFRA activating mutations in gastrointestinal stromal tumors. Science 299:708–710

Heinrich MC, Owzar K, Corless CL, Hollis D, Borden EC, Fletcher CD, Ryan CW, von Mehren M, Blanke CD, Rankin C et al (2008) Correlation of kinase genotype and clinical outcome in the North American Intergroup Phase III Trial of imatinib mesylate for treatment of advanced gastrointestinal stromal tumor: CALGB 150105 Study by Cancer and Leukemia Group B and Southwest Oncology Group. J Clin Oncol 26:5360–5367

Heisterkamp N, Jenster G, ten Hoeve J, Zovich D, Pattengale PK, Groffen J (1990) Acute leukaemia in BCR/ABL transgenic mice. Nature 344:251–253

Hochhaus A, Druker B, Sawyers C, Guilhot F, Schiffer CA, Cortes J, Niederwieser DW, Gambacorti-Passerini C, Stone RM, Goldman J et al (2008) Favorable long-term follow-up results over 6 years for response, survival, and safety with imatinib mesylate therapy in chronic-phase chronic myeloid leukemia after failure of interferon-alpha treatment. Blood 111:1039–1043

Hochhaus A, La Rosee P, Muller MC, Ernst T, Cross NC (2011) Impact of BCR-ABL mutations on patients with chronic myeloid leukemia. Cell Cycle 10:250–260

Hochhaus A, Larson RA, Guilhot F, Radich JP, Branford S, Hughes TP, Baccarani M, Deininger MW, Cervantes F, Fujihara S, Ortmann CE, Menssen HD, Kantarjian H, O'Brien SG, Druker BJ, Investigators IRIS (2017) Long-term outcomes of imatinib treatment for chronic myeloid leukemia. N Engl J Med 376(10):917–927. https://doi.org/10.1056/NEJMoa1609324

Hoeper MM, Barst RJ, Bourge RC, Feldman J, Ghofrani HA, Galié N, Gómez-Sánchez MA, Grimminger F, Grünig E, Hassoun PM et al (2013) Imatinib mesylate as add-on therapy for pulmonary arterial hypertension results of the randomized IMPRES study. Circulation 127 (10):1128–1138

Hughes TP, Kaeda J, Branford S, Rudzki Z, Hochhaus A, Hensley ML, Gathmann I, Bolton AE, van Hoomissen IC, Goldman JM, Radich JP (2003) Frequency of major molecular responses to imatinib or interferon alfa plus cytarabine in newly diagnosed chronic myeloid leukemia. N Engl J Med 349:1423–1432

Joensuu H, Eriksson M, Sundby Hall K, Hartmann JT, Pink D, Schutte J, Ramadori G, Hohenberger P, Duyster J, Al-Batran SE et al (2012) One versus three years of adjuvant imatinib for operable gastrointestinal stromal tumor: a randomized trial. JAMA 307:1265–1272

Jovanovic JV, Score J, Waghorn K, Cilloni D, Gottardi E, Metzgeroth G, Erben P, Popp H, Walz C, Hochhaus A et al (2007) Low-dose imatinib mesylate leads to rapid induction of major molecular responses and achievement of complete molecular remission in FIP1L1-PDGFRA-positive chronic eosinophilic leukemia. Blood 109:4635–4640

Kantarjian H, Sawyers C, Hochhaus A, Guilhot F, Schiffer C, Gambacorti-Passerini C, Niederwieser D, Resta D, Capdeville R, Zoellner U et al (2002a) Hematologic and cytogenetic responses to imatinib mesylate in chronic myelogenous leukemia. N Engl J Med 346:645–652

Kantarjian HM, O'Brien S, Cortes JE, Smith TL, Rios MB, Shan J, Yang Y, Giles FJ, Thomas DA, Faderl S et al (2002b) Treatment of philadelphia chromosome-positive, accelerated-phase chronic myelogenous leukemia with imatinib mesylate. Clin Cancer Res 8:2167–2176

Kerkela R, Grazette L, Yacobi R, Iliescu C, Patten R, Beahm C, Walters B, Shevtsov S, Pesant S, Clubb FJ et al (2006) Cardiotoxicity of the cancer therapeutic agent imatinib mesylate. Nat Med 12:908–916

Konopka JB, Watanabe SM, Witte ON (1984) An alteration of the human c-abl protein in K562 leukemia cells unmasks associated tyrosine kinase activity. Cell 37:1035–1042

Larsen RA, Druker BJ, Guilhot F, O'Brien SG, Riviere GJ, Krahnke T, Gathmann I, Wang Y et al (2008) Imatinib pharmacokinetics and its correlation with response and safety in chronic phase chronic myeloid leukemia: a subanalysis of the IRIS study. Blood 111:4022–4028

Le Coutre P, Mologni L, Cleris L, Marchesi E, Buchdunger E, Giardini R, Formelli F, Gambacorti-Passerini C (1999) In vivo eradication of human BCR/ABL-positive leukemia cells with an ABL kinase inhibitor. J Natl Cancer Inst 92:163–168

Levitzky A, Gazit A (1995) Tyrosine kinase inhibition: an approach to drug development. Science 267:1782–1788

Lugo TG, Pendergast AM, Muller AJ, Witte ON (1990) Tyrosine kinase activity and transformation potency of BCR-ABL oncogene products. Science 247:1079–1082

Lux ML, Rubin BP, Biase TL, Chen CJ, Maclure T, Demetri GD, Xiao S, Singer S, Fletcher CD, Fletcher JA (2000) Kit extracellular and kinase domain mutations in gastrointestinal stromal tumors. Am J Pathol 156:791–795

Lyseng-Williamson K, Jarvis B (2001) Imatinib. Drugs 61:1765–1774

Mahon FX, Rea D, Guilhot J, Guilhot F, Huguet F, Nicolini F, Legros L, Charbonnier A, Guerci A, Varet B et al (2010) Discontinuation of imatinib in patients with chronic myeloid leukaemia who have maintained complete molecular remission for at least 2 years: the prospective, multicentre Stop Imatinib (STIM) trial. Lancet Oncol 11:1029–1035

Mahon FX, Richter J, Guilhot J, Hjorth-Hansen H, Almeida A, Janssen JWM, Mayer J, Porkka K, Panayiotidis P, Stromberg U, Berger MG, Diamond J, Ehrencrona H, Kairisto V, Machova Polakova K, Mueller MC, Mustjoki S, Hochhaus A, Pfirrmann M, Saussele S (2016) Cessation of tyrosine kinase inhibitors treatment in chronic myeloid leukemia patients with deep molecular response: results of the Euro-Ski trial. Blood, 128, abstract 787

Marangon E, Citterio M, Sala F, Barisone E, Lippi AA, Rizzari C, Biondi A, D'Incalci M, Zucchetti M (2009) Pharmacokinetic profile of imatinib mesylate and N-demethyl-imatinib (CGP74588) in children with newly diagnosed Ph + acute leukemias. Cancer Chemother Pharmacol 63:563–566

Mauro MJ, O'Dwyer M, Heinrich MC, Druker BJ (2002) STI571: a paradigm of new agents for cancer therapeutics. J Clin Oncol 20:325–334

Moinzadeh P, Hunzelmann N, Krieg T (2013) Pharmacology and rationale for imatinib in the treatment of scleroderma. J Exp Pharmacol 5:15–22

Mueller BA (2009) Imatinib and its successors: how modern chemistry has changed drug development. Curr Pharm Design 15:120–133

NCCN Practice Guidelines in Oncology, v. 3 (2018). https://www.nccn.org/professionals/physician_gls/pdf/cml.pdf

NCCN_Practice_Guidelines_in_Oncology, v. 1 (2018). https://www.nccn.org/professionals/physician_gls/#site

Nowell PC, Hungerford DA (1960) A minute chromosome in human chronic granulocytic leukemia. Science 132:1497

O'Brien SG, Guilhot F, Goldman J, Hochhaus A, Hughes T, Radich J, Rudoltz M, Filian J, Gathmann I, Druker B et al (2008) International randomized study of interferon versus STI571 (IRIS) 7-year follow-up: sustained survival, low rate of transformation and increased rate of major molecular response (MMR) in patients (pts) with newly diagnosed chronic myeloid leukemia in chronic phase (CML-CP) treated with imatinib (IM). Blood 112:76

O'Brien S, Giles F, Talpaz M, Cortes J, Rios MB, Shan J, Thomas D, Andreeff M, Kornblau S, Faderl S et al (2003a) Results of triple therapy with interferon-alpha, cytarabine, and homoharringtonine, and the impact of adding imatinib to the treatment sequence in patients with Philadelphia chromosome-positive chronic myelogenous leukemia in early chronic phase. Cancer 98:888–893

O'Brien SG, Guilhot F, Larson RA, Gathmann I, Baccarani M, Cervantes F, Cornelissen JJ, Fischer T, Hochhaus A, Hughes T et al (2003b) Imatinib compared with interferon and low-dose cytarabine for newly diagnosed chronic-phase chronic myeloid leukemia. N Engl J Med 348:994–1004

Ogawa A, Miyaji K, Matsubara H (2017) Efficacy and safety of long-term imatinib therapy for patients with pulmonary veno-occlusive disease and pulmonary capillary hemangiomatosis. Respir Med 131:215–219. https://doi.org/10.1016/j.rmed.2017.08.032 Epub 2017 Sep 12

Okuda K, Weisberg E, Gilliland DG, Griffin JD (2001) ARG tyrosine kinase activity is inhibited by STI571. Blood 97:2440–2448

Ottmann OG, Druker BJ, Sawyers CL, Goldman JM, Reiffers J, Silver RT, Tura S, Fischer T, Deininger MW, Schiffer CA et al (2002) A phase 2 study of imatinib in patients with relapsed or refractory Philadelphia chromosome-positive acute lymphoid leukemias. Blood 100: 1965–1971

Pardanani A, Tefferi A (2004) Imatinib targets other than BCR/ABL and their clinical relevance in myeloid disorders. Blood 104:1931–1939

Preudhomme C, Guilhot J, Nicolini FE, Guerci-Bresler A, Rigal-Huguet F, Maloisel F, Coiteux V, Gardembas M, Berthou C, Vekhoff A et al (2010) Imatinib plus peginterferon alfa-2a in chronic myeloid leukemia. N Engl J Med 363:2511–2521

Rea D, Nicolini FE, Tulliez M, Guilhot F, Guilhot J, Guerci-Bresler A, Gardembas M, Coiteux V, Guillerm G, Legros L, Etienne G, Pignon JM, Villemagne B, Escoffre-Barbe M, Ianotto JC, Charbonnier A, Johnson-Ansah H, Noel MP, Rousselot P, Mahon FX; France Intergroupe des Leucémies Myéloïdes Chroniques (2017) Discontinuation of dasatinib or nilotinib in chronic myeloid leukemia: interim analysis of the STOP 2G-TKI study. Blood. 16;129(7):846–854. https://doi.org/10.1182/blood-2016-09-742205 Epub 2016 Dec 8

Rea D, Mahon FX (2018) How I manage relapse of chronic myeloid leukaemia after stopping tyrosine kinase inhibitor therapy. Br J Haematol 180(1):24–32. https://doi.org/10.1111/bjh. 14973 Epub 2017 Oct 19

Rowley JD (1973) A new consistent abnormality in chronic myelogenous leukaemia identified by quinacrine fluorescence and Giemsa staining. Nature 243:290–293

Saußele S, Krauss MP, Hehlmann R, Lauseker M, Proetel U, Kalmanti L, Hanfstein B, Fabarius A, Kraemer D, Berdel WE, Bentz M, Staib P, de Wit M, Wernli M, Zettl F, Hebart HF, Hahn M, Heymanns J, Schmidt-Wolf I, Schmitz N, Eckart MJ, Gassmann W, Bartholom€aus A, Pezzutto A, Leibundgut EO, Heim D, Krause SW, Burchert A, Hofmann WK, Hasford J, Hochhaus A, Pfirrmann M, M€uller MC Schweizerische Arbeitsgemeinschaft fur Klinische Krebsforschung and the German CML Study Group (2015) Impact of comorbidities on overall survival in patients with chronic myeloid leukemia: results of the randomized CML study IV. Blood 126:42–49

Saußele S, Richter J, Hochhaus A, Hochhaus A, Mahon FX (2016) The concept of treatment-free remission in chronic myeloid leukemia. Leukemia 30(8):1638–1647. https://doi.org/10.1038/ leu.2016.115 Epub 2016 May 2

Sawyers CL (1999) Chronic myeloid leukemia. N Engl J Med 340:1330–1340

Sawyers CL, Hochhaus A, Feldman E, Goldman JM, Miller CB, Ottmann OG, Schiffer CA, Talpaz M, Guilhot F, Deininger MW et al (2002) Imatinib induces hematologic and cytogenetic responses in patients with chronic myelogenous leukemia in myeloid blast crisis: results of a phase II study. Blood 99:3530–3539

Schiffer CA (2007) BCR-ABL tyrosine kinase inhibitors in chronic myelogenous leukemia. N Engl J Med 357:258–265

Shah NP, Sawyers CL (2003) Mechanisms of resistance to STI571 in Philadelphia chromosome-associated leukemias. Oncogene 22:7389–7395

Shah NP, Kantarjian HM, Kim DW, Rea D, Dorlhiac-Llacer PE, Milone JH, Vela-Ojeda J, Silver RT, Khoury HJ, Charbonnier A et al (2008) Intermittent target inhibition with dasatinib

100 mg once daily preserves efficacy and improves tolerability in imatinib-resistant and intolerant chronic-phase chronic myeloid leukemia. J Clin Oncol 26:3204–3212

Talpaz M, Silver RT, Druker BJ, Goldman JM, Gambacorti-Passerini C, Guilhot F, Schiffer CA, Fischer T, Deininger MW, Lennard AL et al (2002) Imatinib induces durable hematologic and cytogenetic responses in patients with accelerated phase chronic myeloid leukemia: results of a phase 2 study. Blood 99:1928–1937

Verweij J, Casali PG, Zalcberg J, et al. (2004) Progression-free survival in gastrointestinal stromal tumours with high-dose imatinib: Randomised trial. Lancet 364:1127–1134

von Bubnoff N, Peschel C, Duyster J (2003) Resistance of Philadelphia-chromosome positive leukemia towards the kinase inhibitor imatinib (STI571, Glivec): a targeted oncoprotein strikes back. Leukemia 17:829–838

von Mehren M, Joensuu H. (2018) Gastrointestinal Stromal Tumors. J Clin Oncol. 10; 36(2):136–143. https://doi.org/10.1200/jco.2017.74.9705 Epub 2017 Dec 8

van Oosterom AT, Judson I, Verweij J, et al. (2001) Safety and efficacy of imatinib (STI571) in metastatic gastrointestinal stromal tumours: A phase I study. Lancet 358:1421–1423

Voncken JW, Kaartinen V, Pattengale PK, Germeraad WT, Groffen J, Heisterkamp N (1995) BCR/ABL P210 and P190 cause distinct leukemia in transgenic mice. Blood 86:4603–4611

Dasatinib

Markus Lindauer and Andreas Hochhaus

Contents

M. Lindauer (✉)
Klinik für Innere Medizin III, Klinikum am Gesundbrunnen, Am Gesundbrunnen 20–24,
74078 Heilbronn, Germany
e-mail: markus.lindauer@slk-kliniken.de

A. Hochhaus
Abteilung Hämatologie/Onkologie, Klinik für Innere Medizin II, Universitätsklinikum Jena,
Erlanger Allee 101, 07740 Jena, Germany
e-mail: andreas.hochhaus@med.uni-jena.de

Abstract

Dasatinib is an oral available short-acting inhibitor of multiple tyrosine kinases.
It was designed to inhibit ABL and SRC, but also has activity in multiple other
kinases, including c-KIT, PDGFR-α, PDGFR-β, and ephrin receptor kinases.
Dasatinib is a very potent inhibitor of BCR-ABL and an effective treatment for
the BCR-ABL-driven diseases chronic myeloid leukemia (CML) and
Philadelphia-chromosome-positive acute lymphoblastic leukemia (Ph+ ALL),
characterized by the constitutively active tyrosine kinase, BCR-ABL. Dasatinib
is approved for the treatment of CML (all phases) including children and for the
treatment of Ph+ ALL, resistant or intolerant to prior imatinib treatment.
Randomized trials in CML comparing dasatinib with imatinib show that first-line
dasatinib causes significantly deeper and faster molecular remissions. In
accelerated and blastic phase CML, as well as in Ph+ ALL, dasatinib frequently
induces complete hematologic and cytogenetic remissions even in imatinib
pretreated patients. Remissions however are often short. Dasatinib is administered independent of food intake as a once-daily dose of 100 mg in chronic
phase CML and 140 mg in Ph+ ALL or blastic phase. Side effects of dasatinib
are frequent but mostly moderate and manageable and include cytopenias and
pleural effusions. The review presents the preclinical and clinical activity of
dasatinib with a focus on clinical studies in CML.

Keyword

Chronic myeloid leukemia · Tyrosine kinase inhibitor · Dasatinib

Abbreviations

ALL   Acute lymphoblastic leukemia
AML   Acute myeloid leukemia

AP   Accelerated phase
BID   Twice daily
BP   Blast phase
CCyC   Complete cytogenetic response
CEL   Chronic eosinophilic leukemia
CHR   Complete hematologic response
CLL   Chronic lymphocytic leukemia
CML   Chronic myeloid leukemia
CMML   Chronic myelomonocytic leukemia
CP   Chronic phase
CR   Complete response
CRI   Complete response with incomplete hematologic recovery
CRPC   Castration-resistant prostate cancer
HES   Hypereosinophilic syndrome
MDS   Myelodysplastic syndrome
MMR   Major molecular response
OS   Overall survival
PFS   Progression-free survival
Ph+   Philadelphia chromosome positive
PMF   Primary myelofibrosis
PR   Partial remission
QD   Daily
SD   Stable disease
SM   Systemic mastocytosis
TKI   Tyrosine kinase inhibitor

1 Introduction

Dasatinib is a potent multikinase inhibitor targeting BCR-ABL, the SRC family of kinases (SRC, LCK, HCK, YES, FYN, FGR, BLK, LYN, FRK), receptor tyrosine kinases (c-KIT, PDGFR, DDR1 and 2, c-FMS, ephrin receptors), and TEC family kinases (TEC and BTK). It was discovered in the Bristol-Myers Squibb research laboratories as part of an effort to develop potent inhibitors of SRC family kinases (SFKs). Dasatinib was named after Jagabandhu Das who suggested some crucial improvements in the development of the molecule (Lombardo et al. 2004; Das et al. 2006).

Most important is dasatinib's potent, short-acting inhibition of BCR-ABL. BCR-ABL is a chimeric fusion protein resulting from the chromosomal translocation t(9;22)(q34;q11), the so-called Philadelphia Chromosome (Tokarsky et al. 2006). Functional BCR-ABL is a constitutively active ABL tyrosine kinase and an active driver in chronic myeloid leukemia (CML) and in Philadelphia-chromosome-positive (Ph+) acute Lymphoblastic leukemia (ALL).

Dasatinib as BCR-ABL inhibitor is effective in the treatment of adults with newly diagnosed Philadelphia-chromosome-positive (Ph+) CML in all phases of the disease, e.g., chronic (CP), accelerated (AP), blast phase (BP; myeloid or lymphoid) Ph+ CML, and Ph+ ALL (Sprycel® BMS 2017; Hochhaus and Kantarjian 2013). Only recently it was approved by the FDA for treatment of children in CML-CP.

Dasatinib is also an inhibitor of SRC family kinases. Located closely to the inner side of the plasma membrane, SRC family kinases are involved in complex signal transduction. Via SRC inhibition, dasatinib blocks cell duplication, migration, and invasion, and it triggers apoptosis of tumor cells. It also diminishes metastatic spread of tumor cells and acts on the tumoral microenvironment. In addition, it sensitizes and resensitizes tumor cells to chemotherapy, antiangiogenetic, antihormonal, or epidermal growth factor receptor (EGFR) inhibitor therapy (Montero et al. 2011). Despite those most important effects in oncogenesis and antitumoral therapy, SRC inhibitors have failed to demonstrate benefit in clinical trials so far. This is not only true for dasatinib, but also for other SRC inhibitors like saracatinib, bosutinib, and KX01 (Zhang and Yu 2012; Creedon and Brunton 2012).

Since SRC inhibition in clinical trials is much more difficult than anticipated, there is a need for good biomarkers to select patients who eventually will benefit from SRC inhibitor therapies.

Dasatinib inhibits several receptor tyrosine kinases, including the c-KIT receptor tyrosine kinase, involved in proliferation, differentiation, and survival of cells. Activating mutations of c-KIT are associated with different human neoplasms, including the majority of patients with systemic mast cell disorders, acute myelogenous leukemia (AML), and gastrointestinal stromal tumors (GISTs). Gain-of-function mutations of c-KIT are inhibited by dasatinib (Schittenhelm et al. 2006). Clinical studies to explore the relevance of c-KIT inhibition by dasatinib are underway with focus on acute myeloid leukemia.

2 Structure and Mechanism of Action

Dasatinib (former BMS 354825), or N-(2-chloro-6-methyl-phenyl)-2-(6-(4-(2-hydroxyethyl)-piperazin-1-yl)-2-methylpyrimidin-4-ylamino) thiazole-5-carboxamide monohydrate (C22H26ClN7O2S), is an orally available small-molecule multitargeted kinase inhibitor (Fig. 1).

The compound targets the SRC family of kinases (SRC, LCK, HCK, YES, FYN, FGR, BLK, LYN, FRK). In addition, and clinically more significant, dasatinib inhibits BCR-ABL with greater potency compared to other BCR-ABL inhibitors.

It also inhibits receptor tyrosine kinases (c-KIT, PDGFR, DDR1 and 2, c-FMS, ephrin receptors) and TEC family kinases (TEC and BTK) (Table 1).

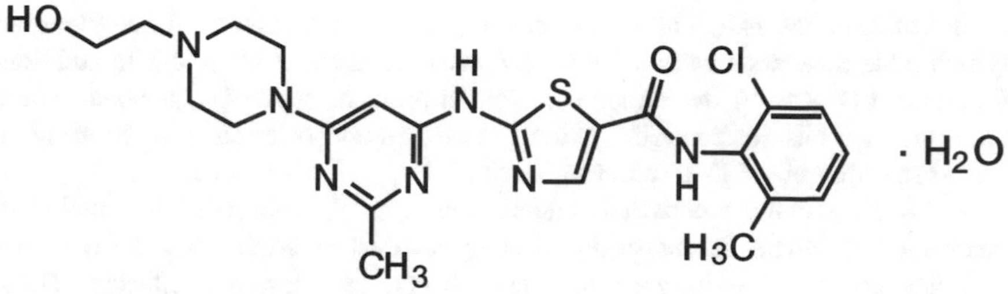

Fig. 1 Chemical structure of dasatinib

Table 1 Inhibitory activity of dasatinib on selected tyrosine kinases and potential clinical applications

Kinase	IC$_{50}$ (nmol)	Potential clinical applications	Reference
Nonreceptor tyrosine kinases			
ABL	0.6	CML, Ph+ ALL	Lombardo et al. (2004)
SRC	0.5	Several tumors, hematopoietic neoplasias	Lombardo et al. (2004) and O'Hare et al. (2005)
LYN	2.8		
LCK	0.4		Lombardo et al. (2004)
YES	0.5		Lombardo et al. (2004)
BTK	5	CLL, B-cell lymphomas	Hantschel et al. (2007)
TEC	14		Hantschel et al. (2007)
Receptor tyrosine kinases			
KIT	5–10	GIST, CML, breast cancer, AML, systemic mastocytosis	Lombardo et al. (2004)
Ephrin A2 receptor kinase	17	Breast cancer, lung cancer	Huang et al. (2007)
Ephrin B2 receptor kinase	17		Chang et al. (2008)
PDGFR-β	4–28	GIST, breast cancer, head and neck cancer	Lombardo et al. (2004)
		Chronic eosinophilic leukemia, hypereosinophilic syndrome	Chen et al. (2006)

Preclinical studies suggest that dasatinib induces apoptosis in only a small subset of cell lines. Inhibition of migration, invasion, and cell adhesion by dasatinib is reported more frequently (Johnson et al. 2005; Nam et al. 2005; Serrels et al. 2006).

It has been demonstrated that dasatinib induces defects in spindle generation, cell cycle arrest, and centrosome alterations in leukemic cells, tumor cell lines, and also in normal cells. These effects are not attributable to the inhibition of a single kinase; rather, it is expression of nonspecific effects on multiple kinases (Fabarius et al. 2008).

In a nude mouse model of prostate cancer, tumor growth and the development of lymph node metastasis were inhibited by dasatinib (Park et al. 2008). In addition, dasatinib acts also on the tumoral microenvironment, especially in bone, where dasatinib inhibits osteoclastic activity and favors osteogenesis, exerting a bone-protecting effect (Metcalf et al. 2002).

Although immunosuppressive effects were initially observed in preclinical studies of dasatinib, recent evidence suggests that dasatinib may activate and mobilize antileukemic immune responses which may improve efficacy. These immunomodulatory effects may also be implicated in the clinically relevant side effects observed with dasatinib treatment (Mustjoki et al. 2013; Kreutzman et al. 2010; Qiu et al. 2014).

3 Preclinical Data

3.1 Inhibition of ABL

Dasatinib was designed as an ATP-competitive inhibitor of SRC and ABL. Abelson kinase (ABL) is the constitutively active tyrosine kinase of the BCR-ABL fusion protein. It is a cytoplasmic nonreceptor tyrosine kinase. Human ABL has a number of structural domains critical for its activity. The major isoform of c-ABL has three SRC homology (SH) domains. The SH1 domain contains the tyrosine kinase activity, while SH2 and SH3 domains allow interaction with other proteins. Under normal conditions, the activity of the ABL tyrosine kinase is tightly regulated.

Like many tyrosine kinases, ABL regulates its catalytic activity via conformational changes, switching between active and inactive forms by opening and closing an activation loop. The sequence available for binding in the inactive conformation varies dramatically between different kinases and provides a potential for binding specificity.

As demonstrated by X-ray crystallography, dasatinib, unlike imatinib, nilotinib, and ponatinib, binds the ATP-binding pocket of the SH1 domain of BCR-ABL in both the active and inactive conformations (Tokarski et al. 2006; Vajpai et al. 2008; O'Hare et al. 2005).

Dasatinib has been shown to be 325-fold more potent than imatinib for inhibiting unmutated BCR-ABL. The concentration required for 50% inhibition [IC50] is 0.6 nmol/L for dasatinib and 280 nmol/L for imatinib (O'Hare et al. 2005). It is suggested that this stronger binding activity of dasatinib over imatinib is at least partially due to its ability to bind to active and inactive conformations of the ABL protein.

Crystal structures of the inhibitors bound to ABL show that dasatinib has fewer interactions with the P-loop, the activation loop, and α-helix compared with imatinib (Tokarski et al. 2006). Mutations resistant to imatinib but sensitive to dasatinib can be found in these regions (Tokarski et al. 2006). This is the basis for the activity of the drug in imatinib-resistant disease, caused by mutated BCR-ABL. Dasatinib demonstrates activity against most imatinib-resistant BCR-ABL mutations (Karaman et al. 2008; Shah et al. 2004).

Based on in vitro assays, outcomes in patients treated with second-line dasatinib after developing a BCR-ABL mutation on imatinib, and emergence of mutations during dasatinib treatment, dasatinib has little or no activity against T315I/A F317L/I/C/V, or V299L, and lower activity against Q252H, E255 V/K, and possibly G250E (O'Hare et al. 2005; Redaelli et al. 2009; Hochhaus et al. 2012; Müller et al. 2009; Soverini et al. 2009; Shah et al. 2007; Cortes et al. 2007a).

3.2 Inhibition of SRC

SRC is a member of a nine-gene family (SRC family kinases, SFK) that includes YES, FYN, LYN, LCK, HCK, FGR, BLK, and YRK.

SRC family kinases are membrane-associated and involved in signal transduction. They integrate and regulate signaling from multiple transmembrane receptor-associated tyrosine kinases, such as the EGFR receptor family, PDGFR, or steroid hormone receptors.

SRC family kinases consist of a unique NH2-terminal region, two SRC homology domains (SH2 and SH3), a highly conserved kinase domain, and a COOH-terminal tail containing a negative regulatory tyrosine residue. SRC and SFK cooperate in several cellular processes including migration, adhesion, invasion, angiogenesis, proliferation, differentiation, and immune function. They play a major role in the development, growth, progression, and metastasis of a wide variety of human cancers (Kopetz et al. 2007; Montero ct al. 2011).

Elevated levels of SRC kinase activity and/or protein expression levels have been found in a variety of human epithelial cancers, including colon, breast, pancreatic, and lung carcinomas, in brain tumors, but also in osteosarcomas, Ewing sarcomas, and acute myeloid leukemia (Dos Santos et al. 2013). The levels of expression or activation generally correlate with disease progression.

Dasatinib inhibits SRC with an IC_{50} of 0.5 nmol/L (Lombardo et al. 2004). Inhibition of SRC activation by dasatinib can suppress tumor growth in human breast cancer cell lines, in human prostate cancer cells, in head and neck, in lung cancer, and in osteosarcoma cell lines (Johnson et al. 2005; Finn et al. 2007; Shor et al. 2007). Pathologic SRC family kinase activity might contribute to BCR-ABL-independent imatinib resistance in CML (Donato et al. 2003; Pene-Dumitrescu and Smithall 2010).

Nuclear translocation of EGFR is mediated by SRC family kinases and may contribute to acquired resistance to cetuximab in solid tumors. Dasatinib treatment of cetuximab-resistant lung cancer cell line samples was found to be associated with loss of nuclear EGFR and resensitization to cetuximab (Li et al. 2009). In a similar manner, SRC is involved in coordinating signaling from the steroid receptors, including estrogen and androgen receptors. SRC inhibition may overcome endocrine resistance in hormonally driven cancers (Mayer and Krop 2010). In the same way, dasatinib improves p53-mediated targeting of human acute myeloid stem cells by chemotherapy (Dos Santos et al. 2013).

Regarding the tumor microenvironment, SRC is involved in bone metabolism. Increased SRC activity has a net bone resorption result, as a consequence of inhibition of osteoclast generation, together with osteoclast stimulation (Metcalf et al. 2002; Garcia-Gomez et al. 2012).

3.3 Inhibition of KIT

KIT (CD117) is a 145-kD transmembrane glycoprotein, which is a member of the type III receptor tyrosine kinase family. Following ligand binding, the receptor dimerizes, is phosphorylated, and activates downstream signaling pathways involved in proliferation, differentiation, and survival. Normally, KIT is activated when bound to its ligand, the stem cell factor (SCF). Ligand-independent activation of KIT can be caused by gain-of-function mutations that have been reported in several malignancies, including GIST (Hirota et al. 1998), systemic mastocytosis (SM), acute myeloid leukemia (AML), especially core-binding factor AML (CBF-AML), lymphomas, and germ cell tumors.

Dasatinib inhibits KIT with an IC_{50} of 5–10 nmol/l for inhibition of autophosphorylation and cellular proliferation (Schittenhelm et al. 2006) (Table 1). Imatinib-resistant KIT mutants are frequent and often occur in the activation loop of KIT, resulting in a constitutively active conformation of c-KIT, to which imatinib cannot bind. These mutations have relevance in mast cell disorders, seminoma, and AML.

Dasatinib is a potent inhibitor of many clinically relevant mutated forms of KIT, including imatinib-resistant KIT activation loop mutations in vitro (Shah et al. 2006). In core-binding factor (CBF)-AML, KIT mutations cluster most frequently within exon 17, which encodes the KIT activation loop in the kinase domain. In addition, CBF-AML is characterized by a higher KIT expression compared with other AML subgroups (Bullinger et al. 2004). Clinical trials with dasatinib in combination with chemotherapy in CBF-AML are ongoing.

3.4 Inhibition of Platelet-Derived Growth Factor Receptor (PDGFR) α and β Tyrosine Kinases

PDGFR-α and PDGFR-β are receptor tyrosine kinases. They are activated by binding of platelet-derived growth factor (PDGF). PDGF signaling has a significant role in the formation of connective tissue and is also important during wound healing in the adult. PDGFR-α and PDGFR-β are expressed mainly on fibroblasts and smooth muscle cells (Heldin and Westermark 1999). Dasatinib inhibits PDGFR-β with an IC_{50} of 4 nmol/L (Chen et al. 2006) (Table 1).

PDGFR-α tyrosine kinase-activating mutations have been described in the pathogenesis of some GISTs (Heinrich et al. 2003). Fusion proteins consisting of PDGFR-α and PDGFR-β receptor tyrosine kinases have constitutive transforming activity. They are found in a subgroup of myeloproliferative disorders associated with eosinophilia (Cross and Reiter 2008). In intima sarcoma, amplification of PDGFR-α is a common finding. Dasatinib was shown to inhibit PDGFR-α in intima sarcoma in vitro (Dewaele et al. 2010).

3.5 Inhibition of Ephrin Receptor Tyrosine Kinases

The ephrin family of receptor tyrosine kinases constitutes the largest subfamily of receptor tyrosine kinases. They are divided into two subclasses (ephrin A and ephrin B) based on sequence similarity and their preferential binding to ligands, which are tethered to the cell surface either by a glycosylphosphatidylinositol-anchor (ephrin A) or by a single transmembrane domain (ephrin B) (Kullander and Klein 2002). Eph receptor tyrosine kinases have important functions in development and diseases. In tumorigenesis, they have been implicated in cellular transformation, metastasis, and angiogenesis. EphA2 is frequently overexpressed and functionally altered in many invasive cancers including metastatic melanoma, as well as cancers of the mammary gland, cervix, ovary, prostate, colon, lung, kidney, esophagus, and pancreas.

Dasatinib was shown to be a potent inhibitor of ephrin A2 receptor kinase with an IC_{50} of 17 nmol/L in various cell lines (Huang et al. 2007; Chang et al. 2008) (Table 1).

3.6 Inhibition of TEC Family Kinases and BTK

TEC kinases are a large group of nonreceptor TKs and are closely related to SRC and ABL. TEC kinases play a pivotal role in the development and signaling of hematopoietic cells (Smith et al. 2001). Bruton tyrosine kinase (BTK) is a member of the TEC family kinases with a well-characterized role in B-cell receptor signaling and B-cell activation. Dasatinib has been shown to inhibit BTK with an IC_{50} of 5 nM and TEC with an IC_{50} of 14 nM (Hantschel et al. 2007) (Table 1).

The irreversible strong BTK inhibitor ibrutinib with an IC_{50} of 0.5 nM (Pan et al. 2007) has been shown to be very effective not only in CLL (Byrd et al. 2013), but also in other lymphomas (Badar et al. 2014). Ibrutinib is approved for the treatment of CLL, mantle cell lymphoma, and marginal zone lymphoma. Clinical trials with dasatinib in CLL only showed modest activity.

4 Clinical Data

4.1 Pharmacokinetic Profile

Dasatinib is administered orally. The drug is rapidly absorbed, and peak plasma concentrations occur 0.5–3 h after administration. The intake of food is not relevant for pharmacokinetics of dasatinib. In a dose range of 25–120 mg twice daily, the area under the plasma concentration–time curve (AUC) increased proportionally. The drug is extensively metabolized in the liver, predominantly by cytochrome P450 (CYP) 3A4; only 30% remains unchanged. The metabolites of the compound are unlikely to play a pharmacologic role. There were linear elimination characteristics over the above-mentioned dose range with a terminal elimination half-life of 5–6 h.

Elimination occurs mostly in the feces (85%) only little in urine (4%). Dasatinib is excreted as metabolites, and only 19% of a dose was recovered as unchanged drug in the feces (Sprycel® BMS 2017).

4.2 Clinical Trials with Dasatinib

More than 300 clinical trials in almost all tumor entities have been performed so far with dasatinib, and about 60 are still ongoing. Dasatinib treatment is most effective in the BCR-ABL-driven diseases CML and Ph+ ALL. Dasatinib is approved for the treatment of all phases of CML and Ph+ ALL, and therefore, treatment of these diseases will be discussed in more detail, followed by a short overview of trials in other malignancies.

4.3 Clinical Trials with Dasatinib in CML Patients

4.3.1 Chronic Myeloid Leukemia

Chronic myeloid leukemia (CML) is a malignant clonal disorder of hematopoietic stem cells caused by a chromosomal aberration, the Philadelphia (Ph) chromosome. The Ph-chromosome is formed by the chromosomal translocation t(9;22)(q34;q11). This translocation juxtaposes the ABL gene (chromosome 9) and the BCR gene (chromosome 22) creating a BCR-ABL fusion gene. The resulting chimeric protein is a constitutively active ABL tyrosine kinase (Hehlmann et al. 2007). Knowledge of the molecular pathogenesis of CML has allowed development of molecular targeted therapy, which has considerably changed the management and outcome of patients (Wong et al. 2004; Hehlmann et al. 2007). Treatment options for CML include BCR-ABL tyrosine kinase inhibitors (TKIs), interferon alpha, chemotherapy, stem cell transplantation, or clinical trials of novel therapies (Baccarani et al. 2013; NCCN v2 2018).

Actually, three TKIs are approved for first-line treatment of CML: imatinib, the first BCR-ABL targeted therapy, and the second-generation TKIs dasatinib and nilotinib. Second-generation TKIs have a stronger activity and are able to induce faster and deeper molecular remissions. However, they did not show a survival benefit (Cortes et al. 2016; Hochhaus et al. 2016).

Since early, deep molecular responses ($\leq 10\%$ BCR-ABL at 3 months) are associated with significantly improved survival, and this goal can be achieved more often with second-generation TKIs; this might argue for those substances, especially in younger patients.

This threshold ($\leq 10\%$ BCR-ABL at 3 months) is also prognostic for reaching very deep molecular remissions, with a 4.5log reduction of the BCR-ABL transcript, the so-called $MR^{4.5}$. A $MR^{4.5}$ is prerequisite for eventually stopping the TKI treatment. About 50% of the patients stopping the TKI treatment remain in remission provided they had a very deep molecular remission for a long time (Mahon et al. 2010).

Treatment-free remission is a new goal in the treatment of CML patients. Ongoing clinical trials evaluating the criteria necessary for securely cease TKI treatment have shown that besides other criteria like treatment duration for at least 8 years, a deep molecular remission (at least MR^4) has to be obtained (Hughes and Ross 2016).

Actually, three TKIs are approved for first-line treatment of CML: imatinib, and the second-generation TKIs dasatinib and nilotinib. The choice of first-line treatment is based on the aim of therapy, i.e., achievement of treatment-free remission, risk of transformation, and toxicity profile.

4.3.2 Clinical Trials with Dasatinib in CML: Overview

The clinical efficacy of dasatinib in CML patients was first studied in patients, resistant or intolerant to imatinib. A pivotal phase I trial (Talpaz et al. 2006) was followed by five phase II trials, termed START (**S**RC–ABL **T**yrosine kinase inhibition **A**ctivity **R**esearch **T**rials). These trials were consecutively performed in all phases of CML in patients resistant or intolerant to imatinib (Kantarjian et al. 2007; Hochhaus et al. 2007; Ottmann et al. 2007; Guilhot et al. 2007a; Cortes et al. 2007a).

Dose-optimization phase III trials have been performed in chronic phase CML (Shah et al. 2008a) and in advanced phases of the disease (Kantarjian et al. 2009b; Saglio et al. 2010a, b).

First-line treatment of CML patients with dasatinib was assessed in two phase II trials (Pemmaraju et al. 2011; Radich et al. 2012) and two phase III trials (Cortes et al. 2016; O'Brien et al. 2014).

4.3.3 Phase I Clinical Trial of Dasatinib in CML, ALL Phases and Ph+ ALL

The efficacy of oral dasatinib was first assessed in a phase I, open-label, dose-escalation study. Patients ($n = 84$) with various phases of CML or Ph+ ALL intolerant or resistant to imatinib received oral dasatinib (15–240 mg/d) once or

Table 2 Chronic phase CML: efficacy of dasatinib in second line after imatinib failure

Trial	No. patients/type of treatment	CHR (%)	MCyR (%)	CCyR (%)	MMR (%)	OS (%)	PFS (%)	Reference
START-C[a]	387 (dasatinib 70 mg BID)	90	62	53	–	94	80	Hochhaus et al. (2008)
START-R[a]	101 (dasatinib 70 mg BID)	93	53	44	29	nr	86	Kantarjian et al. (2009b)
	49 (high-dose imatinib 800 mg)	82	33	18	12	nr	65	
Dose optimizing study	167 (dasatinib 100 mg QD)	92	63	50	43	71	49	Rea et al. (2012)
CA180-034[b]	168 (dasatinib 70 mg BID)	88	61	53	70	70	47	Shah et al. (2016)
	167 (dasatinib 140 mg QD)	87	63	50	40	77	40	
	168 (dasatinib 50 MG BID)	92	61	49	40	74	51	

QD once daily; BID twice daily, CHR complete hematologic remission, MCyR major cytogenetic response: ≤ 35% Ph+ cells in metaphase in bone marrow, CCyR complete cytogenetic response: 0% Ph+ cells in metaphase in bone marrow, MMR major molecular response: defined as a BCR-ABL transcript level of 0.1% or lower, corresponding to a reduction in the BCR-ABL transcript level by at least 3 log from the standardized baseline level, OS overall survival, PFS progression-free survival
[a]At 2-year follow-up
[b]At 7-year follow-up

twice daily in 4-week treatment cycles (Talpaz et al. 2006). Dasatinib had clinical activity in all CML phases and Ph+ ALL. Complete hematologic response (CHR) was achieved in 92% of patients (37/40) with CML-CP, and major hematologic response (MHR) was seen in 70% of patients (31/44) with CML-AP, CML-BP, or Ph+ ALL. The rates of major cytogenetic response (MCyR) were 45% in patients with CML-CP (18/40) and 43% in patients with CML-AP (19/44), CML-BP, or Ph+ ALL. Of note, imatinib-associated side effects including muscle cramps and nausea were infrequently observed with dasatinib and patients intolerant to imatinib did not have recurrence of the same nonhematologic adverse events (AEs) (e.g., rash and live-function abnormalities) with dasatinib treatment. The major AE associated with dasatinib was reversible myelosuppression.

4.3.4 Phase II Clinical Trials in Chronic Phase CML

A series of phase II trials, the pivotal START trial program, followed the phase I dose-escalation study. The primary objective for these trials was to treat patients with resistance or intolerance to imatinib treatment and who therefore had a life-threatening medical need. As the pharmacokinetics of the dasatinib 70 mg twice-daily regimen were better understood, it was selected for these trials. These open-label, multicenter trials established the efficacy and safety of second-line dasatinib (70 mg twice-daily) in the treatment of imatinib-resistant or imatinib-intolerant patients with CML (all phases) or Ph+ ALL (Tables 2 and 4). Data from this program led to the initial approval of dasatinib in these indications.

Two START studies assessed second-line dasatinib 70 mg twice daily in patients with CML-CP. START-C trial was a single-arm study, and START-R was a randomized, parallel-arm study of dasatinib versus high-dose imatinib (800 mg/day) in patients resistant to standard-dose imatinib (Hochhaus et al. 2008, Kantarjian et al. 2009b). In START-C ($n = 387$), dasatinib-induced MCyR (primary endpoint) in 62% of patients after a minimum follow-up of 24 months (Mauro et al. 2008). The corresponding CCyR rate was 53%. In START-R, rates of MCyR were 53% in the dasatinib 70 mg twice-daily arm ($n = 101$) and 33% in the high-dose imatinib arm ($n = 49$) ($P = 0.017$) after a minimum follow-up of 24 months (Kantarjian et al. 2009a). CCyR rates were 44 and 18%, respectively ($P = 0.0025$) (Kantarjian et al. 2009a). These responses were also durable, as a pooled analysis ($n = 387$) of the START-C and START-R studies showed that 90% of patients achieving a CCyR maintained this level of response after 24 months (Baccarani et al. 2008).

4.3.5 Dose-Optimization Study

The recommended starting dose for dasatinib in patients with CML in chronic phase is 100 mg once daily (Sprycel® BMS 2017; EMA 2012). This dose is the result of a phase III dose-optimization study (NCT00123474; CA180-034) showing that 100 mg once daily was associated with similar efficacy as the twice-daily regimen, but with a reduction in toxicity (Shah et al. 2008a). The rationale for this study was based on observations from the phase I study that once-daily and twice-daily dose schedules were associated with similar response rates (Talpaz et al. 2006). Although dasatinib has a half-life of 3–5 h (Sprycel® BMS 2017), transient exposure of CML cell lines to dasatinib has been demonstrated to induce apoptosis (Shah et al. 2008b), supporting once-daily dosing. Furthermore, due to dose reductions in the START-C and START-R studies, the median total daily dose delivered to patients approximated 100 mg/day (Hochhaus et al. 2007; Kantarjian et al. 2007). It was therefore proposed to compare the 100 mg once schedule with other schedules. In this dose-optimization study, patients ($n = 670$) were randomized to receive dasatinib at 100 mg once daily ($n = 167$), 140 mg once daily ($n = 167$), 50 mg twice daily ($n = 168$), or 70 mg twice daily ($n = 168$) (Shah et al. 2008a) (Table 2). After a minimum follow-up of 2 years, rates of CCyR and MMR were similar across the different dosing schedules (CCyR 50–54%; MMR 37–38%) (Shah et al. 2010). In the 100 mg once-daily arm, the 24-month rates of CCyR and MMR were 50 and 37%, respectively. Rates of progression-free survival (PFS), overall survival (OS), and transformation to AP/BP by 24 months were 80, 91, and 3%, respectively. The 100 mg once-daily arm was associated with improved safety. Rates of all-grade pleural effusion ($P = 0.049$), grade $\geq$ 3 thrombocytopenia ($P = 0.003$), all-grade neutropenia ($P = 0.034$), and all-grade leukocytopenia ($P = 0.017$) were significantly lower for patients treated with dasatinib 100 mg once daily compared with other schedules (Shah et al. 2010). After a minimum follow-up of 7 years, PFS, OS, and rates of transformation to AP/BP were 49, 71, and 5%, respectively, in the 100 mg once-daily arm (Shah et al. 2016).

4.3.6 First-Line Treatment of CML with Dasatinib

First-line treatment of CML with dasatinib was investigated in the MDACC phase II trial (Pemmaraju et al. 2011) comparing two dosing schemes of dasatinib.

Three randomized trials have been reported so far, comparing dasatinib first line 100 mg once daily with imatinib 400 mg once daily: These are the randomized phase II SWOG S0325 study (NCT00070499) (Radich et al. 2012), the randomized phase III DASSISION trial (NCT 00481247; Kantarjian et al. 2010; Cortes et al. 2016), and the randomized phase III Spirit-2 trial (ISRCTN 54923521, O'Brien et al. 2014) (Table 3).

The first trial investigating dasatinib as first-line treatment was a phase II, open-label study (Cortes et al. 2010). Patients with newly diagnosed CML-CP were randomized to receive dasatinib 100 mg once daily ($n = 66$) or 50 mg twice daily ($n = 33$) (Pemmaraju et al. 2011). Because of results from a phase III multinational randomized study of first-line dasatinib (discussed in the previous section) and trends in favor of the 100 mg once-daily schedule of dasatinib seen in this study, the 50 mg twice-daily arm of this trial was closed after 66 patients were enrolled and all subsequent patients were randomized to the 100 mg once-daily arm. The

Table 3 Randomized first-line therapy trials in chronic phase CML: dasatinib versus imatinib

	DASSISION[a]		SWOG[b]		Spirit 2[c]	
	Imatinib	Dasatinib	Imatinib	Dasatinib	Imatinib	Dasatinib
Patients	260	260	123	123	407	407
Treatment discontinued [%]	15.5	18.6	28	20	20.7	18.3
BCR-ABL levels of ≤10% at 3 months [%]	64	84				
CCyR 12 Mo [%]	72*	83*	69*	84*	40**	51**
MMR 12 Mo [%]	28*	46*	44	59	43**	58**
1 year OS [%]	97	99	97	97		
5 year OS [%]	90	90				

CCyR: complete cytogenetic remission, MMR: major molecular response, BCR-ABL <0.1% or >3 log reduction from baseline
*Difference statistically significant, **Difference statistically significant but missing analyses in 367 of 812 (45.2%) patients
[a]NCT 00481247, Kantarjian et al. (2010), Cortes et al. (2016)
[b]NCT00070499, Radich et al. (2012)
[c]ISRCTN 54923521, O'Brien et al. (2014)

study continued with the once-daily schedule (Pemmaraju et al. 2011). After a median follow-up of 29 months, in patients with ≥ 3 months follow-up ($n = 87$), rates of CCyR and MMR were 95 and 86%, respectively. BCR-ABL levels of 0.0032% ($MR^{4.5}$) were achieved in 67% of patients. Responses were achieved rapidly with 94 and 95% of patients achieving a CCyR after 6 and 12 months, respectively. Similarly, MMR rates at 6 and 12 months were 68 and 73%, respectively. These data compared favorably with historic response data for imatinib (Pemmaraju et al. 2011).

The first randomized trial in the first-line setting was the pivotal, open-label, multinational, randomized phase III trial of Dasatinib versus Imatinib Study in Treatment-Naïve CML Patients (DASISION) (Kantarjian et al. 2010; Cortes et al. 2016). In this study, 519 patients newly diagnosed with CML-CP were randomized to receive dasatinib 100 mg once daily ($n = 259$) or imatinib 400 mg once daily ($n = 260$) (Kantarjian et al. 2010). Efficacy data are shown in Table 3. The primary endpoint of this study was confirmed CCyR (cCCyR; CCyR on two consecutive assessments) by 12 months. For the dasatinib versus imatinib arms, the rate of cCCyR by 12 months was 77 versus 66% ($P = 0.007$), respectively (Kantarjian et al. 2010).

Cumulative MMR and $MR^{4.5}$ rates were higher for dasatinib over the whole 5-year period (Cortes et al. 2016). In the fifth year, MMR and $MR^{4.5}$ rates for dasatinib and imatinib were 76% versus 64% and 42% versus 33% ($p = 0.0022$, and $p = 0.0251$, respectively).

Estimated 5-year OS was 91% for dasatinib and 90% for imatinib (HR, 1.01; 95%CI, 0.58–1.73). More imatinib-treated patients died as a result of CML-related causes ($n = 17$) compared with dasatinib-treated patients ($n = 9$). Transformation to accelerated or blast phase occurred in 4.6% in the dasatinib arm and in 7.3% in the imatinib arm (Cortes et al. 2016).

Deeper levels of response were achieved earlier with dasatinib compared with imatinib as equivalent BCR-ABL transcript levels were achieved 6 months earlier with dasatinib. Rapid molecular responses were associated with lower transformation rates and better long-term outcomes. A higher percentage of dasatinib-treated patients achieved BCR-ABL levels of ≤ 10% at 3 months compared with imatinib-treated patients (84 and 64%, respectively) (Jabbour et al. 2014; Saglio et al. 2012).

An early molecular response (BCR-ABL transcript levels of ≤ 10%) at 3 months was associated with lower transformation rates (dasatinib 1.5 vs. 8.1%; imatinib 2.6 vs. 9.4%), better long-term outcomes (5 year OS: dasatinib 93.8 vs. 80.6%, imatinib 95.4 vs. 80.5%), and improved response (5-year $MR^{4.5}$ rates: dasatinib 54 vs. 5%, imatinib 48 vs. 12%) in both treatment arms (Cortes et al. 2016).

In total, 61% of dasatinib-treated patients and 63% of imatinib-treated patients remained on study treatment in DASISION for the whole study period of five years (Cortes et al. 2016). 11 and 14% discontinued treatment in the dasatinib and the imatinib group, respectively, due to progression or treatment failure (defined as any of the following: doubling of white cell count to >20 × 10^9/L in the absence of

CHR; loss of CHR; increase in Ph-positive metaphases to >35%; transformation to AP/BP; death from any cause), 16 and 7% due to intolerance (Cortes et al. 2016). In patients who discontinued treatment, BCR-ABL mutations were found in 15 patients treated with dasatinib and in 19 patients treated with imatinib.

Except for pleural effusions, drug-related nonhematologic AEs were reported less frequently with dasatinib than imatinib or were comparable.

Similar levels of response have been observed in additional studies of first-line dasatinib. In the SWOG S0325 phase II study, newly diagnosed patients were randomized to receive dasatinib 100 mg once daily ($n = 123$) or imatinib 400 mg once daily ($n = 123$) (Radich et al. 2012). At 12 months, median reductions in BCR-ABL transcript levels were greater with dasatinib compared with imatinib (3.3 vs. 2.8 log, p = 0.063), as were the rates of >3-log BCR-ABL reductions (59 vs. 44%, p = 0.059). Rate of CCyR was significantly different between the dasatinib and imatinib arms (84 and 69%, respectively, p = 0.040), although cytogenetic responses were only assessed in 53% of patients (Radich et al. 2012).

The largest first-line trial comparing dasatinib 100 mg once daily and imatinib 400 mg once daily in 814 randomized patients is the spirt 2 trial. The results are published as abstract only (O'Brien et al. 2014), and final results will be presented in 2018, says the trial homepage. After one year on treatment, the rate of BCR-ABL levels <0.1% (major molecular remission, MMR) is significantly higher ($p < 0.001$) in the dasatinib group (236/406, 58.1%) compared to 173/406 (42.6%) with imatinib. The rate of complete cytogenetic responses at 12 months is also significantly better in dasatinib-treated patients (dasatinib 207/406 patients (51.0%) versus imatinib 163/406 patients (40.1%)). Due to missing analyses in 367 of 812 patients, these data have to be interpreted with caution (Table 3).

More patients discontinued treatment with imatinib by reason of suboptimal response [imatinib 37/406 (9.1%); dasatinib 3/406 (0.7%)]. Of note, more patients developing pleural effusions in the dasatinib arm (51 patients) had BCR-ABL levels <0.1% (65.1%) compared to those without pleural effusions (56.4%).

In the phase II OPTIM study, association of dasatinib (100 mg once daily) pharmacokinetics with safety and response is being investigated. Dose adjustments were made as needed to achieve optimal minimal dasatinib concentrations (C_{min}) in order to reduce the rates of AEs. Interim data for the first 125 patients are available (Rousselot et al. 2012). For all patients enrolled with at least 12 months follow-up, the rates of CCyR at 3, 6, and 12 months were 60, 82, and 95%, and rates of MMR were 21, 46, and 62%, respectively. At 12 months, the rate of $MR^{4.5}$ was 25%, of which 80% had undetectable BCR-ABL transcript levels (Rousselot et al. 2010, 2012).

4.3.7 Treatment of Chronic Phase CML in Children

CML in children is a rare disease. Two clinical trials evaluated the efficacy of dasatinib in children and adolescents.

A phase I/II trial established a dose of 60 mg/m^2 for treatment in chronic phase and 80 mg/m^2 in accelerated phase or Ph+ ALL. In subsequent trials, a total of 91 patients were treated with 60 mg/m^2. Of them 46 patients, median age 13.5 years, were imatinib-resistant/intolerant, and 51 patients, median age 12.8 years, were newly diagnosed. Median duration of follow-up was 5.2 years for patients, resistant or intolerant to imatinib, and 4.5 years for newly diagnosed patients. At 24 months, the rates for CCyR and MMR in the newly diagnosed patients were 96.1 and 74.5%, respectively. For patients imatinib-resistant/intolerant, the respective numbers were 82.6 and 52.2%.

The median time to MMR was 8.3 months (95% CI: 5.0 months, 11.8 months) in the pooled imatinib-resistant/intolerant CP-CML patients, and 8.9 months (95% CI: 6.2 months, 11.7 months) in the newly diagnosed treatment-naïve CP-CML patients. In the phase II pediatric study, one of the newly diagnosed patients and two imatinib-resistant or -intolerant patients progressed to blast phase CML (Gore et al. 2017; Zwaan et al. 2013).

These data led to FDA approval of dasatinib in pediatric patients with Ph+ CML in chronic phase.

4.3.8 Treatment of Advanced Stages of CML

The natural course of CML begins typically with a chronic phase. The duration of chronic phase usually is several years. Eventually, the disease progresses to accelerated phase (AP) and later blastic phase (BP). Accelerated phase is characterized by increasing blast cells in the peripheral blood, basophilia, thrombocytopenia, and additional clonal cytogenetic abnormalities. Blast crisis or blast phase is defined by a blast count above 20% in peripheral blood or bone marrow or extramedullary blast proliferations, also called chloromas. Blast phase can be discerned in myeloid blast phase (MBP, approximately two-thirds) and lymphatic blast phase (LBP, approximately one-third) depending on the nature of blasts involved. Prognosis of accelerated phase and blast phase is dismal. Overall survival from the onset of BC is approximately 3–6 months.

Three studies out of the START program, assessing dasatinib in imatinib-resistant disease, were dedicated to advanced stages of CML.

START-A, START-B, and START-L were single-arm studies of second-line dasatinib 70 mg twice daily in patients with CML-AP, CML-BP, and CML-BP/Ph+ ALL, respectively (Apperley et al. 2009; Guilhot et al. 2007b; Cortes et al. 2008; Porkka et al. 2007; Ottmann et al. 2007; Saglio et al. 2008) (Table 4).

In the START-A trial, including 174 patients with CML in accelerated phase (CML-AP), after a median follow-up of 14.1 months, 64% of patients achieved the primary endpoint of MHR (Apperley et al. 2009).

START-B included patients with myeloid blast phase (CML-BP) ($n = 109$), and START-L included patients with lymphoid CML-BP ($n = 48$) and a subset of patients with Ph+ ALL (Cortes et al. 2007b, 2008; Porkka et al. 2007; Ottmann et al. 2007). After a minimum follow-up of 24 months, a CHR was achieved in 26% of patients with myeloid CML-BP, in 29% of patients with lymphoid CML-BP, and in 35% of patients with Ph+ ALL. The median overall survival in myeloid blast phase, lymphoid blast phase, and Ph+ ALL was 11.8, 5.3, and 3 months, respectively (Table 4).

Table 4 Advanced stages of CML including blast crisis and Ph+ ALL (START-trials): efficacy of dasatinib second line after imatinib in phase II single-arm clinical studies

Trial	Disease/phase	n	Follow-up [months]	Mutated BCR-ABL [% pts.]	Response [% of patients]				Survival				References
					MHR	CHR	MCyR	CCyR	1 year PFS [%]	1 year OS [%]	Median PFS [mo]	Median OS [mo]	
START-A	Accelerated phase	174	14.1		64	45	39	32	66	82			Guilhot et al. (2007a, b) Apperley et al. (2009)
START-B	Myeloid blast phase	109	>12	42	34	27	33	26			6.7	11.8	Cortes et al. 2008
START-L	Lymphoid blast phase	49	>12	65	35	29	52	46			3.0	5.3	Cortes et al. (2008)
START-L	Ph+ ALL	46	>12	78	41	35	57	54				3	Porkka et al. (2007) Ottmann et al. (2007)

CHR complete hematologic response: normal white blood cell count, platelets $< 450,000/\mu l$, no blasts or promyelocytes in peripheral blood, $< 5\%$ myelocytes and metamyelocytes in peripheral blood, normal basophil count, no extramedullary involvement, *MHR* major hematologic response: CHR or neutrophil count between 500 and 1000/μl, and/or platelets between 20,000 and 100,000/μl, *MCyR* major cytogenetic response: $\leq 35\%$ Ph+cells in metaphase in bone marrow, *CCyR* complete cytogenetic response: 0% Ph+cells in metaphase in bone marrow, *PFS* progression-free survival, *OS* overall survival

A large phase III dose-optimization study in patients with CML-AP (Kantarjian 2009b) and CML-BP (Saglio et al. 2010a, b) led to a recommended dasatinib dose of 140 mg once daily in these indications (Sprycel® BMS 2017). Patients were randomized to receive dasatinib 70 mg twice daily (n = 159, AP; n = 74, myeloid BP; n = 28, lymphoid BP) or 140 mg once daily (n = 158, AP; n = 75 myeloid BP; n = 33, lymphoid BP). In patients with CML-AP, similar rates of MHR (68 vs. 66%) and MCyR (43 vs. 39%) were observed in both treatment arms after a median follow-up of 15 months. Significantly fewer patients in the once-daily arm had pleural effusion compared with the twice-daily arm (P < 0.001) (Kantarjian et al. 2009b). After 2 years of follow-up, for patients with myeloid BP, the MHR rates in both arms were 28%; for those with lymphoid BP, the corresponding rates were 42% in the once-daily arm and 32% in the twice-daily arm. AE rates were suggestive of improved safety for dasatinib 140 mg once daily (Saglio et al. 2010a, b).

4.4 Dasatinib in Ph+ Acute Lymphoblastic Leukemia (Ph+ ALL)

Acute lymphoblastic leukemia is a rare malignant disease. It is characterized by the proliferation and accumulation of immature lymphatic blast cells in bone marrow, blood, and other organs. Without treatment, patients typically die within months. Treatment of ALL is intended to be curative. Long-term survival in adults is about 50%.

Philadelphia (Ph) chromosome is the most frequent recurrent cytogenetic abnormality in elderly ALL patients. Its incidence increases with age, accounting for 12–30% in patients 18–35 years of age, 40–45% in patients 36–50 years of age, and reaching approximately 50% in ALL patients aged 60 years and older. For patients with Ph+ ALL, imatinib in combination with chemotherapy is still the standard first-line treatment.

The effect of dasatinib in the treatment of Ph+ ALL was examined in three first-line phase II clinical trials, and one trial in relapsed or refractory disease, depicted in Table 5.

A phase II study in adults evaluated the combination of dasatinib with alternating hyper-CVAD (hyperfractioned cyclophosphamide, doxorubicin, vincristine, and dexamethasone alternating with high-dose cytarabine and methotrexate) (Kantarjian et al. 2000). Dasatinib was administered for the first 14 days of 8 cycles.

Seventy-two patients were treated with a median age of 55 years, and 96% of them achieved complete remission. A CCyR was observed in 83% after 1 cycle of treatment, and a major molecular response occurred at a median of 4 weeks in 93% of patients. After a median follow-up of 67 months, 33 patients (46%) were alive, 30 patients (43%) in complete remission. Allogeneic stem cell transplantation was performed in 12 patients. Median disease-free survival was 31 months, median overall survival 47 months (Ravandi et al. 2015).

Table 5 Clinical trials with dasatinib in Ph+ acute lymphoblastic leukemia in adults

Trial	No. of pts.	Age	CHR [%]	MMR [%]	3y OS [%]	5y OS [%]	Median OS [months]	
First-line treatment								
Hyper-CVAD + Dasatinib	72	55 (21–80)	96	93		46	47 (0.2–97)	Ravandi et al. (2015)
Dasatinib + Steroids	55	53.6 (23.8–76.5)	92.5	22.7			30.8	Foa et al. (2011)
Dasatinib + EWALL-PH01	71	69 (59–83)	96	60	41	36	25.8	Rousselot et al. (2016)
Relapsed/refractory								
Hyper-CVAD + Dasatinib	19 ALL 15 CML-LB	52 (21–77) 47 (26–71)	68 73	35 36	26 70			Benjamini et al. (2014)

CHR complete hematologic response, *MMR* major molecular response, *BCR-ABL* < 0.1%, *EWALL-PH01* age adapted chemotherapy backbone, including vincristine, dexamethasone, asparaginase, methotrexate, cytarabine. *Hyper-CVAD* complex chemotherapy regimen, consisting of odd 3 week courses (1, 3, 5, and 7) of hyperfractionated cyclophosphamide, doxorubicin, vincristine, and dexamethasone with alternating even courses (2, 4, 6, and 8) of high-dose cytarabine and methotrexate (Kantarjian et al. 2000)

In a second study, dasatinib as single agent was combined with steroids for 84 days and free post-remission therapy (Foa et al. 2011). Of 53 evaluable patients, all achieved complete hematologic remission, of which 92.5% at day 22, and at this time point, 10 patients achieved 3-log reduction in the BCR-ABL transcript. Twenty-month OS and DFS were 69 and 51%, with better results in terms of DFS for patients who showed a molecular response at day 22. No deaths or relapses occurred during induction therapy: 23 out of 53 patients relapsed after completing induction and of these 12 with the T315I mutation, resistant to most TKIs. Overall, treatment was well tolerated: Four patients discontinued due to toxicity (only one case of pleural effusion grades 1–2) (Foa et al. 2011).

The third trial assessed the effect of dasatinib in combination with chemotherapy first line in elderly patients. Patients with Ph+ acute lymphoblastic leukemia (ALL) older than age 55 years were treated in the EWALL study number 01 with dasatinib and low-intensity chemotherapy. Dasatinib dose was 140 mg per day with a dose reduction to 100 mg/day for those over 70 years. Chemotherapy consisted of an induction phase of 7 weeks in combination with dexamethasone, vincristine, and intrathecal chemotherapy, followed by consolidation treatments with intermediate-dose cytarabine, asparaginase, and methotrexate for 6 months. A maintenance treatment for the following 18 months consisted of oral 6

Table 6 Dasatinib in hematologic malignancies other than CML and Ph+ ALL

Indication	No. of Pts	Treatment	outcome	Reference
SM AML MDS/CMML HES CEL PMF	33 9 6 5 3 11	Dasatinib 140 mg QD	Overall response rate in SM 33% 1 CR in AML and hypereosinophilic syndrome, no response 1 CR 1 CR SM-CEL 1 CR SM-PMF, other: no response	Verstovsek et al. (2008)
Primary myelofibrosis	6	Dasatinib 50 mg BID	2 bone marrow remissions, 5 clinical responses, 1 SD	
CLL	13	Dasatinib 50 mg BID	1 SD for 12 weeks	Garg et al. (2008)
CLL	15	Dasatinib 140 mg QD	PR in 3 of 15 Pts Additional 5 Pts with clinical response	Amrein et al. (2011)
High-risk MDS	18	Dasatinib 100 mg QD	3 PR 4 SD 10 Progress	Duong et al. (2008)

SM systemic mastocytosis, *AML* acute myeloid leukemia, *MDS/CMML* myelodysplastic syndrome/chronic myelomonocytic leukemia, *HES* hypereosinophilic syndrome, *CEL* chronic eosinophilic leukemia, *PMF* primary myelofibrosis; *CLL* chronic lymphocytic leukemia, *CR* complete response, *PR* partial remission, *SD* stable disease

mercaptopurine and methotrexate in combination with dasatinib, with reinductions with vincristine/dexamethasone. Subsequently patients received dasatinib until disease progression or death. The study enrolled 71 patients with a median age of 69 years (Rousselot et al. 2016).

Sixty-seven patients achieved a complete remission, which was persistent in 31 patients. Thirty-six patients relapsed. Twenty-four of these were tested for mutation by Sanger sequencing, and 75% were T315I-positive. Ten of the relapsing patients achieved a second complete remission. At 5 years, overall survival was 36% and up to 45% taking into account deaths unrelated to disease or treatment as competitors.

A further trial reported treatment of patients with relapsed or refractory Ph+ ALL or with CML-LB with a combination of hyper-CVAD and dasatinib (Benjamini et al. 2014). Results are depicted in Table 6. Nineteen patients with Ph+ ALL and 15 with CML-LB were treated. After one treatment cycle, a high rate of complete hematologic remissions of 68% (Ph+ ALL) and 73% (CML-LB) was reported, with major molecular remissions in 35 and 36%. The overall response rate was 91%, with 24 patients (71%) achieving complete response (CR), and 7 (21%) CR with incomplete platelet recovery (CRp). Two patients died during induction, and one had progressive disease. Twenty-six patients (84%) achieved complete cytogenetic remission after one cycle of therapy. Overall survival for patients with Ph+ ALL at 3 years was 26%, in patients with CML-LB 70%.

4.4.1 Central Nervous System Disease of CML with Lymphoid BP or Ph+ ALL

Substantial activity of dasatinib in patients with Ph+ ALL or blast phase CML and central nervous system (CNS) involvement has been shown. Eleven adult and pediatric patients were treated with dasatinib as first-line treatment for CNS leukemia, whereas three patients experienced a CNS relapse while on dasatinib therapy for other reasons. All of the eleven patients responded with seven complete responders, four after dasatinib monotherapy. Three patients achieved a partial response. Responses were generally durable, and response durations of more than 26 months have been reported (Porkka et al. 2008).

4.5 Dasatinib in Philadelphia-Chromosome-Negative Acute and Chronic Myeloid Diseases, Including Systemic Mastocytosis

Few studies have been reported with dasatinib in Philadelphia-chromosome-negative myeloid diseases. The largest study included a total number of 67 patients, with various hematologic disorders including 33 patients with SM, nine patients with AML, six patients with myelodysplastic syndromes, five patients with hypereosinophilic syndrome (HES), three patients with chronic eosinophilic leukemia (CEL), and 11 patients with primary myelofibrosis (PMF) (Verstovsek et al. 2008) (Table 6).

Most patients with SM presented with the D816 V KIT mutation, which confers imatinib resistance. Since dasatinib has been shown to be active against the KIT D816 V mutation in vitro, activity of the drug in SM was expected. The D816 V was present in 28 of the 33 patients with SM. Patients were treated with dasatinib with different doses and schedules. In SM patients, an overall response rate of 33% was reported, mostly symptomatic improvements including two complete responses, none of them with the D816 V.

The authors concluded that it is questionable, whether the use of dasatinib provides any advantage over other treatment options in SM, and that dasatinib therapy does not seem to have significant activity in patients with MDS, PMF, and HES/CEL (Verstovsek et al. 2008).

However, complete remissions were reported in the same study in four patients: one patient with a SM-AML, one with SM-CEL, a patient with HES, and one patient with AML. The patient with HES had a complex karyotype with an aberrant signaling via PDGFR-β. The patient with AML was KIT mutation positive.

An additional case with HES, characterized by the FIP1L1-PDGFR-α gene fusion, intolerant to imatinib was successfully treated with dasatinib 20 mg/day (Imagawa et al. 2011).

A recent study found a beneficial effect of dasatinib in patients with primary myelofibrosis. A Chinese group treated six patients for 15 weeks with 50 mg dasatinib twice daily. They report a significant and rapid improvement of performance status and quality of life, together with a reduction in spleen size in 5 out of

6 treated patients. Bone marrow, examined in two of the patients under dasatinib, showed a remission (Song et al. 2017). This is in contrast to findings of a group at MD Anderson (Verstovsek et al. 2008). They treated 11 patients with primary myelofibrosis with dasatinib and found no objective clinical response.

Patients with high-risk MDS have been treated with dasatinib monotherapy in another phase II clinical study. Few responses to dasatinib monotherapy were reported (Table 6). The authors conclude that the treatment was safe but with only limited clinical efficacy (Duong et al. 2008).

4.5.1 Dasatinib in the Treatment of Chronic Lymphocytic Leukemia (CLL)

Dasatinib is an inhibitor of BTK. Dasatinib monotherapy has modest clinical activity in CLL, as shown in two phase II studies and one case report, documenting dasatinib-induced CR in a CLL patient (Garg et al. 2008; Pittini et al. 2009; Amrein et al. 2011).

In an approach to overcome chemotherapy resistance to fludarabine in CLL patients with dasatinib, 18 patients have been treated with a combination of dasatinib 100 mg/day and fludarabine, 40 mg/m2 day 1–3 of a 28-day cycle. Most of the patients experienced a slight reduction of lymph node size; only 3 patients reached formal PR (Kater et al. 2014).

However, since ibrutinib as irreversible and stronger BTK inhibitor is much more effective in clinical trials, dasatinib has no role in this setting (Badar et al. 2014).

4.5.2 Dasatinib in the Treatment of Acute Myeloid Leukemia (AML)

Core-binding factor (CBF) AML is characterized by overexpression or mutation of c-KIT. Dasatinib inhibits both mutated and unmutated forms of KIT. Clinical trials with dasatinib in CBF-AML are ongoing.

Individual cases have been reported so far with promising results (Ustun et al. 2009; Verstovsek et al. 2008).

A phase II trial found the combination of dasatinib after standard chemotherapy is feasible (Marcucci et al. 2013). The study included 61 patients out of 779 prescreened patients with confirmed *RUNX1/RUNX1T1* or *CBFB/MYH11* transcripts, the fusion genes in CBF-AML. They received a standard chemotherapy consisting of cytarabine 200 mg/m^2/day continuous intravenous infusion day 1–7, daunorubicin 60 mg/m^2/day IV bolus day 1–3, and consecutively dasatinib 100 mg/day PO day 8–21. The CR rate was 90%, two-year overall survival 87%. The authors concluded that chemotherapy followed by dasatinib is tolerable in CBF-AML patients of all ages. Clinical outcomes for CBF-AML patients receiving chemotherapy followed by dasatinib are at least comparable to those historically observed in CBF-AML patients who received chemotherapy alone. Older CBF-AML patients seem to benefit from this intensive approach. The outcomes of

Table 7 Phase III study of dasatinib in combination with docetaxel and prednisolon in the treatment of metastatic CRPC (READY trial)

	Docetaxel-Prednisolon-Dasatinib	Docetaxel-Prednisolon-Placebo	HR
No. of patients	762	766	
Median overall survival	21.5 months	21.2 months	0.99
Overall response rate	31.9%	30.5%	
PFS	11.8 months	11.1 months	0.92
Median time to PSA-progression	8.0 months	7.6 months	0.91
Pain reduction	66.6%	71.5%	

Median follow-up 19 months; *CRPC* castration-resistant prostate cancer; (Araujo et al. 2013)

patients with KIT-mutated AML are usually worse. Dasatinib in combination with chemotherapy seems to compensate for this; patients achieve similar outcomes as KIT-WT patients (Marcucci et al. 2014).

A phase I study in high-risk AML was reported using dasatinib in combination with standard chemotherapy. The rationale for this approach is the preclinical finding that dasatinib by inhibition of SRC enhances expression of p53, hereby sensitizing leukemic stem cell to chemotherapy (Dos Santos et al. 2013). Eighteen patients with high-risk AML were enrolled. They received dasatinib concomitantly with a standard "7 + 3" protocol with cytarabine and idarubicin for the seven days of chemotherapy. The CR/Cri rate is promising with 77%. Correlative studies on blood samples documented a significant decrease of SRC activity and a higher expression of p53 (Aribi et al. 2015).

4.6 Dasatinib in the Treatment of Solid Tumors

Due to its ability to inhibit SRC family kinases and further receptor TKIs, a huge number of clinical phase I and phase II trials with dasatinib in different solid tumors have been performed so far (Montero et al. 2011; Lindauer and Hochhaus 2014).

In summary, dasatinib as monotherapy has only modest activity in solid tumors. Combinations of dasatinib and other agents have been investigated intensively. Only few remissions have been reported in singular patients.

Since SRC is involved in bone metabolism and has the potency to resensitize tumor cells to antihormonal treatment, the SRC inhibitor dasatinib was expected to be especially effective in metastatic castration-resistant prostate cancer (CRPC). However a multinational, double-blinded, placebo-controlled READY trial randomized 1522 patients with metastatic CRPC 1:1 to receive either docetaxel 75 mg/m^2 every three weeks plus prednisone with dasatinib 100 mg every day ($n = 762$) or docetaxel plus prednisone with placebo ($n = 760$). The primary endpoint was overall survival (Table 7) (Araujo et al. 2013).

Despite the large number of patients, the study failed to show any significant improvement in dasatinib-treated patients with respect to overall survival, progression-free survival, or reduction of pain. Treatment-related AEs were more frequent in the dasatinib arm: 18% versus 9% for placebo. Serious AEs were reported in 30% of patients in both arms of the study. The rate of death occurring within 30 days of the last study drug was 10% in the dasatinib arm versus 6% in the placebo arm (Araujo et al. 2013).

In a more recent trial, women with metastatic breast cancer were treated in a gene signature-guided approach with a dasatinib monotherapy. Patients were planned to receive oral dasatinib, stratified to either a dasatinib sensitivity signature, a SRC pathway activity signature, or a dasatinib target index. Thirty of 97 patients were positive for at least one of the signatures and received treatment. There was only one patient with stable disease, receiving dasatinib for more than 300 days. All tree arms were closed early for futility (Pusztai et al. 2014).

Based on the big number of negative trials in solid tumors with dasatinib alone and in different combinations with chemotherapy and other treatments, it can be concluded that the drug has no role in the treatment of solid tumors.

5 Toxicity

Dasatinib has a unique safety profile, and since early clinical trials, some AEs have been consistently reported in patients receiving dasatinib including myelosuppression, fluid retention, pleural effusion, gastrointestinal disorders, fatigue, headache, musculoskeletal disorders, rash, and infection (Table 8). Some bleeding events and cases of pulmonary arterial hypertension (PAH), a subcategory of pulmonary hypertension (PH), have been reported in a small number of patients receiving dasatinib (Galie et al. 2009; McLaughlin et al. 2009; Fang et al. 2012). In clinical trials of first-line and second-line dasatinib, most AEs occurred within 12–24 months of treatment and were managed with dose modifications (Kantarjian et al. 2012; Sprycel® BMS 2017).

In the early phase I and II studies, dasatinib was applied twice daily, resulting in higher toxicity. The second-line, phase III dose-optimization study indicated that dasatinib 100 mg once daily was associated with reduced frequency of AEs in patients with CML-CP, while efficacy was maintained (Shah et al. 2008a; Porkka et al. 2010).

In the first-line treatment-related AEs led to the discontinuation of dasatinib in 16% of patients over a treatment time of five years in the DASISION trial (Cortes et al. 2016).

Grade 3–4 hematologic AEs were common in patients with CML-CP receiving dasatinib (100 mg once daily) (neutropenia 24%, thrombocytopenia 19%, anemia 11%) (Kantarjian et al. 2012).

Severe biochemical abnormalities were uncommon with the exception of grade 3–4 hypophosphatemia (7%) (Kantarjian et al. 2012).

Table 8 Adverse drug reactions reported $\geq 5\%$ in clinical trials ($n = 2.182$)

	All Grades	Grades 3/4
Gastrointestinal disorders		
Diarrhea	**32**	**4**
Nausea	22	1
Vomiting	13	1
Abdominal pain	10	1
Gastrointestinal bleeding	8	4
Mucosal inflammation (including mucositis/stomatitis)	7	<1
Dyspepsia	5	0
Abdominal distension	5	0
Respiratory, thoracic and mediastinal disorders		
Pleural effusion	**25**	6
Dyspnoea	21	4
Cough	10	<1
Nervous system disorders		
Headache	**25**	1
Neuropathy (including peripheral neuropathy)	6	<1
Skin and subcutaneous tissue disorders		
Skin rash	**22**	1
Pruritus	7	<1
General disorders and administration site conditions		
Superficial edema	**21**	**<1**
Fatigue	21	2
Pyrexia	13	1
Pain	7	<1
Asthenia	**9**	**1**
Chest pain	5	1
Vascular disorders		
Hemorrhage	**15**	**2**
Musculoskeletal and connective tissue disorders		
Musculoskeletal pain	**14**	1
Arthralgia	8	1
Myalgia	8	<1
Infections and infestations		
Infection (including bacterial, viral, fungal, nonspecific)	**10**	**3**
Metabolism and nutrition disorders		
Anorexia	**9**	**<1**
Blood and lymphatic system disorders		
Febrile neutropenia	5	5

Percent of patients (Sprycel® 2017)

The most common nonhematologic AEs in dasatinib-treated patients in DASI-SION (all grades) were pleural effusion (28%), myalgia (22%), diarrhea (19%), headache (13%), superficial edema (11%), rash (11%), nausea (10%), and pulmonary hypertension (5%) (Kantarjian et al. 2012).

Grade 3–4 nonhematologic AEs associated with dasatinib were uncommon at 0–2% (fluid retention 2%, pleural effusion 2%, diarrhea < 1%, fatigue < 1%) (Kantarjian et al. 2012).

A subanalysis of DASISION demonstrated no substantial effects of baseline cardiovascular conditions, other comorbidities, or use of baseline medications on the general safety profile of dasatinib (Cortes et al. 2016).

5.1 Pleural Effusion

In DASISION, at 5-year follow-up, 66 patients (26%) had pleural effusion grade 1 or 2, seven patients (3%) grade 3 or 4 (Cortes et al. 2016). Pleural effusions developed in approximately 8% of at-risk patients per year. The percentage of patients who developed pleural effusions was higher in patients age over 65 years (15 of 25 patients; 60%) compared with patients younger than age 65 years (58 of 233 patients; 25%).

Events were largely manageable with treatment interruption (62%), dose reduction (41%), or the use of diuretics (47%), corticosteroids (32%), or therapeutic thoracocentesis (12%). At 5-year follow-up, 15 patients (6%) had discontinued dasatinib due to pleural effusion. Notably, the occurrence and management of pleural effusion appeared not to affect the efficacy of dasatinib (Cortes et al. 2016).

An analysis of risk factors for pleural effusion in patients treated with second-line dasatinib identified prior history of cardiac disease (p = 0.02), hypertension (p = 0.01), and twice-daily dosing schedule (p = 0.05) was associated with an increased risk of pleural effusion (Quintás-Cardama et al. 2007). In a separate analysis, older age was the only baseline characteristic associated with an increased risk of pleural effusion (Porkka et al. 2010). The development of lymphocytosis during dasatinib treatment was associated with a 1.7-fold increased risk of pleural effusion (95% CI, 1.1–2.5) (Porkka et al. 2010).

In approximately 30% of patients receiving dasatinib, large granular lymphocyte (LGL) expansions carrying clonal T-cell receptor gene arrangements occur resulting in LGL lymphocytosis (Kreutzman et al. 2010, Qiu et al. 2014). LGL cells represent activated T or NK cells. This is unique to dasatinib compared to other TKIs. It has been shown that dasatinib induces the expansion of already-present LGL clones. A discrimination of dasatinib-induced LGL expansion versus real T- or NK-LGL is possible only by stopping dasatinib.

Data from a retrospective analysis of patients enrolled in DASISION suggested that dasatinib-treated patients with lymphocytosis had higher rates of any-grade pleural effusion and lower rates of myalgias and arthralgias compared with patients without lymphocytosis (Schiffer et al. 2010a). In a separate analysis of pooled study data, 31% of patients with CML-CP had lymphocytosis, which was associated with a higher rate of CCyR and longer PFS in patients with advanced disease (Schiffer et al. 2010b). However, no formal statistical testing has been reported for either of these analyses. The beneficial effect of pleural effusion on MMR and CCyR has been reported in several papers with only few patients, some of them with statistical significance (Eskazan et al. 2014; Qiu et al. 2014).

5.2 Pulmonal Arterial Hypertension (PAH)

More recently, rare cases of PAH in patients receiving dasatinib for CML and Ph+ ALL have been reported in the literature ($n = 16$) (Mattei et al. 2009; Rasheed et al. 2009; Hennigs et al. 2011; Orlandi et al. 2011; Dumitrescu et al. 2011; Philibert et al. 2011; Montani et al. 2012; Sano et al. 2012). By 5-year follow-up of the phase III DASISION, 14 patients receiving dasatinib developed PAH (5%); nine patients had pleural effusions as well. However, no cases of PAH diagnosed by RHC were recorded (Cortes et al. 2016). Of the 14 PAH diagnoses, 12 were drug-related. PAH observed in patients receiving dasatinib is not typical as this disease is normally progressive, including cases with a drug-induced etiology which do not reverse on treatment withdrawal (Galie et al. 2009; McLaughlin et al. 2009) To date, however, the typical clinical course for dasatinib-associated cases of PAH is improvement or complete resolution in the majority of cases upon withdrawal of treatment.

5.3 Pregnancy Outcomes Under Treatment with Dasatinib

In the BMS pharmacovigilance database, 147 pregnancies under treatment with dasatinib were identified: Seventy-eight in dasatinib-treated women and 69 in female partners of dasatinib-treated men.

Of the 78 pregnant women, pregnancy outcomes were known in 46. Of these, 33% had a normal pregnancy and delivered a healthy child, 11% had an abnormal pregnancy, and one child with hydrops fetalis was born. Almost all female patients stopped or interrupted dasatinib upon confirmation of pregnancy.

Thirty-nine percent of patients electively terminated pregnancy, and spontaneous abortion occurred in 17%. Documented abnormalities in spontaneous abortion were hydrops fetalis and CNS abnormality (Cortes et al. 2015)

Outcomes of pregnancies conceived by men treated with dasatinib have been provided for 33 of 69 (48%) pregnancies. Of these, 30 (91%) resulted in normal deliveries of normal infants, two (6%) resulted in spontaneous abortions, and one (3%) resulted in the birth of an infant at term with syndactyly (Cortes et al. 2015).

5.4 Management of Adverse Events

Most AEs occurring in patients receiving dasatinib treatment are manageable through dose interruption or dose reduction (Sprycel® BMS 2017). If hematologic AEs occur in patients receiving dasatinib, treatment should be interrupted until the absolute neutrophil count is $\geq 1.0 \times 10^9$/L and platelets $\geq 50 \times 10^9$/L. Dasatinib can then be resumed at the original dose if recovery occurs within 7 days or at a reduced dose of 80/50 mg/day if recovery takes longer than seven days or if the event was a second/third recurrence. Growth factor support may also be considered (Sprycel® BMS 2017). If a severe nonhematologic AE (grade 3/4) develops, dasatinib should be withheld until resolution or improvement. Treatment can then be resumed at a reduced dose dependent on initial severity of the event (Sprycel® BMS 2017).

Pleural effusion events are largely manageable through dose reduction or interruption, and/or corticosteroids and diuretics. Once resolved, a reduced dasatinib dose can be resumed. Rare cases of severe pleural effusion may require thoracentesis and oxygen therapy (Kantarjian et al. 2012). Other fluid retention events can be managed with diuretics and supportive care.

To reduce the risk of PAH, patients should be evaluated for signs and symptoms of underlying cardiopulmonary disease before initiating dasatinib treatment. Upon confirmation of a PAH diagnosis based on RHC, dasatinib should be permanently discontinued (Sprycel® BMS 2017). PAH may be at least partially reversible upon treatment discontinuation.

For bleeding events, management steps include dose interruption and transfusion (Quintás-Cardama et al. 2009; Sprycel® BMS 2017). Rash may be managed with topical or systemic steroids in addition to dose reduction, interruption, or discontinuation. In cases of gastrointestinal upset, the NCCN guidelines suggest that dasatinib be taken with a meal and a large glass of water. Specific supportive medication is also indicated in case of headache and diarrhea (Sprycel® BMS 2017; NCCN v2 2018). A subanalysis of DASISION showed that dose modifications taken to manage AEs had no apparent effect on response (Jabbour et al. 2011).

Toxicity can be reduced, if necessary, by changing the dose schedule. An analysis indicated that intermittent dosing of dasatinib at 100 mg per day for five days per week, including a weekend drug holiday where dasatinib was not taken, led to reductions in the rate and severity of AEs including fluid retention and pleural effusion, while efficacy and disease control were maintained (La Rosée et al. 2013).

6 Drug Interactions

Dasatinib is a substrate and an inhibitor of CYP3A4. Therefore, there is a potential for interaction with other concomitantly administered drugs that are metabolized primarily by or modulate the activity of CYP3A4.

Systemic exposure to dasatinib is increased if it is coadministered with drugs that are inhibitors of CYP 3A4 (e.g., clarithromycin, erythromycin, itraconazole, ketoconazole).

If coadministered with drugs that induce CYP 3A4 (e.g., dexamethasone, phenytoin, carbamazepine, rifampicin, phenobarbital, or *Hypericum perforatum*, also known as St. John's Wort), dasatinib AUC is reduced. It was reduced by 82% when coadministered with rifampicin.

Dasatinib AUC was reduced when coadministered with H2-blockers/proton-pump inhibitors, or antacids. Concomitant administration of famotidine reduced dasatinib AUC by 61%, coadministration of aluminum hydroxide by 55%.

Dasatinib is an inhibitor of CYP3A4. Substrates of CYP3A4 with a narrow therapeutic index should be administered with caution in patients receiving dasatinib. Drugs that rank among that list are alfentanil, astemizole, terfenadine, cyclosporine, fentanyl, pimozide, quinidine, sirolimus, tacrolimus, or ergot alkaloid (ergotamine, dihydroergotamine) (Sprycel® BMS 2017).

7 Biomarkers

7.1 Biomarkers for BCR-ABL

In CML and Ph+ ALL, the presence of the BCR-ABL fusion gene not only determines the diagnosis. BCR-ABL transcript levels under TKI treatment are a good biomarker for prognosis. In chronic phase CML scheduled response checkpoints have been published, describing minimal requirements, expressed as BCR-ABL transcript levels or the extent of cytogenetic response at a given time. Treatment results are categorized as "optimal response," "warning," or "failure." Warnings imply that the patient should be monitored very carefully and may become eligible for other treatments. Failure implies that the patient should be moved to other treatments whenever available (Baccarani et al. 2013).

Mutation analysis of the BCR-ABL in these cases frequently identifies mutations, and due to a known activity profile of the available BCR-ABL inhibitors, recommendations can be made on further treatment with an alternative TKI or even stem cell transplantation.

A good marker for prognosis is early, deep molecular response ($\leq 10\%$ BCR-ABL at 3 months) since it has been shown that this is associated with achieving a deeper molecular remission and better overall survival (Jabbour et al. 2014).

7.2 Biomarkers for KIT

At present, there are no biomarkers for clinical response with dasatinib in KIT-driven diseases. KIT expression can be detected immunohistologically by the presence of the CD117 antigen. Mutation analysis of KIT is possible by PCR and Sanger or next-generation sequencing.

7.3 Biomarkers for SRC

At the moment, there are no reliable biomarkers to predict clinical outcomes in tumors treated with dasatinib and other SRC inhibitors although several attempts have been made. A SRC oncogenic pathway signature predicting sensitivity to dasatinib in vitro had been described (Bild et al. 2006; Huang et al. 2007). In addition, a dasatinib sensitivity signature was found by analyzing gene expression profiles in 23 breast cancer cell lines. A six-gene profile was identified that predicted dasatinib sensitivity in breast and lung cancer cell lines. Furthermore, a gene expression signature related to dasatinib resistance was described (Huang et al. 2007). A SRC pathway activity index has been defined to select patients that may respond to dasatinib (Moulder et al. 2010).

However, in a clinical trial evaluating a gene signature-guided therapy using three different approaches to predict dasatinib response, no significant effect of dasatinib was recorded, in none of the cohorts, and the trial was closed due to futility (Pusztai et al. 2014).

8 Summary and Perspectives

Dasatinib has superior efficacy over imatinib and an acceptable safety profile in first- and second-line treatment of patients with CML. The potent, multitargeted activity of dasatinib may contribute to the depth and speed of response achieved with this agent. Dasatinib's potential immune activity may play a role in the observed potency and requires further investigation. These factors may also play a role in the unique safety profile and the AEs observed in patients receiving dasatinib.

Dasatinib was shown to induce faster and deeper molecular remissions in comparison with imatinib. Early, deep molecular responses ($\leq 10\%$ BCR-ABL at 3 months) were associated with significantly improved survival (Cortes et al. 2016).

Since deep molecular remission with an $MR^{4.5}$ is prerequisite for eventually stopping TKI treatment for treatment-free remission, more patients treated with dasatinib first line will eventually become treatment-free—and eventually be cured.

With changing treatment goals supporting earlier, deeper responses, it is reasonable to suggest that dasatinib and other second-generation BCR-ABL inhibitors are likely to be used more frequently as a first-line treatment option in patients with newly diagnosed disease, dependent on existing patient comorbidities and BCR-ABL mutation status (if known). The speed of response achieved with second-generation BCR-ABL inhibitors may also allow the early identification of a subset of patients resistant to BCR-ABL inhibitor treatment who may benefit from alternate TKI, stem cell transplant, or clinical trials.

In addition, second-generation BCR-ABL inhibitors have demonstrated some activity against CML stem cells, providing support for future investigation of dasatinib in achieving a functional cure (Bocchia et al. 2010; Hiwase et al. 2010).

The loss of patent exclusivity for imatinib, however, is likely to influence first-line treatment selection. With the potential for increased use of imatinib, it will be important to closely monitor patient response to ensure early milestones are achieved. Data are emerging to support a change in treatment for patients failing to reach certain levels of response ($\leq 10\%$ BCR-ABL by 3 months) (Marin et al. 2012; Hanfstein et al. 2012; Neelakantan et al. 2013). A phase II study comparing dasatinib 100 mg once daily to imatinib standard of care in patients failing to achieve an optimal response of $\leq 10\%$ BCR-ABL after 3 months of imatinib 400 mg/day is currently in progress. This study will prospectively test the hypothesis that changing to dasatinib treatment in this patient population will induce an improved response rate (primary endpoint, MMR at 12 months) compared with continuing imatinib at any dose.

With the growing number of BCR-ABL inhibitors available for patients with CML-CP and the lack of head-to-head clinical trials with second-generation BCR-ABL inhibitors, choosing a treatment requires consideration on a patient-to-patient basis and therefore information regarding the efficacy and use of these agents in the real-world setting is of increasing interest. An observational 5-year prospective cohort study (SIMPLICITY: NCT01244750) has been initiated to further understand the use of dasatinib, imatinib, and nilotinib in patients with newly diagnosed CML-CP including real-world response, outcomes, treatment adherence, and patient quality of life. Data on early molecular monitoring patterns in the first year of treatment show that NCCN and ELN recommendations on response monitoring have not been consistently translated into routine clinical practice. Appropriate molecular monitoring in the first year of treatment was performed in only 80% of patients (Goldberg et al. 2017).

A role of dasatinib as SRC inhibitor in cancer is still not defined. All clinical trials so far have found no benefit for the treatment with SRC inhibitors—not only for dasatinib. This is true not only for monotherapy studies, but also for many different combinations. One big obstacle is that there are still no reliable biomarkers for clinical use. At the moment, it is not clear in which combination SRC inhibition might improve the outcome of cancer patients.

Few clinical trials with dasatinib in solid tumors are still ongoing. Anyway it is questionable—whether dasatinib's potential to inhibit SRC will have a role in the treatment of cancer in the future.

References

Amrein PC, Attar EC, Takvorian T et al (2011) Phase II study of dasatinib in relapsed or refractory chronic lymphocytic leukemia. Clin Cancer Res 17:2977–2986

Apperley JF, Cortes JE, Kim DW et al (2009) Dasatinib in the treatment of chronic myeloid leukemia in accelerated phase after imatinib failure: the START a trial. J Clin Oncol 27: 3472–3479

Araujo JC, Trudel GC, Saad F et al (2013) Docetaxel and dasatinib or placebo in men with metastatic castration-resistant prostate cancer (READY): a randomised, double-blind phase 3 trial. Lancet Oncol 14:1307–1316

Aribi A, Dos Santos C, O' Donnell M et al (2015) Combination of dasatinib with conventional chemotherapy is associated with a high response rate in high risk acute myeloid leukemia (AML). Blood 126:3743

Baccarani M, Rosti G, Saglio G et al (2008) Dasatinib time to and durability of major and complete cytogenetic response (MCyR and CCyR) in patients with chronic myeloid leukemia in chronic phase (CML-CP). Blood 112(Suppl.):450

Baccarani M, Deininger MW, Rosti G et al (2013) European LeukemiaNet recommendations for the management of chronic myeloid leukemia: 2013. Blood 122:872–884

Badar T, Burger JA, Wierda WG et al (2014) Ibrutinib: a paradigm shift in management of CLL. Expert Rev Hematol 7:705–717

Benjamini O, Dumlao TL, Kantarjian H et al (2014) Phase II trial of hyper CVAD and dasatinib in patients with relapsed Philadelphia chromosome positive acute lymphoblastic leukemia or blast phase chronic myeloid leukemia. Am J Hematol 89:282–287

Bild AH, Yao G, Chang JT et al (2006) Oncogenic pathway signatures in human cancers as a guide to targeted therapies. Nature 439:353–357

Bocchia M, Defina M, Ippoliti M et al (2010) Evaluation of residual CD34+/Ph+ stem cells in chronic myeloid leukemia patients in complete cytogenetic response during first line nilotinib therapy. Blood 116:1398

Bullinger L, Döhner K, Bair E et al (2004) Use of gene expression profiling to identify prognostic subclasses in adult acute myeloid leukemia. New Engl J Med 350:1605–1616

Byrd JC, Furman RR, Coutre SE et al (2013) Targeting BTK with ibrutinib in relapsed chronic lymphocytic leukemia. N Engl J Med 369:32–42

Chang Q, Jorgensen C, Pawson T, Hedley DW (2008) Effects of dasatinib on EphA2 receptor tyrosine kinase activity and downstream signaling in pancreatic cancer. Br J Cancer 99:1074–1082

Chen Z, Lee FY, Bhalla KN et al (2006) Potent inhibition of platelet-derived growth factor-induced responses in vascular smooth muscle cells by BMS-354825 (Dasatinib). Mol Pharmacol 69:1527–1533

Cortes J, Jabbour E, Kantarjian H et al (2007a) Dynamics of BCR-ABL kinase domain mutations in chronic myeloid leukemia after sequential treatment with multiple tyrosine kinase inhibitors. Blood 110:4005–4011

Cortes J, Rousselot P, Kim DW et al (2007b) Dasatinib induces complete hematologic and cytogenetic responses in patients with imatinib-resistant or—intolerant chronic myeloid leukemia in blast crisis. Blood 109:3207–3213

Cortes J, Kim DW, Raffoux E et al (2008) Efficacy and safety of dasatinib in imatinib-resistant or intolerant patients with chronic myeloid leukemia in blast phase. Leukemia 22:2176–2183

Cortes JE, Jones D, O'Brien S et al (2010) Results of dasatinib therapy in patients with early chronic-phase chronic myeloid leukemia. J Clin Oncol 28:398–404

Cortes JE, Abruzzese E, Chelysheva E et al (2015) The impact of dasatinib on pregnancy outcomes. Am J Hematol 90:1111–1115

Cortes JE, Saglio G, Kantarjian HM, Baccarani M et al (2016) Final 5-year study results of DASISION: the dasatinib versus imatinib study in treatment-naïve chronic myeloid leukemia patients trial. J Clin Oncol 34:2333–2340

Creedon H, Brunton VG (2012) Src kinase inhibitors: promising cancer therapeutics? Crit Rev Oncog 17:145–159

Cross NCP, Reiter A (2008) Fibroblast growth factor receptor and platelet-derived growth factor receptor abnormalities in eosinophilic myeloproliferative disorders. Acta Haematol 119: 199–206

Das J, Chen P, Norris D et al (2006) 2-aminothiazole as a novel kinase inhibitor template. Structure-activity relationship studies toward the discovery of N-(2-chloro-6-methylphenyl)-2-[[6-[4-(2-hydroxyethyl)-1-piperazinyl)]-2-methyl-4-pyrimidinyl]amino)]-1,3-thiazole-5-carboxamide (dasatinib, BMS-354825) as a potent pan-Src kinase inhibitor. J Med Chem 49:6819–6832

Dewaele B, Floris G, Finalet-Ferreiro J et al (2010) Coactivated platelet-derived growth factor receptor alpha and epidermal growth factor receptor are potential therapeutic targets in intimal sarcoma. Cancer Res 70:7304–7314

Donato NJ, Wu JY, Stapley G et al (2003) BCR-ABL independence and LYN kinase overexpression in chronic myelogenous leukemia cells selected for resistance to ST571. Blood 101:690–698

Dos Santos C, McDonald T, Ho YW et al (2013) The Src and c-Kit kinase inhibitor dasatinib enhances p53-mediated targeting of human acute myeloid leukemia stem cell by chemotherapeutic agents. Blood 122:1900–1913

Dumitrescu D, Seck C, Ten FH et al (2011) Fully reversible pulmonary arterial hypertension associated with dasatinib treatment for chronic myeloid leukaemia. Eur Respir J 38:218–220

Duong VH, Jaglal MV, Zhang L et al (2008) Phase II pilot study of oral dasatinib in patients with higher-risk myelodysplastic syndrome (MDS) who failed conventional therapy. Blood 112 (Suppl) (abstract 4197)

Eskazan AE, Eyice D, Kurt EA et al (2014) Chronic myeloid leukemia patients who develop grade I/II pleural effusion under second-line dasatinib have better responses and outcomes than patients without pleural effusion. Leuk Res 8:781–787

European Medicines Agency (2012) Sprycel (dasatinib) summary of product characteristics. Uxbridge, UK, Bristol-Myers Squibb Pharma EEIG. Nov 2012. http://www.ema.europa.eu/docs/en_GB/document_library/EPAR_-_Product_Information/human/000709/WC500056998.pdf

Fabarius A, Giehl M, Rebacz B et al (2008) Centrosome aberrations and G1 phase arrest after in vitro and in vivo treatment with the SRC/ABL inhibitor dasatinib. Haematologica 93: 1145–1154

Fang JC, DeMarco T, Givertz MM et al (2012) World Health Organization pulmonary hypertension group 2: pulmonary hypertension due to left heart disease in the adult—a summary statement from the pulmonary hypertension council of the international society for heart and lung transplantation. J Heart Lung Transpl 31:913–933

Finn RS, Dering J, Ginther C et al (2007) Dasatinib, an orally active small molecule inhibitor of both the src and abl kinases, selectively inhibits growth of basal-type/"triple-negative" breast cancer cell lines growing in vitro. Breast Cancer Res Treat 105:319–326

Foa R, Vitale A, Vignetti M et al (2011) Dasatinib as first-line treatment for adult patients with Philadelphia chromosome-positive acute lymphoblastic leukemia. Blood 118:6521–6528

Galie N, Hoeper MM, Humbert M et al (2009) Guidelines for the diagnosis and treatment of pulmonary hypertension: the task force for the diagnosis and treatment of pulmonary hypertension of the European Society of Cardiology (ESC) and the European Respiratory Society (ERS), endorsed by the International Society of Heart and Lung Transplantation (ISHLT). Eur Heart J 30:2493–2537; Eur Respir J 34:1219–1263

Garcia-Gomez A, Ocio EM, Crusoe E et al (2012) Dasatinib as a bone-modifying agent: anabolic and anti-resorptive effects. PLoS ONE 7(4):e34914

Garg RJ, Wierda W, Fayad L et al (2008) Phase II study of dasatinib in patients with relapsed CLL abstract. Blood 112(Suppl) (abstract 4197)

Goldberg SL, Cortes JE, Gambacorti-Passerini C et al (2017) First-line treatment selection and early monitoring patterns in chronic phase-chronic myeloid leukemia in routine clinical practice: SIMPLICITY. Am J Hematol 92:1214–1223

Gore L, Kearns P, Lee ML et al (2017) Phase II trial of dasatinib (DAS) in pediatric patients (pts) with chronic myeloid leukemia in chronic phase (CML-CP). J Clin Oncol 35(Suppl) (10511)

Guilhot F, Apperley J, Kim D-W et al (2007a) Dasatinib induces significant hematologic and cytogenetic responses in patients with imatinib-resistant or—intolerant chronic myeloid leukemia in accelerated phase. Blood 109:4143–4150

Guilhot F, Apperley JF, Kim DW et al (2007b) Efficacy of dasatinib in patients with. Accelerated-phase chronic myelogenous leukemia with resistance or intolerance to imatinib: 2-year follow-up data from START-A (CA180-005). Blood 110(Suppl) (abstract 470)

Guilhot F, Kantarjian H, Shah NP et al (2010) Dasatinib (versus imatinib) in patients (pts) with newly diagnosed chronic myeloid leukemia in chronic phase (CML-CP): analysis of safety and efficacy by use of baseline medications in the DASISION trial. Blood 116(Suppl) (abstract 2295)

Hallaert DYH, Jaspers A, van Noesel CJ et al (2008) c-Abl kinase inhibitors overcome CD40-mediated drug resistance in CLL: implications for therapeutic targeting of chemoresistant niches. Blood 112:5141–5149

Hanfstein B, Muller MC, Hehlman R et al (2012) Early molecular and cytogenetic response is predictive for long-term progression-free and overall survival in chronic myeloid leukemia (CML). Leukemia 26:2096–2102

Hantschel O, Rix U, Schmidt U et al (2007) The Btk tyrosine kinase is a major target of the Bcr-Abl inhibitor dasatinib. Proc Natl Acad Sci USA 104:13283–13288

Hehlmann R, Hochhaus A, Baccarani M (2007) Chronic myeloid leukaemia. Lancet 370:342–350

Heinrich MC, Corless CL, Duensing A et al (2003) PDGFRA activating mutations in gastrointestinal stromal tumors. Science 299:708 710

Heldin CH, Westermark B (1999) Mechanism of action and in vivo role of platelet-derived growth factor. Physiol Rev 79:1283–1316

Hennigs JK, Keller G, Baumann HJ et al (2011) Multi tyrosine kinase inhibitor dasatinib as novel cause of severe pre-capillary pulmonary hypertension? BMC Pulm Med 11:30

Hirota S, Isozaki K, Moriyama Y et al (1998) Gain-of-function mutations of c-kit in human gastrointestinal stromal tumors. Science 279:577–580

Hiwase DK, White DL, Powell JA et al (2010) Blocking cytokine signaling along with intense Bcr-Abl kinase inhibition induces apoptosis in primary CML progenitors. Leukemia 24: 771–778

Hochhaus A, Kantarjian HM (2013) The development of dasatinib as a treatment for chronic myeloid leukemia (CML): from initial studies to application in newly diagnosed patients. J Cancer Res Clin Oncol 139:1971–1984

Hochhaus A, Kantarjian HM, Baccarani M et al (2007) Dasatinib induces notable hematologic and cytogenetic responses in chronic-phase chronic myeloid leukemia after failure of imatinib therapy. Blood 109:2303–2309

Hochhaus A, Baccarani M, Deininger M et al (2008) Dasatinib induces durable cytogenetic responses in patients with chronic myelogenous leukemia in chronic phase with resistance or intolerance to imatinib. Leukemia 22:1200–1206

Hochhaus A, Shah NP, Cortes JE et al (2012) Dasatinib versus imatinib in newly diagnosed chronic myeloid leukemia in chronic phase (CML-CP): DASISION 3-year follow-up. J Clin Oncol 30(Suppl) (abstract 6504)

Hochhaus A, Saglio G, Hughes TP et al (2016) Long-term benefits and risks of frontline nilotinib vs imatinib for chronic myeloid leukemia in chronic phase: 5-year update of the randomized ENESTnd trial. Leukemia 30:1044–1054

Huang F, Reeves K, Han X et al (2007) Identification of candidate molecular markers predicting sensitivity in solid tumors to dasatinib: rationale for patient selection. Cancer Res 67: 2226–2238

Hughes TP, Ross DM (2016) Moving treatment-free remission into mainstream clinical practice in CML. Blood 128:17–23

Imagawa J, Harada Y, Yoshida T et al (2011) Successful treatment with low-dose dasatinib in a patient with chronic eosinophilic leukemia intolerant to imatinib. Rinsho Ketsueki 52:546–550

Jabbour E, Kantarjian HM, Saglio G et al (2014) Early response with dasatinib or imatinib in chronic myeloid leukemia: 3-year follow-up from a randomized phase 3 trial (DASISION). Blood 123:494–500

Johnson FM, Saigal B, Talpaz M et al (2005) Dasatinib (BMS-354825) tyrosine kinase inhibitor suppresses invasion and induces cell cycle arrest and apoptosis of head and neck squamous cell carcinoma and non-small cell lung cancer cells. Clin Cancer Res 11:6924–6932

Kantarjian HM, O'Brien S, Smith TL et al (2000) Results of treatment with hyper-CVAD, a dose-intensive regimen, in adult acute lymphocytic leukemia. J Clin Oncol 18:547–561

Kantarjian HM, Pasquini R, Hamerschlak N et al (2007) Dasatinib or high-dose imatinib for chronic-phase chronic myeloid leukemia after failure of first-line imatinib: a randomized phase 2 trial. Blood 109:5143–5150

Kantarjian H, Cortes J, Kim D-W et al (2009a) Phase 3 study of dasatinib 140 mg once daily versus 70 mg twice daily in patients with chronic myeloid leukemia in accelerated phase resistant or intolerant to imatinib: 15-month median follow-up. Blood 113:6322–6329

Kantarjian H, Pasquini R, Levy V et al (2009b) Dasatinib or high-dose imatinib for chronic-phase chronic myeloid leukemia resistant to imatinib at a dose of 400 to 600 milligrams daily: two-year follow-up of a randomized phase 2 study (START-R). Cancer 115:4136–4147

Kantarjian H, Shah NP, Hochhaus A et al (2010) Dasatinib versus imatinib in newly diagnosed chronic-phase chronic myeloid leukemia. N Engl J Med 362:2260–2270

Kantarjian HM, Shah NP, Cortes JE et al (2012) Dasatinib or imatinib in newly diagnosed chronic phase chronic myeloid leukemia: 2-year follow-up from a randomized phase 3 trial (DASISION). Blood 119:1123–1129

Karaman MW, Herrgard S, Treiber DK et al (2008) A quantitative analysis of kinase inhibitor selectivity. Nat Biotechnol 26:127–132

Kater AP, Spiering M, Liu RD et al (2014) Dasatinib in combination with fludarabine in patients with refractory chronic lymphocytic leukemia: a multicenter phase 2 study. Leuk Res 38:34–41

Kopetz S, Shah AN, Gallick GE (2007) Src continues aging: current and future clinical directions. Clin Cancer Res 13:7232–7236

Kreutzman A, Juvonen V, Kairisto V et al (2010) Mono/oligoclonal T and NK cells are common in chronic myeloid leukemia patients at diagnosis and expand during dasatinib therapy. Blood 116:772–782

Kullander K, Klein R (2002) Mechanisms and functions of Eph and ephrin signalling. Nat Rev Mol Cell Biol 3:475–486

La Rosée P, Martiat P, Leitner, A et al (2013) Improved tolerability by a modified intermittent treatment schedule of dasatinib for patients with chronic myeloid leukemia resistant or intolerant to imatinib. Ann Hematol. April 28 (Epub ahead of print)

Li C, Lida M, Dunn EF et al (2009) Nuclear EGFR contributes to acquired resistance to cetuximab. Oncogene 28:3801–3813

Lindauer M, Hochhaus A (2014) Dasatinib. Recent Results Cancer Res 201:27–65

Lombardo LJ, Francis YL, Chen P et al (2004) Discover of N-(2-chloro-6-methyl-phenyl)-2-(6-(4-(2-hydroxyethyl)-piperazin-1-yl)-2-methylpyrimidin-4-ylamino)thiazole-5-carboxamide (BMS-354825), a dual Src/Abl kinase inhibitor with potent antitumor activity in preclinical assays. J Med Chem 47:6658–6661

Mahon FX, Réa D, Guilhot J et al, Intergroupe Francais des Leucémies Myéloïdes Chroniques (2010) Discontinuation of imatinib in patients with chronic myeloid leukaemia who ave maintained complete molecular remission for at least 2 years: the prospective, multicentre Stop Imatinib (STIM) trial. Lancet Oncol 11:1029–1035

Marcucci G, Geyer S, Zhao J et al (2013) Adding the KIT inhibitor dasatinib (DAS) to standard induction and consolidation therapy for newly diagnosed patients with core binding factor (CBF) acute myeloid leukemia (AML): initial results of the CALGB 10801 (alliance) study. Blood 123:357

Marcucci G, Geyer S, Zhao W et al (2014) Adding KIT inhibitor dasatinib (DAS) to chemotherapy overcomes the negative impact of KIT mutation/over-expression in core binding factor (CBF) acute myeloid leukemia (AML): results from CALGB 10801 (alliance). Blood 124:8

Marin D, Hedgley C, Clark RE et al (2012) The predictive value of early molecular response in chronic phase CML patients treated with dasatinib first line therapy. Blood 120:291–294

Mattei D, Feola M, Orzan F et al (2009) Reversible dasatinib-induced pulmonary arterial hypertension and right ventricle failure in a previously allografted CML patient. Bone Marrow Transplant 43:967–968

Mauro MJ, Baccarani M, Cervantes F et al (2008) Dasatinib 2-year efficacy in patients with chronic-phase chronic myelogenous leukemia (CML-CP) with resistance or intolerance to imatinib (START-C). J Clin Oncol 26(Suppl) (abstract 7009)

Mayer EL, Krop IE (2010) Advances in targeting Src in the treatment of breast cancer and other solid malignancies. Clin Cancer Res 16:3526–3532

McLaughlin VV, Archer SL, Badesch DB et al (2009) ACCF/AHA 2009 expert consensus document on pulmonary hypertension a report of the American College of Cardiology Foundation task force on expert consensus documents and the American Heart Association developed in collaboration with the American College of Chest Physicians; American Thoracic Society, Inc.; and the Pulmonary Hypertension Association. J Am Coll Cardiol 53:1573–1619; Circulation 119:2250–2294

Metcalf CA 3rd, van Schravendijk MR, Dalgarno DC, Sawyer TK (2002) Targeting protein kinases for bone disease: discovery and development of Src inhibitors. Curr Pharm Des 8:2049–2075

Montani D, Bergot E, Gunther S (2012) Pulmonary arterial hypertension in patients treated by dasatinib. Circulation 125:2128–2137

Montero JS, Seoane S, Ocaña A et al (2011) Inhibition of Src family kinases and receptor tyrosine kinases by dasatinib: possible combinations in solid tumors. Clin Cancer Res 17:5546–5552

Moulder S, Yan K, Huang F et al (2010) Development of candidate genomic markers to select breast cancer patients for dasatinib therapy. Mol Cancer Ther 9:1120–1127

Müller MC, Cortes JE, Kim DW et al (2009) Dasatinib treatment of chronic-phase chronic myeloid leukemia: analysis of responses according to preexisting BCR-ABL mutations. Blood 114:4944–4953

Mustjoki S, Auvinen K, Kreutzman A et al (2013) Rapid mobilization of cytotoxic lymphocytes induced by dasatinib therapy. Leukemia 27:914–924

Nam S, Kim D, Cheng JQ et al (2005) Action of the Src family kinase inhibitor, dasatinib (BMS-354825), on human prostate cancer cells. Cancer Res 65:9185–9189

National Comprehensive Cancer Network. NCCN Clinical Practice Guidelines in Oncology™. Chronic myelogenous leukemia v.2.2018. http://www.nccn.org/professionals/physician_gls/f_guidelines.asp#site

Neelakantan P, Gerrard G, Lucas C et al (2013) Combining BCR-ABL1 transcript levels at 3 and 6 months in chronic myeloid leukemia: implications for early intervention strategies. Blood 121:2739–2742

O'Brien SG, Hedgley C, Adams S et al (2014) Spirit 2: An NCRI randomised study comparing dasatinib with imatinib in patients with newly diagnosed CML. Blood 124:517

O'Hare T, Walters DK, Stoffregen EP et al (2005) In vitro activity of Bcr-Abl inhibitors AMN107 and BMS-354825 against clinically relevant imatinib-resistant Abl kinase domain mutants. Cancer Res 65:4500–4505

O'Hare T, Shakespeare WC, Zhu X et al (2009) AP24534, a pan-BCR-ABL inhibitor for chronic myeloid leukemia, potently inhibits the T315I mutant and overcomes mutation-based resistance. Cancer Cell 16:401–412

Orlandi EM, Rocca B, Pazzano AS et al (2011) Reversible pulmonary arterial hypertension likely related to long-term, low-dose dasatinib treatment for chronic myeloid leukaemia. Leuk Res 36 (1):e4–e6

Ottmann O, Dombret H, Martinelli G et al (2007) Dasatinib induces rapid hematologic and cytogenetic responses in adult patients with Philadelphia chromosome positive acute lymphoblastic leukemia with resistance or intolerance to imatinib: interim results of a phase 2 study. Blood 110:2309–2315

Pan Z, Scheerens H, Li SJ et al (2007) Discovery of selective irreversible inhibitors for Bruton's tyrosine kinase. ChemMedChem 2:58–61

Park SI, Zhang JZ, Phillips KA et al (2008) Targeting Src family kinases inhibits growth and lymph node metastases of prostate cancer in an orthotopic nude mouse model. Cancer Res 68:3323–3333

Pemmaraju N, Kantarjian H, Luthra R et al (2011) Results of a phase II trial of dasatinib as frontline therapy for chronic myeloid leukemia (CML) in chronic phase (CP). Blood 118 (Suppl) (abstract 1700)

Pene-Dumitrescu T, Smithall TE (2010) Expression of a Src family kinase in chronic myelogenous leukemia cells induces resistance to imatinib in a kinase-dependent manner. J Biol Chem 285:21446–21457

Philibert L, Carzola C, Peyriere H et al (2011) Pulmonary arterial hypertension induced by dasatinib: positive reintroduction with nilotinib. Fundam Clin Pharmacol 25(Suppl):95 (abstract 476)

Pittini V, Arrigo C, Altavilla G et al (2009) Dasatinib induces a response in chronic lymphocytic leukemia. Blood 113(Suppl) (abstract 498)

Porkka K, Simonsson B, Dombret H et al (2007) Efficacy of dasatinib in patients with Philadelphia-chromosome-positive acute lymphoblastic leukemia who are resistant or intolerant to imatinib: 2-year follow-up data from START-L (CA180-015). Blood 110(Suppl) (abstract 2810)

Porkka K, Koskenvesa P, Lundan T et al (2008) Dasatinib crosses the blood-brain barrier and is an efficient therapy for central nervous system Philadelphia chromosome–positive leukaemia. Blood 112:1005–1012

Porkka K, Khoury HJ, Paquette RL et al (2010) Dasatinib 100 mg once daily minimizes the occurrence of pleural effusion in patients with chronic myeloid leukemia in chronic phase and efficacy in unaffected in patients who develop pleural effusion. Cancer 116:377–386

Pusztai L, Moulder S, Altan M et al (2014) Gene signature-guided dasatinib therapy in metastatic breast cancer. Clin Cancer Res 20:5265–5271

Qiu ZY, Xu W, Li JY (2014) Large granular lymphocytosis during dasatinib therapy. Cancer Biol Ther 15:247–255

Quintás-Cardama A, Kantarjian H, O'Brien S et al (2007) Pleural effusion in patients with chronic myelogenous leukemia treated with dasatinib after imatinib failure. J Clin Oncol 25:3908–3914

Quintás-Cardama A, Kantarjian H, Ravandi F et al (2009) Bleeding diathesis in patients with chronic myelogenous leukemia receiving dasatinib therapy. Cancer 115:2482–2490

Radich JP, Kopecky KJ, Applebaum FR et al (2012) A randomized trial of dasatinib 100 mg versus imatinib 400 mg in newly diagnosed chronic phase chronic myeloid leukemia in chronic phase (CML-CP). Blood 120:3898–3905

Rasheed W, Flaim B, Seymour JF (2009) Reversible severe pulmonary hypertension secondary to dasatinib in a patient with chronic myeloid leukemia. Leuk Res 33:861–864

Ravandi F, O'Brien SM, Cortes JE et al (2015) Long-term follow-up of a phase 2 study of chemotherapy plus dasatinib for the initial treatment of patients with Philadelphia chromosome-positive acute lymphoblastic leukemia. Cancer 121:4158–4164

Rea D, Vellenga E, Junghan C et al (2012) Six-year follow-up of patients with imatinib-resistant or imatinib-intolerant chronic phase chronic myeloid leukemia (CML-CP) receiving dasatinib. Haematologica 97(Suppl 1) (abstract 199)

Redaelli S, Piazza R, Rostagno R et al (2009) Activity of bosutinib, dasatinib and nilotinib against 18 imatinib-resistant BCR/ABL mutants. J Clin Oncol 27:469–471

Ren CL, Morio T, Fu SM, Geha RS (1994) Signal transduction via CD40 involves activation of lyn kinase and phosphatidylinositol-3-kinase, and phosphorylation of phospholipase C gamma 2. J Exp Med 179:673–680

Rousselot P, Boucher S, Etienne G et al (2010) Pharmacokinetics of dasatinib as a first line therapy in newly diagnosed CML patients (OPTIM dasatinib trial): correlation with safety and response. Blood 116(Suppl) (abstract 3432)

Rousselot P, Mollica L, Etienne G et al (2012) Pharmacologic monitoring of dasatinib as first line therapy in newly diagnosed chronic phase chronic myelogenous leukemia (CP-CML) identifies patients at higher risk of pleural effusion: a sub-analysis of the OPTIM-dasatinib trial. Blood 120(Suppl) (abstract 3770)

Rousselot P, Coudé MM, Gokbuget N et al (2016) Dasatinib and low-intensity chemotherapy in elderly patients with Philadelphia chromosome-positive ALL. Blood 128:774–782

Saglio G, Dombret H, Rea D et al (2008) Dasatinib efficacy in patients with imatinib-resistant/-intolerant chronic myeloid leukemia in blast phase: 24-month data from the START program. Haematologica 93 (abstract 0880)

Saglio G, Hochhaus A, Cortes JE et al (2010A) Safety and efficacy of dasatinib versus imatinib by baseline cardiovascular comorbidity in patients with chronic myeloid leukemia in chronic phase (CML-CP): analysis of the DASISION trial. Blood 116(Suppl) (abstract 2286)

Saglio G, Hochhaus A, Goh YT et al (2010b) Dasatinib in imatinib-resistant or imatinib-intolerant chronic myeloid leukemia in blast phase after 2 years of follow-up in a phase 3 study. Cancer 116:3852–3861

Saglio G, Kantarjian HM, Shah N et al (2012) Early response (molecular and cytogenetic) and long-term outcomes in newly diagnosed chronic myeloid leukemia in chronic phase (CML-CP): exploratory analysis of DASISION 3-year data. Blood 120(Suppl) (abstract 1675)

Sano M, Saotome M, Urushida T et al (2012) Pulmonary arterial hypertension caused by treatment with dasatinib for chronic myeloid leukemia: critical alert. Intern Med 51:2337–2340

Schiffer CA, Cortes JE, Saglio G et al (2010a) Lymphocytosis following first-line treatment for CML in chronic phase with dasatinib is associated with improved responses: a comparison with imatinib. Blood 116(Suppl) (abstract 358)

Schiffer CA, Cortes JE, Saglio G et al (2010b) Lymphocytosis following treatment with dasatinib is associated with improved response and outcome. J Clin Oncol 28:15s (abstract 6553)

Schittenhelm MM, Shiraga S, Schroeder A et al (2006) Dasatinib (BMS-354825), a dual SRC/ABL kinase inhibitor, inhibits the kinase activity of wild-type, juxtamembrane, and activation loop mutant KIT isoforms associated with human malignancies. Cancer Res 66:473–481

Serrels A, Macpherson IRJ, Evans TRJ et al (2006) Identification of potential biomarkers for measuring inhibition of Src kinase activity in colon cancer cells following treatment with dasatinib. Mol Cancer Ther 5:3014–3022

Shah NP, Tran C, Lee FY et al (2004) Overriding imatinib resistance with a novel ABL kinase inhibitor. Science 305:399–401

Shah NP, Lee FY, Luo R et al (2006) Dasatinib (BMS-354825) inhibits KITD816 V, an imatinib-resistant activating mutation that triggers neoplastic growth in most patients with systemic mastocytosis. Blood 108:286–291

Shah NP, Skaggs BJ, Branford S et al (2007) Sequential ABL kinase inhibitor therapy selects for compound drug-resistant BCR-ABL mutations with altered oncogenic potency. J Clin Invest 117:2562–2569

Shah NP, Kantarjian HM, Kim DW et al (2008a) Intermittent target inhibition with dasatinib 100 mg once daily preserves efficacy and improves tolerability in imatinib-resistant and—intolerant chronic-phase chronic myeloid leukemia. J Clin Oncol 26:3204–3212

Shah NP, Kasap C, Weier C et al (2008b) Transient potent BCR-ABL inhibition is sufficient to commit chronic myeloid leukemia cells irreversibly to apoptosis. Cancer Cell 14:485–493

Shah NP, Kim DW, Kantarjian H et al (2010) Potent, transient inhibition of BCR-ABL with dasatinib 100 mg daily achieves rapid and durable cytogenetic responses and high transformation-free survival rates in chronic phase chronic myeloid leukemia patients with resistance, suboptimal response or intolerance to imatinib. Haematologica 95:232–240

Shah NP, Rousselot P, Schiffer C et al (2016) Dasatinib in imatinib-resistant or -intolerant chronic-phase, chronic myeloid leukemia patients: 7-year follow-up of study CA180-034. Am J Hematol 91:869–874

Shor AC, Keschman EA, Lee FY et al (2007) Dasatinib inhibits migration and invasion in diverse human sarcoma cell lines and induces apoptosis in bone sarcoma cells dependent on Src kinase for survival. Cancer Res 67:2800–2808

Smith CI, Islam TC, Mattsson PT et al (2001) The Tec family of cytoplasmic tyrosine kinases: mammalian Btk, Bmx, Itk, Tec, Txk and homologs in other species. BioEssays 23:436–446

Song QL, Zhang B, Xu Y et al (2017) Treatment of patients with primary myelofibrosis using dasatinib. Eur Rev Med Pharmacol Sci 21:3312–3319

Soverini S, Gnani A, Colarossi S et al (2009) Philadelphia-positive patients who already harbor imatinib-resistant Bcr-Abl kinase domain mutations have a higher likelihood of developing additional mutations associated with resistance to second- or third-line tyrosine kinase inhibitors. Blood 114:2168–2171

Sprycel® (dasatinib) capsules prescribing information. Princeton, NJ, Bristol-Myers Squibb Company, Nov 2017. http://packageinserts.bms.com/pi/pi_sprycel.pdf

Talpaz M, Shah NP, Kantarjian H et al (2006) Dasatinib in imatinib-resistant Philadelphia chromosome-positive leukemias. N Engl J Med 354:2531–2541

Tokarski JS, Newitt JA, Chang CY et al (2006) The structure of dasatinib (BMS-354825) bound to activated ABL kinase domain elucidates its inhibitory activity against imatinib-resistant ABL mutants. Cancer Res 66:5790–5797

Ustun C, Corless CL, Savage N et al (2009) Chemotherapy and dasatinib induce long-term hematologic and molecular remission in systemic mastocytosis with acute myeloid leukemia with KIT D816V. Leuk Res 33:735–741

Vajpai N, Strauss A, Fendrich G et al (2008) Solution conformations and dynamics of ABL kinase-inhibitor complexes determined by NMR substantiate the different binding modes of imatinib/nilotinib and dasatinib. J Biol Chem 283:18292–18302

Verstovsek S, Tefferi A, Cortes J et al (2008) Phase II study of dasatinib in Philadelphia chromosome-negative acute and chronic myeloid diseases, including systemic mastocytosis. Clin Cancer Res 14:3907–3915

Wong S, Witte ON (2004) The BCR-ABL story: bench to bedside and back. Annu Rev Immunol 22:247–306

Zhang S, Yu D (2012) Targeting Src family kinases in anti-cancer therapies: turning promise into triumph. Trends Pharmacol Sci 33:122–128

Zwaan CM, Rizzari C, Mechinaud F et al (2013) Dasatinib in children and adolescents with relapsed or refractory leukemia: results of the CA180-018 phase I dose-escalation study of the Innovative Therapies for Children with Cancer Consortium. J Clin Oncol 31:2460–2468

Nilotinib

Martin Gresse, Theo D. Kim and Philipp le Coutre

Contents

M. Gresse (✉) · T. D. Kim · P. le Coutre
Division of Hematology and Oncology, Medical Department, Charité Universitätsmedizin Berlin,
Campus Charité Mitte, Charitéplatz 1, 10117 Berlin, Germany
e-mail: martin.gresse@charite.de

© Springer International Publishing AG, part of Springer Nature 2018
U. M. Martens (ed.), *Small Molecules in Hematology*, Recent Results
in Cancer Research 211, https://doi.org/10.1007/978-3-319-91439-8_3

Abstract

With imatinib still being linked to the breakthrough in CML therapy and probably being the most prescribed drug, second-generation TKIs are increasingly gaining importance. Showing higher response rates while not leading to more adverse events, nilotinib has become an attractive option in the first-line treatment of chronic-phase chronic myeloid leukemia. By reaching deep and long-lasting molecular remissions, discontinuation of TKIs is becoming one of the central topics of future CML therapy. Stopping nilotinib seems safe and provides a stable remission in about half of the eligible patients, though long-term data are still missing.

Keywords

CML · TKI · Nilotinib

1 Introduction

Since the beginning of the century, treatment of chronic-phase Philadelphia-chromosome-positive chronic myeloid leukemia (CML) is largely based on tyrosine kinase inhibitors (TKIs) targeting the oncogenic origin of the disease. After the discovery of the Philadelphia chromosome more than fifty years ago, understanding of the underlying oncogenic mechanism started to grow. This reciprocal chromosomal translocation was found to form a fusion protein identified as the dysregulated BCR-ABL tyrosine kinase. After proving that this kinase leads to unregulated growth of the leukemia cells, approaches to pharmacologically counteract it arose (Nowell and Hungerford 1960; Rowley 1973; Druker et al. 1996).

The introduction of imatinib, a potent inhibitor of the BCR-ABL kinase, led to a change of pace in treating CML, showing high rates of cytogenetic and even molecular remission (Druker et al. 2006). Thus, it quickly became the new standard in CML therapy. Despite this success, some patients showed primary or secondary resistance or insufficient response to imatinib. The main mechanism was found to be additional point mutations of the kinase domain, preventing the optimal effect of imatinib on a molecular level (Gorre et al. 2001; O'Hare et al. 2007). In other cases, failure of imatinib therapy could not be further characterized (Apperley 2007). Additionally, relevant side effects could not be tolerated in some cases and could even lead to discontinuation of the targeted therapy, especially in light of a daily administration (Druker et al. 2006). Therefore, the need for second-generation BCR-ABL inhibitors followed the initial excitement after the introduction of imatinib.

Nowadays, second-generation TKIs for the treatment of CML have been used for over ten years, one of them being nilotinib. The drug not only shows superior effectiveness in both first- and second-line CML but also leads to deep and long-lasting remissions (Kantarjian et al. 2007; Hochhaus et al. 2016a, b). Therefore, the focus increasingly shifts to tolerability in light of high rates of disease control. Furthermore, questions are raised, if and which patients are able to maintain their remission status even after discontinuation of TKI.

With growing experience in the use of nilotinib even in a first-line setting, emphasis will be put on recent clinical data instead of known preclinical findings.

2 Structure and Mechanism of Action

After clinical proof of the antileukemic effect of imatinib, research for further substances with increased activity started. The crystallographic analysis of imatinib interacting with the kinase domain of the BCR-ABL fusion protein was the basis for further development. Nilotinib, formerly known as AMN107, was designed by replacing an *N*-methylpiperazine group in the imatinib molecule (Manley et al. 2004; Weisberg et al. 2005). The molecular structure is displayed in Fig. 1. This novel molecule was found to have a 10- to 50-fold higher BCR-ABL kinase inhibition activity compared to imatinib. Besides this effect against unmutated BCR-ABL, nilotinib was also proven to show sufficient activity against most kinase domain mutations known at that time to cause imatinib resistance (Weisberg et al. 2005). The inhibiting effect is accomplished by preventing the BCR-ABL kinase from switching to an active conformation.

Of note in this context, nilotinib was also shown to have an inhibitory effect on KIT, PDGFR, DDR1, and NQO2 (Rix et al. 2007).

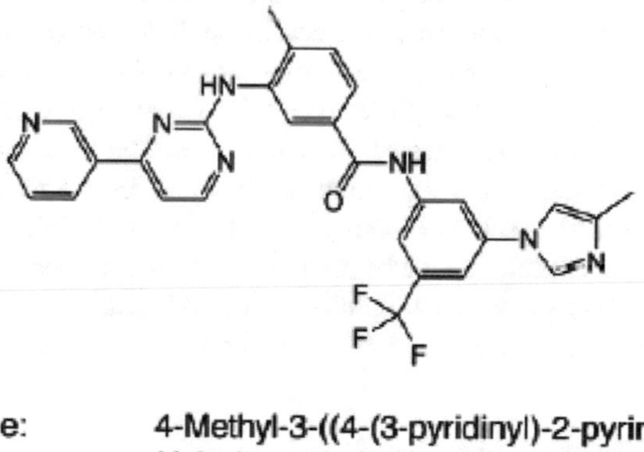

Chemical name:	4-Methyl-3-((4-(3-pyridinyl)-2-pyrimidinyl)amino)-N-(5-(4-methyl-1H-imidazol-1-yl)-3-(trifluoromethyl)phenyl)benzamide
Synonym:	AMN107
Molecular weight:	529.52
Molecular formula:	$C_{28}H_{22}F_3N_7O$

Fig. 1 Molecular structure and chemical characteristics of nilotinib. Adopted from O'Hare et al. (2005)

Table 1 Comparison of IC_{50} values of imatinib and nilotinib in wild-type and mutated BCR-ABL

Mutation of BCR-ABL	IC_{50} (nM) imatinib	IC_{50} (nM) nilotinib
Wild type	260–678	<10–25
M244V	1600–3100	38–39
G250E	1350 to >20,000	48–219
Y253F	6400–8953	182–725
Y253H	6400–17,700	450–1300
E255K	3174–12,100	118–566
E255V	6111–8953	430–725
F311L	480–1300	23
T315I	6400 to >20,000	697 to >10,000
V379I	1000–1630	51
F359V	1400–1825	91–175

Baccarani et al. (2013), Bradeen et al. (2006), von Bubnoff et al. (2006), Gorre et al. (2001), Hochhaus et al. (2013), O'Hare et al. (2005), Ray et al. (2007), Redaelli et al. (2012), Soverini et al. (2006), Weisberg et al. (2006)

3 Preclinical Data

As noted above, nilotinib was found to be more potent in inhibiting BCR-ABL as imatinib. These findings could be confirmed by studies both on murine and human cell lines in vitro. Additionally, nilotinib led to fewer rates of BCR-ABL autophosphorylation in exposed cells compared to imatinib (Golemovic et al. 2005; Weisberg et al. 2005). When tested in a mouse model with an induced CML, nilotinib was able to significantly prolong survival and reduce the overall burden of tumor cells in imatinib-resistant clones (Weisberg et al. 2005). Thus, most mutations of the kinase domain could be overcome, important exceptions being, for example, T315I, T315V, and L248R. IC_{50} values of some mutations are shown in Table 1. Maximum plasma concentration of nilotinib was 2329 ± 1233 nM.

4 Clinical Data

4.1 Nilotinib Phase I Trial

After demonstration of a superior effect in both unmutated and mutated BCR-ABL-positive CML cells in vitro, a Phase I trial in CML patients resistant to imatinib was conducted. In this dose escalation study, patients of all stages of disease (chronic, accelerated, and blastic phase), who developed resistance to prior imatinib therapy, were randomly assigned to receive 100–1200 mg of nilotinib once per day or 400–600 mg twice daily. A steady-state level of the drug in blood serum was reached after eight days of intake. At this level, the exposure to the drug was higher when administered at 400 mg twice daily than at 800 mg once per day, thus making two doses per day favorable. Furthermore, peak concentrations and the area under the curve were found to rise in increasing dosages up to 400 mg and then steadied. The half-life of nilotinib was about 15 h.

Toxicity was found to be reasonable up to doses of 600 mg twice per day.

In this highly heterogenous study population, a notable response to therapy could be noted. Of 33 patients in blastic phase at the beginning of treatment, 13 developed a complete hematological response (CHR) with 9 patients showing cytogenetic response. In the accelerated phase cohort, 33 out of 46 patients achieved CHR and 22 showed any cytogenetic response. Of patients in chronic phase, 11 out of 12 with active disease at baseline achieved CHR, whereas 9 out of the total 17 showed cytogenetic response (Kantarjian et al. 2006).

Tanaka et al. could show that the intestinal absorption of nilotinib is altered depending on the kind of food intake. For example, it could be shown that the area under the curve of nilotinib was increased up to 50% after a meal with high content of fat (Tanaka et al. 2009). These findings were consistent with previous data of healthy volunteers (Kagan et al. 2005; Tanaka et al. 2009). Thus, intake of nilotinib is recommended at least two hours after the last meal; afterwards, the patient should be fasting for another hour.

4.2 Nilotinib Second- and Third-Line Therapy

After successful use of nilotinib in patients resistant to imatinib, the only approved TKI at that time, controlled studies were initiated for further investigations of the drugs effects.

In 2007, Kantarjian et al. first published a study of 280 patients with Philadelphia-positive CML in chronic phase resistant or intolerant to imatinib, treated with nilotinib 400 mg twice daily in a single arm. A first analysis after six months of treatment revealed a rate of 31% of patients with a complete cytogenetic remission (CCyR). Almost half of the study population (48%) achieved at least a major cytogenetic remission (MCyR), defined as <35% Philadelphia-positive cells. With the exception of the T315I mutation, a majority of mutational and non-mutational mechanisms of imatinib resistance were overcome (Kantarjian et al. 2007).

The four-year update of the same Phase II trial showed that 31% of patients were still under the study drug at 48 months. Furthermore, the median administered daily dose of nilotinib was found to be 789 mg, which comes close to the optimal dose of 800 mg split up in 400 mg twice daily according to the study protocol. Thus, nilotinib was found to be safe and tolerable. After four years, 59% of patients had reached a MCyR with 45% being in CCyR. Interestingly, rates of MCyR were identical after 24 and 48 months, indicating that an early response is associated with better outcome (Kantarjian et al. 2011a, b; Giles et al. 2013). This fact was supported by an analysis, showing that deep molecular remissions after 3 and 6 months were associated with better overall survival and progression-free survival. Nilotinib had to be discontinued in the first 48 months mainly because of disease progression (30%), but it has to be noted that only 3% of patients progressed to accelerated or blastic phase of CML. Another 21% of patients had to stop nilotinib because of adverse events.

Parallel to nilotinib, another second-generation TKI, dasatinib, was developed. Giles et al. investigated the effectiveness of nilotinib after failure of imatinib and dasatinib. A majority of patients (67%) previously treated with dasatinib had to discontinue this drug due to intolerance instead of resistance. Interestingly, 79% of patients switching from dasatinib had not reached MCyR before. After switching to nilotinib, 43% reached MCyR, while 79% reached CHR (Giles et al. 2010).

Further studies have been conducted, investigating the efficacy of nilotinib in the second or further line of therapy for patients in accelerated or blastic phase. After 24 months of therapy, patients in accelerated phase showed any hematologic response in 55% of cases with 31% achieving CHR and 32% achieving MCyR (le Coutre et al. 2008; le Coutre et al. 2012). After the same period of time, patients in myeloid blastic phase and lymphoid blastic phase achieved a major hematologic response in 60 and 59% and MCyR in 38 and 52%, respectively (Giles et al. 2008).

Thus, nilotinib was proven to be effective in all stages of CML after failure of prior TKI therapy. Usual dosages applied were 400 mg of nilotinib twice per day, while today's standard is 300 mg twice daily.

Recently, the ENESTfreedom extension trial could show that switching to a higher dosed nilotinib regimen (400 mg twice daily) leads to sufficient response rates in patients with non-optimal disease control under treatment with imatinib 400 mg once daily or nilotinib 300 mg twice daily. After change of treatment, 32% of patients pre-treated with imatinib and 39% pre-treated with regular doses of nilotinib reached major molecular response (MMR). However, estimated progression-free survival and overall survival were worse in the group switching from imatinib. Toxicity rates were not significantly higher compared to the standard dose nilotinib group (Hughes et al. 2014a, b). Thus, dose escalation of nilotinib is an option for patients not eligible for another second-generation or third-generation TKI.

On the other hand, Cortes et al. could show that in a case of an insufficient response to first-line imatinib, switching the TKI to nilotinib at a dose of 400 mg twice a day might lead to better rates of remission than a dose escalation of imatinib. Among the 191 patients enrolled, who had not reached a complete cytogenetic remission (CCyR) yet, 50% of the nilotinib group reached this endpoint after six months. Of patients escalated to 600 mg imatinib once per day in the other arm, only 42% reached CCyR at the same point of time (Cortes et al. 2016). Statistically, these findings were not significant, but they raise interest in further studies in this field covering a longer study interval.

In summary, nilotinib stays a potent option for second or further line therapy of CML, enabling decent rates of remission after failure of prior TKI therapy.

4.3 Nilotinib First-Line Therapy

The first and most relevant study of frontline nilotinib usage was ENESTnd. In this randomized open-label multicentre Phase III trial, nilotinib was tested against the standard therapy with imatinib in patients with newly diagnosed chronic myeloid leukemia in chronic phase. Patients in the control arm received 400 mg of imatinib once per day, whereas patients in the study arms received 300 mg or 400 mg of nilotinib twice daily, respectively.

The first data were published by Saglio et al. in 2010 after a 12-month treatment period. The primary endpoint was defined as the rate of major molecular remission (MMR), equaling $\leq 0.1\%$ BCR-ABL according to the International Scale. Rates of MMR were 44% for the group treated with 300 mg nilotinib twice a day, 42% at 400 mg nilotinib twice daily, and 22% in the imatinib group. These findings were highly significant in favor of nilotinib. Reinforcing these facts, rates of complete cytogenetic remission were significantly higher in the nilotinib groups (80% in the 300 mg arm and 78% in the 400 mg arm) compared to patients treated with imatinib (65%). Furthermore, time to progression of the disease was notably longer under treatment with nilotinib ($p = 0.01$ in the nilotinib 300 mg group, $p = 0.004$ in the 400 mg group), while toxicity rates were comparable between imatinib and nilotinib groups (Saglio et al. 2010).

These findings led to the approval of nilotinib as first-line therapy in the USA and the European Union at the end of 2010 and the beginning of 2011, respectively.

In the 2016 update of the ENESTnd trial, both 300 mg and 400 mg of nilotinib administered twice daily were found to lead to rates of deep molecular remission ($MR^{4,5}$, see below) in more than 50% of patients (54 and 52%, respectively) after a study period of five years. In contrast, 31% of patients treated with imatinib reached the same milestone. Since toxicity was significantly higher in the group receiving 400 mg twice a day, the dosage of 300 mg twice daily should be considered standard in first-line therapy, especially in light of the excellent results (Hochhaus et al. 2016a, b). Table 2 shows further details retrieved from the 5-year update.

This work confirmed that nilotinib leads to faster responses, even on the molecular level. Previously, Jain et al. were already able to show that early responses are an individual prognostic factor, as earlier responses to therapy are associated with better outcome, e.g., regarding progression or overall survival (Jain et al. 2013). These findings were confirmed by Hughes et al., who could prove another advantage of nilotinib versus imatinib: Whereas a high Sokal risk score was associated with lower rates of early molecular response (here defined as $\leq 10\%$ BCR-ABL at 3 or 6 months), the same was not true in the nilotinib group.

In the ENEST1st study, a remarkable number of 1089 patients were treated in a single arm with nilotinib 300 mg twice per day in the first-line setting. For the first time, molecular remission was not only set as a primary endpoint in a trial of this size, but the cutoff was set to $\leq 0.01\%$ BCR-ABL according to the International Scale. This milestone was reached by 38.4% of all patients after a treatment interval of 18 months. This endpoint was especially important as it leads a way to a possible discontinuation of the drug after successful primary therapy (Hochhaus et al. 2016a, b).

Table 2 Five-year outcome of patients treated with nilotinib or imatinib in first line

Parameter	Imatinib 1 × 400 mg/day (%)	Nilotinib 2 × 300 mg/day (%)	Nilotinib 2 × 400 mg/day (%)
MMR	60.4	77.0	77.2
MR^4	41.7	65.6	63.0
MR$^{4.5}$	31.4	53.5	52.3
Progression of CML	7.4	3.5	2.1
New mutations of BCR-ABL	7.8	4.3	3.9
New T315I Mutation	1.4	0.7	1.1
Grade 3/4 AE	58.9	60.6	71.5
Cardiovascular events	2.1	7.5	13.4
Deaths	7.7	6.4	3.6

Adopted from Hochhaus et al. (2016a, b)

Concluding, nilotinib has not only reached the status of a first-line option for patients with newly diagnosed CML in chronic phase. It has even proven a higher efficacy in terms of response rates as well as time to response compared to the established therapy with imatinib.

4.4 Nilotinib Discontinuation

As mentioned above, nilotinib is able to achieve faster and deeper remissions than imatinib in the majority of patients. With growing experience and a large number of patients in deep molecular remissions, aspirations of stopping the medication came up. Initially, this idea was realized for patients treated with imatinib, showing continuous remission rates between 39 and 51.9% after discontinuation of the drug (Mahon et al. 2010; Mori et al. 2015).

The ENESTfreedom study was the first to determine the outcome of controlled discontinuation in patients in deep molecular remission treated with nilotinib (Hochhaus et al. 2017). The patient population had to be treated with nilotinib for at least two years and was required to be in deep molecular remission (MR$^{4.5}$, see below) for at least one year. After discontinuing nilotinib, 51.6% of these patients were found to stay in major molecular remission during the first 48 weeks. Relapsing patients were retreated with nilotinib with 98.8% reaching at least MMR again. The most common adverse event during the study was musculoskeletal pain, which had been described after imatinib discontinuation before (Mahon et al. 2010; Mori et al. 2015; Hochhaus et al. 2017).

The rates of treatment-free remission, defined as maintaining at least MMR, are similar to the findings with imatinib mentioned above. However, since more patients are able to achieve remission levels necessary for discontinuation when

Table 3 Sustained molecular remission after discontinuation of TKI therapy

Trial	Drug	TF interval	MMR rate[a] (%)	MMR rate after reinitiation[b] (%)	Reference
EURO-SKI	Ima	18 months	53	–	Mahon et al. (2016)
STIM	Ima	12 months	41	62	Mahon et al. (2010)
ISAV	Ima	36 months	51.9	100	Mori et al. (2015)
ENESTfreedom	Nil	48 weeks	51.6	99	Hochhaus et al. (2017)
ENESTop	Nil	48 weeks	57.9	98	Hughes et al. (2016)
STOP 2G-TKI	Nil	48 months	61.4	–	Rea et al. (2016)

Ima Imatinib; *Nil* Nilotinib; TF interval: (median) treatment-free follow-up (i.e., time after TKI discontinuation)
[a]Percentage of patients with sustained MMR (or better) after TKI discontinuation
[b]Percentage of patients regaining MMR after TKI re-exposition following molecular relapse

treated with nilotinib, in total numbers more patients are getting the chance of discontinuation and treatment-free remission.

Table 3 shows success rates of different trials testing the discontinuation of imatinib and nilotinib after achieving deep molecular remission. Noteworthy are the very high numbers of patients, who were able to re-gain MMR or better after restart of TKI therapy following relapse. Therefore, discontinuation seems safe even considering that nearly half of patients are relapsing.

The ongoing ENESTpath trial is the first to have the objective of determining optimal conditions for a possible stop of therapy after reaching a deep molecular remission. A first analysis showed that 30.5% of patients with prior imatinib therapy and non-optimal molecular response were able to achieve $MR^{4,5}$ after 12 months (Rea et al. 2015). Thus, switching to nilotinib might be favorable for an intended TKI discontinuation. On the other hand, this study is making nilotinib the only TKI available at publishing date with a noted possibility of discontinuation at start of therapy.

4.5 Resistance to Nilotinib

Resistance to tyrosine kinase inhibitors in the treatment of CML is largely based on additional mutations of the kinase domain, leading to ineffective binding of the drug. These mechanisms were first identified in the context of imatinib resistance (Shah et al. 2002). In most cases, these mutations are not present at the time of diagnosis but develop over the course of treatment (Soverini et al. 2006; Ernst et al. 2011). In total, nilotinib was found to develop fewer kinase domain (KD) mutations than imatinib (Hochhaus et al. 2013). Furthermore, mutations were mainly identified in the p-loop of KD, contrasting the findings of imatinib (Bradeen et al. 2006; Ray et al. 2007). This can partly explain the efficacy of switching TKIs after developing resistance (Giles et al. 2013).

In a sub-analysis of the ENESTnd trial, the incidence and character of developing mutations under TKI therapy was investigated (Hochhaus et al. 2013). Shortly summarized, additional mutations emerged more seldom under treatment with nilotinib than imatinib; furthermore, progression to advanced stages of CML was not as frequent. The rate of new mutations when treated with nilotinib was 4.9% during the first three years. The most common mutations developing under nilotinib therapy were Y253H, E255K/V, and F359C/V. The European Leukemia Net recently released guidelines including an overview of the most frequent kinase domain mutations and their resistance to individual TKIs. Interestingly, mutations often acquired under imatinib treatment are usually sensitive to nilotinib, whereas the aforementioned frequent mutations developing under nilotinib are mostly resistant to imatinib as well (Baccarani et al. 2013).

An exception stays the crucial T315I mutation, which shows resistance to both first- and second-generation TKIs, emphasizing the status of ponatinib and research for further generation drugs. By changing amino acids at the binding site of nilotinib (as well as imatinib and dasatinib), this exact binding is hindered, leading to resistance to the drug (Gorre et al. 2001).

Shortly, nilotinib therapy leads to fewer mutations of BCR-ABL conferring drug resistance compared to imatinib. Furthermore, most mutations acquired under treatment with imatinib can be overcome by further treatment with nilotinib. One of the most significant resistances still is the T315I mutation.

5   Toxicity

Despite being closely related to the first-generation drug imatinib, nilotinib shows quite a distinct profile in terms of toxicity (Kantarjian et al. 2006).

Already in early studies it was shown, that treatment discontinuation because of higher grade (grade 3/4) adverse events (AEs) was noticeably low with nilotinib. Further investigation even noted lower rates of the mentioned events as in a comparable study population treated with imatinib, thus making nilotinib an overall well-tolerated drug (Giles et al. 2012, 2013; Larson et al. 2012; le Coutre et al. 2012).

As typical in nearly all antileukemic drugs, hematological toxicity was most common. Grade 3 or 4 anemia could be noted in 3.9% of cases with neutropenia and thrombocytopenia showing rates of 11.8 and 10.4% of the same grades, respectively (Larson et al. 2012). Dose reductions or interruptions of the drug were common, whereas discontinuation was rare.

Among the non-hematological AEs, rash and fluid retentions were most common with both of these rarely occurring in higher grades. Even more important, fluid retention rates were significantly lower than with imatinib with the same percentage of clinical relevant effusions (1.8%). Other clinical side effects included pancreatitis, hepatotoxicity, and significant bleeding.

Interestingly, Kim et al. could show high rates of thyroid dysfunction in patients treated with nilotinib. Both hypo- and hyperthyroidism were common. The mechanism still is unclear, and discontinuation of nilotinib was very rare in the study population. The same effect was found under treatment with imatinib and dasatinib. Thyroid dysfunction was noted in 25% of patients treated with imatinib, 55% of patients treated with nilotinib, and 70% of patients under dasatinib treatment, respectively (Kim et al. 2010).

Preclinical analyses hinted at a prolongation of the QTc interval by nilotinib; thus, electrocardiographic controls had to be conducted during all studies. Recent findings state no higher rate of relevant QTc prolongation under nilotinib than under imatinib with absolute numbers being considerably low (Larson et al. 2013). Nevertheless as the induction of cardiac arrhythmias could lead to severe complications up to cardiac death, the recent NCCN guidelines demand further precaution. Blood levels of potassium and magnesium should be taken care of and elevated to normal if necessary. Furthermore, the combination of additional drugs prolonging the QTc interval should be avoided (see below). During treatment, ECG should be performed regularly, in case of a prolonged QTc interval nilotinib should be either reduced in dosage or discontinued (Radich et al. 2017).

An increasing attention was paid to cardiovascular diseases and events in recent years. These were not obvious in the first years of nilotinib usage but emerged as distinct risks of the drug. Aischberger et al. and le Coutre et al. first described the increased risk of developing peripheral artery occlusive disease (PAOD) under treatment with nilotinib (Aichberger et al. 2011; le Coutre et al. 2011). These findings were later confirmed by analyses of the ENESTnd study, revealing a newly diagnosed PAOD in 1.4% and 1.8% of patients treated with nilotinib 300 mg twice daily and 400 mg twice daily. In contrast, no patient in the imatinib arm developed PAOD during the study course (Larson et al. 2013). Even prospective analyses were able to show significantly higher rates of PAOD and early stages of peripheral circulation disorders revealed by ankle–brachial index (ABI) (Kim et al. 2013). Most cases were found to occur in the first 48 months of nilotinib therapy. As a pathogenetic correlate, elevated levels of glucose and LDL were found in patients with nilotinib, pointing at a general role in atherosclerosis. Supporting these findings, other atherosclerotic-driven events such as ischemic heart attack or stroke were also more common in patients treated with nilotinib (Quintás-Cardama et al. 2012). The 2016 update of the ENESTnd trial revealed a rate of 4.7% of grade 3/4 cardiovascular events in patients treated with nilotinib 300 mg twice daily and 8.7% of patients treated with nilotinib 400 mg twice daily. In contrast, these events occured only in 1.8% of patients in the imatinib arm (Hochhaus et al. 2016a, b).

Giles et al. could recently show that age has a relevant effect on the cardiovascular toxicity of nilotinib (Giles et al. 2017). Details are shown in Table 4.

Steegmann et al. suggest regular assessment of cardiovascular risk profiles in their ELN toxicity recommendations. When treating with nilotinib, laboratory tests and the ABI should be performed every six to twelve months. In patients with a

Table 4 Rates of cardiovascular events in different age groups treated with nilotinib

Cardiovascular events	18–39 years (%)	40–59 years (%)	60–74 years (%)	≥ 75 years (%)
Total	0.8	5.3	10	13.5
Ischemic heart disease	0.4	2.8	5.7	9.6
PAOD	0.4	1.8	3.0	1.9
Ischemic cerebrovascular event	0	0.8	1.3	1.9

PAOD peripheral artery occlusive disease
Adopted from Giles et al. (2017)

high cardiovascular risk, nilotinib initiation is not recommended. In case of newly diagnosed PAOD, the drug should be discontinued (Steegmann et al. 2016).

In summary, nilotinib stays a favorable option in both first- and second-line treatment of CML with less overall toxicity compared to imatinib. Nevertheless, the distinct toxicity profile needs to be considered. Prolongation of the QTc interval and cardiovascular events might be rare but are of great risk concerning morbidity and mortality.

6 Drug Interactions

Two factors should be taken into account when thinking about the interaction of nilotinib with other drugs: On the one hand, the majority of patients of patients still requires a lifelong CML therapy, and on the other hand, most patients are diagnosed in the middle to elderly age. Thus, prescription of other medication and polypharmacy are common in CML patients.

As described above, nilotinib is known to prolong the QTc interval. Therefore, physicians need to take care of concomitant intake of other drugs with the same side effect. Known substances are amiodarone, digoxin or several opioids such as methadone (Radich et al. 2017).

Nilotinib was found to be metabolized via the cytochrome P450 system (CYP), precisely CYP3A4. Thus, induction or inhibition of this metabolization pathway has a significant effect on the patients' exposure to nilotinib. For example, it could be shown that ketoconazole and even grapefruit juice, known inhibitors of CYP3A4, are able to increase the exposure to nilotinib (Tanaka et al. 2011; Yin et al. 2010). Following the same principle, induction of CYP3A4, e.g., by rifampicin, leads to faster metabolization of nilotinib. As infections are a common complication in CML patients, these interactions need to be taken into account before starting an antimicrobial therapy.

Furthermore, Haouala et al. could show that nilotinib is a possible inhibitor of other cytochrome enzymes, namely CYP2C8, CYP2C9, CYP2D6, CYP3A4. Other inhibited systems include UGT1A1 and P-glycoprotein. Possible drug interactions should therefore be considered when combining a broad variety of common substances, for example, vitamin K-antagonists (Haouala et al. 2011).

7   Biomarkers

Among the earliest markers for therapy response in CML was hematologic response in regard to peripheral blood count. After the introduction of the far more potent TKIs, precise markers were of need. These were identified as cytogenetic remission and molecular remission. The former describes the percentage of Philadelphia chromosome-positive cells in bone marrow tissue or the total absence, respectively (complete cytogenetic remission, CCyR). The latter refers to the percentage of BCR-ABL detected in a specimen on a standardized metering system, the International Scale (IS). An important milestone is the molecular remission[4,5] ($MR^{4,5}$) defined as $\leq 0.0032\%$ IS. Defining this cutoff is especially important for a possible discontinuation of any CML-specific drug and increasingly displacing the older marker major molecular remission (MMR, more precise: $MR^3 \leq 0.1\%$ BCR-ABL) (Baccarani et al. 2009; Jain et al. 2013; Hochhaus et al. 2017).

The European Leukemia Net nowadays defines optimal response to any TKI in a first-line setting as achieving partial remissions in terms of cytogenetic and molecular marker with $\leq 35\%$ Philadelphia-positive cells and/or $\leq 10\%$ BCR-ABL three months after therapy initiation. At six months, either a CCyR or a BCR-ABL count <1% should be noted with the 12-month mark requiring a MR^3 defined as BCR-ABL $\leq 0.1\%$. The latter stays the minimum goal for optimal response to treatment at any time. If the first-line drug has to be discontinued for adverse events, the same numbers apply to the second-line treatment (Baccarani et al. 2013).

As technical progress goes on, even deeper molecular remissions can be distinguished, thus quantifying the BCR-ABL-count is becoming the most important biomarker for assessing treatment response in CML patients. Being able to perform this test on peripheral blood makes it even easier in contrast to the classic chromosome banding analysis performed on bone marrow tissue.

8   Summary and Perspective

Summarizing, nilotinib is a potent second-generation TKI for the treatment of chronic myeloid leukemia with growing importance over the last decade. Currently, it is not only approved as a first-line treatment for newly diagnosed CML in CP, it is even superior to the established therapy with imatinib in regard to rates of deep cytogenetic and molecular remission. Additionally, rates of disease progression are notably lower under treatment with nilotinib. However, the drug shows quite a different profile in terms of side effects, especially cardiovascular diseases and events are still among the most severe ones. Therefore, cardiovascular risk factors need to be monitored regularly during nilotinib treatment. A history of cardiovascular events or a high cardiovascular risk profile still are contraindications for an initiation of the drug, even more in light of equivalent TKIs available.

With growing experience with potent second-generation TKIs, more and more patients reach long-term deep remissions, thus raising claims of therapy discontinuation. Recent studies have proven the latter to be a safe possibility, with about half of the eligible patients staying in the mentioned remission without therapy. Further studies will have to determine the long-term outcome of these cases.

References

Aichberger KJ, Herndlhofer S, Schernthaner G-H et al (2011) Progressive peripheral arterial occlusive disease and other vascular events during nilotinib therapy in CML. Am J Hematol 86:533–539

Apperley JF (2007) Part I: mechanisms of resistance to imatinib in chronic myeloid leukaemia. Lancet Oncol 8:1018–1029

Baccarani M, Cortes J, Pane F (2009) Chronic myeloid leukemia: an update of concepts and management recommendations of European LeukemiaNet. J Clin Oncol 27:6041–6051

Baccarani M, Deininger MW, Rosti G et al (2013) European LeukemiaNet recommendations for the management of chronic myeloid leukemia: 2013. Blood 122:872–894

Bradeen HA, Eide CA, O'Hare T et al (2006) Comparison of imatinib mesylate, dasatinib (BMS-354825), and nilotinib (AMN107) in an N-ethyl-N-nitrosourea (ENU)-based mutagenesis screen: high efficacy of drug combinations. Blood 108:2332–2338

Cortes JE, De Souza CA, Ayala M et al (2016) Switching to nilotinib versus imatinib dose escalation in patients with chronic myeloid leukaemia in chronic phase with suboptimal response to imatinib (LASOR): a randomised, open-label trial. Lancet Haematol 3:e581–e591

Druker BJ, Tamura S, Buchdunger E, Ohno S (1996) Effects of a selective inhibitor of the Abl tyrosine kinase on the growth of Bcr-Abl positive cells. Nat Med 2:561–566

Druker BJ, Guilhot F, O'Brien S et al (2006) Long-term benefits of imatinib (IM) for patients newly diagnosed with chronic myelogenous leukemia in chronic phase (CML-CP): the 5-year update from the IRIS study. J Clin Oncol 24:338S–338S

Ernst T, La Rosee P, Mueller MC, Hochhaus A (2011) Bcr-Abl mutations in chronic myeloid leukemia. Hematol Oncol Clin North Am 25:997–1008

Giles FJ, Larson RA, Kantarjian HM (2008) Nilotinib in patients with Philadelphia chromosome-positive chronic myelogenous leukemia in blast crisis (CML-BC) who are resistant or intolerant to imatinib—Giles et al. 26 (15 supplement): 7017—ASCO meeting abstracts. J Clin Oncol 26:7017

Giles FJ, Abruzzese E, Rosti G et al (2010) Nilotinib is active in chronic and accelerated phase chronic myeloid leukemia following failure of imatinib and dasatinib therapy. Leukemia 24:1299–1301

Giles FJ, Kantarjian HM, le Coutre PD et al (2012) Nilotinib is effective in imatinib-resistant or -intolerant patients with chronic myeloid leukemia in blastic phase. Leukemia 26:959–962

Giles FJ, le Coutre PD, Pinilla-Ibarz J et al (2013) Nilotinib in imatinib-resistant or imatinib-intolerant patients with chronic myeloid leukemia in chronic phase: 48-month follow-up results of a phase II study. Leukemia 27:107–112

Giles FJ, Rea D, Rosti G et al (2017) Impact of age on efficacy and toxicity of nilotinib in patients with chronic myeloid leukemia in chronic phase: ENEST1st subanalysis. J Cancer Res Clin Oncol 143:1585–1596

Golemovic M, Verstovsek S, Giles F et al (2005) AMN107, a novel aminopyrimidine inhibitor of Bcr-Abl, has in vitro activity against imatinib-resistant chronic myeloid leukemia. Clin Cancer Res 11:4941–4947

Gorre ME, Mohammed M, Ellwood K et al (2001) Clinical resistance to STI-571 cancer therapy caused by Bcr-Abl gene mutation or amplification. Science 293:876–880

Haouala A, Widmer N, Duchosal MA et al (2011) Drug interactions with the tyrosine kinase inhibitors imatinib, dasatinib, and nilotinib. Blood 117:E75–E87

Hochhaus A, Saglio G, Larson RA et al (2013) Nilotinib is associated with a reduced incidence of Bcr-Abl mutations vs imatinib in patients with newly diagnosed chronic myeloid leukemia in chronic phase. Blood 121:3703–3708

Hochhaus A, Saglio G, Hughes TP et al (2016a) Long-term benefits and risks of frontline nilotinib vs imatinib for chronic myeloid leukemia in chronic phase: 5-year update of the randomized ENESTnd trial. Leukemia 30:1044–1054

Hochhaus A, Rosti G, Cross NCP et al (2016b) Frontline nilotinib in patients with chronic myeloid leukemia in chronic phase: results from the European ENEST1st study. Leukemia 30:57–64

Hochhaus A, Masszi T, Giles FJ et al (2017) Treatment-free remission following frontline nilotinib in patients with chronic myeloid leukemia in chronic phase: results from the ENESTfreedom study. Leukemia 31:1525–1531

Hughes P, Hochhaus A, Kantarjian H et al (2014a) Safety and efficacy of switching to nilotinib 400 mg twice daily for patients with chronic myeloid leukemia in chronic phase with suboptimal response or failure on front-line imatinib or nilotinib 300 mg twice daily. Hematologica 99(7):1204–1211

Hughes TP, Saglio G, Kantarjian H et al (2014b) Early molecular response predicts outcomes in patients with chronic myeloid leukemia in chronic phase treated with frontline nilotinib or imatinib. Blood 123:1353–1360

Hughes TP, Boquimpani C, Takahashi N et al (2016) Results from ENESTop: Treatment-free remission (TFR) following switch to nilotinib in patients with chronic myeloid leukemia in chronic phase. ASCO 2016 abstract #7054

Jain P, Kantarjian H, Nazha A et al (2013) Early responses predicts for better outcomes in patients with newly diagnosed CML: results with four TKI modalities. Blood 121:4867–4874

Kagan M, Tran P, Fischer V et al (2005) Safety, pharmacokinetics (PK), metabolism, and mass balance of [C-14]-AMN107, a novel aminopyrimidine inhibitor of Bcr-Abl tyrosine kinase, in healthy subjects. Blood 106:302B–302B

Kantarjian H, Giles F, Wunderle L et al (2006) Nilotinib in imatinib-resistant CML and Philadelphia chromosome-positive ALL. N Engl J Med 354:2542–2551

Kantarjian HM, Giles F, Gattermann N et al (2007) Nilotinib (formerly AMN107), a highly selective Bcr-Abl tyrosine kinase inhibitor, is effective in patients with Philadelphia chromosome-positive chronic myelogenous leukemia in chronic phase following imatinib resistance and intolerance. Blood 110:3540–3546

Kantarjian HM, Giles FJ, Bhalla KN et al (2011a) Nilotinib is effective in patients with chronic myeloid leukemia in chronic phase after imatinib resistance or intolerance: 24-month follow-up results. Blood 117:1141–1145

Kantarjian HM, Hochhaus A, Saglio G et al (2011b) Nilotinib versus imatinib for the treatment of patients with newly diagnosed chronic phase, Philadelphia chromosome-positive, chronic myeloid leukaemia: 24-month minimum follow-up of the phase 3 randomised ENESTnd trial. Lancet Oncol 12:841–851

Kim TD, Schwarz M, Nogai H et al (2010) Thyroid dysfunction caused by second-generation tyrosine kinase inhibitors in Philadelphia chromosome-positive chronic myeloid leukemia. Thyroid 20(11):1209–1214

Kim TD, Rea D, Schwarz M et al (2013) Peripheral artery occlusive disease in chronic phase chronic myeloid leukemia patients treated with nilotinib or imatinib. Leukemia 27:1316–1321

Larson RA, Hochhaus A, Hughes TP et al (2012) Nilotinib vs imatinib in patients with newly diagnosed Philadelphia chromosome-positive chronic myeloid leukemia in chronic phase: ENESTnd 3-year follow-up. Leukemia 26:2197–2203

Larson RA, Hochhaus A, Saglio G et al (2013) Nilotinib vs imatinib in patients with newly diagnosed chronic myeloid leukemia in chronic phase (CML-CP): ENESTnd 4-year update. J Clin Oncol (suppl) 31:abstr. 7052

le Coutre P, Ottmann OG, Giles F et al (2008) Nilotinib (formerly AMN107), a highly selective Bcr-Abl tyrosine kinase inhibitor, is active in patients with imatinib-resistant or -intolerant accelerated-phase chronic myelogenous leukemia. Blood 111:1834–1839

le Coutre P, Rea D, Abruzzese E et al (2011) Severe peripheral arterial disease during nilotinib therapy. J Natl Cancer Inst 103:1347–1348

le Coutre PD, Giles FJ, Hochhaus A et al (2012) Nilotinib in patients with Ph+ chronic myeloid leukemia in accelerated phase following imatinib resistance or intolerance: 24-month follow-up results. Leukemia 26:1189–1194

Mahon F-X, Rea D, Guilhot J et al (2010) Discontinuation of imatinib in patients with chronic myeloid leukaemia who have maintained complete molecular remission for at least 2 years: the prospective, multicentre stop imatinib (STIM) trial. Lancet Oncol 11:1029–1035

Mahon FX, Richter J, Guilhot J et al (2016) Cessation of tyrosine kinase inhibitors treatment in chronic myeloid leukemia patients with deep molecular response: results of the euro-ski trial. Blood 128:787

Manley PW, Breitenstein W, Brüggen J et al (2004) Urea derivatives of STI571 as inhibitors of Bcr-Abl and PDCFR kinases. Bioorg Med Chem Lett 14:5793–5797

Mori S, Vagge E, le Coutre P et al (2015) Age and dPCR can predict relapse in CML patients who discontinued imatinib: the ISAV study. Am J Hematol 90(10):910–914

Nowell PC, Hungerford DA (1960) A minute chromosome in human chronic granulocytic leukemia. Science 142:1497

O'Hare T, Walters DK, Stoffregen EP et al (2005) In vitro activity of Bcr-Abl inhibitors AMN107 and BMS-354825 against clinically relevant imatinib-resistant Abl kinase domain mutants. Cancer Res 65:4500–4505

O'Hare T, Eide CA, Deininger MWN (2007) Bcr-Abl kinase domain mutations, drug resistance, and the road to a cure for chronic myeloid leukemia. Blood 110:2242–2249

Quintás-Cardama A, Kantarjian H, Cortes J (2012) Nilotinib-associated vascular events. Clin Lymphoma Myeloma Leuk 12:337–340

Radich JP, Deininger M, Abboud CN et al (2017) NCCN guidelines version 1.2018 chronic myeloid leuemia. NCCN, Professionals, Physician Guidelines, Chronic Myeloid Leukemia. Accessed on Sept 10 2017

Ray A, Cowan-Jacob SW, Manley PW et al (2007) Identification of Bcr-Abl point mutations conferring resistance to the Abl kinase inhibitor AMN107 (nilotinib) by a random mutagenesis study. Blood 109:5011–5015

Rea D, Rosti G, Cross N et al (2015) Enestpath: a phase III study to assess the effect of nilotinib treatment duration on treatment-free remission (TFR) in chronic phase-chronic myeloid leukemia (CP-CML) patients (pts) previously treated with imatinib: interim analysis from the first year of induction phase. Blood 126:4040

Rea D, Nicolini FE, Tulliez M et al (2016) Discontinuation of dasatinib or nilotinib in chronic myeloid leukemia: interim analysis of the STOP 2G-TKI study. Blood 129:846–854

Redaelli S, Mologni L, Rostagno R et al (2012) Three novel patient-derived BCR/ABL mutants show different sensitivity to second and third generation tyrosine kinase inhibitors. Am J Hematol 87:E125–E128

Rix U, Hantschel O, Duernberger G et al (2007) Chemical proteomic profiles of the Bcr-Abl inhibitors imatinib, nilotinib, and dasatinib, reveal novel kinase and nonkinase targets. Blood 110:4055–4063

Rowley JD (1973) A new consistent chromosomal abnormality in chronic myelogenous leukaemia identified by quinacrine fluorescence and Giemsa staining. Nature 243(5405):290–293

Saglio G, Kim D-W, Issaragrisil S et al (2010) Nilotinib versus imatinib for newly diagnosed chronic myeloid leukemia. N Engl J Med 362:2251–2259

Shah NP, Nicoll JM, Nagar B et al (2002) Multiple Bcr-Abl kinase domain mutations confer polyclonal resistance to the tyrosine kinase inhibitor imatinib (STI571) in chronic phase and blast crisis chronic myeloid leukemia. Cancer Cell 2:117–125

Soverini S, Colarossi S, Gnani A et al (2006) Contribution of ABL kinase domain mutations to imatinib resistance in different subsets of Philadelphia-positive patients: by the GIMEMA working party on chronic myeloid leukemia. Clin Cancer Res 12(24):7374–7379

Steegmann JL, Baccarani M, Breccia M et al (2016) European leukemia net recommendations for the management and avoidance of adverse events of treatment in chronic myeloid leukaemia. Leukemia 30:1648–1671

Tanaka C, Yin OQP, Sethuraman V et al (2009) Clinical pharmacokinetics of the Bcr-Abl tyrosine kinase inhibitor nilotinib. Clin Pharmacol Ther 87:197–203

Tanaka C, Yin OQP, Smith T et al (2011) Effects of rifampin and ketoconazole on the pharmacokinetics of nilotinib in healthy participants. J Clin Pharmacol 51:75–83

von Bubnoff N, Manley PW, Mestan J et al (2006) Bcr-Abl resistance screening predicts a limited spectrum of point mutations to be associated with clinical resistance to the Abl kinase inhibitor nilotinib (AMN107). Blood 108:1328–1333

Weisberg E, Manley PW, Breitenstein W et al (2005) Characterization of AMN107, a selective inhibitor of native and mutant Bcr-Abl. Cancer Cell 7:129–141

Weisberg E, Manley P, Mestan J et al (2006) AMN107 (nilotinib): a novel and selective inhibitor of Bcr-Abl. Br J Cancer 94:1765–1769

Yin OQP, Gallagher N, Li A et al (2010) Effect of grapefruit juice on the pharmacokinetics of nilotinib in healthy participants. J Clin Pharmacol 50:188–194

Bosutinib: A Potent Second-Generation Tyrosine Kinase Inhibitor

Susanne Isfort, Martina Crysandt, Deniz Gezer,
Steffen Koschmieder, Tim H. Brümmendorf and Dominik Wolf

Contents

S. Isfort (✉) · M. Crysandt · D. Gezer · S. Koschmieder · T. H. Brümmendorf
Department of Hematology, Oncology, Hemostaseology and Stem Cell Transplantation,
University Hospital RWTH Aachen, Pauwelsstraße 30, 52074 Aachen, Germany
e-mail: sisfort@ukaachen.de

D. Wolf
Department of Oncology, Hematology, Immunoncology and Rheumatology, University
Hospital Bonn, Sigmund-Freud-Str. 25, 53127 Bonn, Germany

© Springer International Publishing AG, part of Springer Nature 2018
U. M. Martens (ed.), *Small Molecules in Hematology*, Recent Results
in Cancer Research 211, https://doi.org/10.1007/978-3-319-91439-8_4

Abstract

Bosutinib is one of the five tyrosine kinase inhibitors which are currently approved for the treatment of chronic myeloid leukemia. By its dual inhibition of Src and ABL kinase and also targeting further kinases, it creates a unique target portfolio which also explains its unique side effect profile. The approval of bosutinib in 2013 made the drug available for patients previously treated with one or more tyrosine kinase inhibitor(s) and for whom imatinib, nilotinib, and dasatinib are not considered appropriate treatment options. As initially the first-line clinical trial comparing bosutinib with imatinib in CML patients in chronic phase did not reach its primary endpoint and therefore the product was not licensed for first-line therapy, a second first-line trial, the so-called BFORE study, was performed and just recently the promising results have been published predicting a quick expansion of the existing label. In comparison with the other approved TKIs, bosutinib harbors a distinct side effect profile with only very few cardiovascular and thromboembolic events and minimal long-term safety issues with most adverse events happening during the first months of treatment. On the other hand, gastrointestinal side effects are very common (e.g., diarrhea rates in more than 80% of the patients) with bosutinib surprising some of the investigators during the early clinical trials evaluating bosutinib. Until then, several approaches have been used to face this problem resulting in extensive supportive efforts (such as early loperamid treatment) as well as new trials testing alternative dosing strategies with early dose adjustment schedules. This article reports preclinical and clinical data available for bosutinib both in hematologic diseases such as CML or ALL and solid tumours as well as other diseases and envisions future perspectives including additional patient groups in which bosutinib might be of clinical benefit.

Keywords · CML · Tyrosine kinase inhibitor · Bosutinib

1   Structure and Mechanism of Action

1.1   Chemical Structure

Bosutinib (SKI-606), 4-[(2,4-dichloro-5-methoxyphenyl)amino]-6-methoxy-7-[3-(4-methyl-1-piperazinyl) propoxy]-3-quinolinecarbonitrile monohydrate is a competitive inhibitor of both Src and ABL tyrosine kinases (Golas et al. 2003). Originally, it was synthesized as a specific Src kinase family inhibitor. However, target screening demonstrated also potent ABL tyrosine kinase inhibition. The small molecule inhibitor is of low weight (548.46 kDa) and orally bioavailable.

1.2 Mechanism of Action (Target Profile)

Bosutinib inhibits Src with an IC50 of 1.2 nM, inhibits anchorage-independent growth of Src-transformed fibroblasts with an IC50 of 100 nM, and inhibits Src-dependent protein tyrosine phosphorylation at comparable or lower concentrations (Boschelli et al. 2001). Bosutinib however does not inhibit growth factor receptor tyrosine kinases such as platelet-derived growth factor receptor, insulin-like growth factor I receptor, epidermal growth factor receptor, fibroblast growth factor receptor, and serine–threonine kinases such as Akt and Cdk4 (Boschelli et al. 2001). The success of the compound in BCR-ABL positive disease relays on its bosutinib potent dual inhibitory effect on Src and ABL tyrosine kinases (Puttini et al. 2006). In addition to those main target kinases, more than 45 other tyrosine and serine/threonine kinases have been identified as potential targets of bosutinib.

1.3 ABL and BCR-ABL Inhibition

c-ABL belongs to an evolutionary conserved protein family and encodes a ubiquitously expressed non-receptor protein tyrosine kinase localized in both the cytoplasm and the nucleus (Laneuville 1995; Pendergast 1996). Oncogenic transformation leading to ABL-induction is mediated by genomic alterations including genomic rearrangements (e.g. by the Philadelphia (Ph+)-Chromosome in chronic myeloid leukemia (CML) or acute lymphocytic leukemia (ALL) leading to the fusion of the BCR with the ABL genes (Nowell and Hungerford 1961; Heisterkamp et al. 1985) or by enhanced ABL expression [e.g. in solid cancer (Greuber et al. 2013)]. In case of the reciprocal translocation between the proto-oncogene *c-ABL* from chromosome 9 to the breakpoint cluster region *(BCR)* of chromosome 22, high expression levels of a constitutively activated tyrosine kinase are induced which directly or indirectly phosphorylates a broad spectrum of binding substrates. Many of these activated downstream signaling components are a crucial driver of cellular proliferation, migration, and apoptosis (Ren 2005). Interestingly, the efficacy between imatinib and bosutinib as inhibitor of v-ABL phosphorylation is within the same range (approximately, 200 nM are required to inhibit the non-translocated v-ABL), whereas substantially lower concentrations of bosutinib (25 and 50 nM) are required to reduce BCR-ABL phosphorylation (Golas et al. 2003). Concerning IC50 values, it is important to realize that those concentrations substantially depend on the cell system used to address this issue. Exemplarily, bosutinib inhibits BCR-ABL kinase activity at 1 nM in a non-cellular in vitro enzymatic assay, whereas an IC50 of 90 nM is required to inhibit ABL kinase activity and consequently the growth of ABL-MLV-transformed fibroblasts. The extent of tyrosine phosphorylation inhibition by bosutinib in ABL-MLV-transformed fibroblasts correlates with the degree of anti-proliferative activity. In addition, incubation of ABL-MLV-transformed Rat 2 fibroblasts with comparable concentrations of bosutinib and imatinib results in quantitatively similar reductions of tyrosine phosphorylation of cellular proteins (Golas et al. 2003). In cell line models for Ph+ leukemias, bosutinib inhibited the proliferation of all three cell lines, with IC50s ranging from 5 nm in the KU812 cells to 20 nm in K562 and MEG-01 cell lines. The IC50s for imatinib to inhibit proliferation of these cell lines were higher, ranging from 88 nm (KU812), 180 nm (MEG-01) to 210 nm (K562) (Golas et al. 2005). The emergence of TKI resistance is a major clinical problem during TKI therapy with imatinib (and later nilotinib, dasatinib, or bosutinib) (Patel et al. 2017). Approximately, half of the resistance cases are conferred by specific mutations in the BCR-ABL fusion gene. This may lead to varying degrees of resistance to first-generation (imatinib), second-generation (nilotinib, dasatinib, and bosutinib), and third-generation (ponatinib) TKIs. It is essential for optimized and individualized treatment to screen for BCR-ABL mutations to select (in case one or more mutations are detected) the most appropriate TKI, as all TKIs have a highly specific in vitro resistance profile (shown for bosutinib and the other TKIs, as studied in Ba/F3 cell lines, in Fig. 9.1 (Redaelli et al. 2012)). More advanced structural and spectroscopic analyses revealed the mode of action and explain even efficacy in most imatinib-resistant mutants as well as inefficacy in T315I-mutated CML or ALL (Levinson and Boxer 2012). As mentioned before, the IC50 values are also impacted by the leukemia cells' capability to in- and export TKIs. This is largely mediated by drug transporter such as ATP-binding cassette transporters (ABC transporters). While the mechanisms are not fully understood, Hegedus et al. (2009) were able to identify a significant difference between second-generation TKIs dasatinib and nilotinib in comparison with bosutinib, as neither ABCB1 nor ABCG2 induced resistance to bosutinib. The potential clinical impact of this finding has to be further evaluated, e.g., by quantification of intracellular drug levels in TKI-treated patients.

1.4 Src Kinase Inhibition

The tyrosine kinase Src is a member of a family of related kinases known as the Src family kinases (SFKs) that share a common structural organization and function as key regulators of signal transduction pathways triggered by a wide variety of surface receptors, including receptor tyrosine kinases, integrins, G protein-coupled receptors and antigen receptors (Thomas and Brugge 1997). Various studies and clinical observations point to a key role of Src kinases in malignant cell transformation, tumor progression, and metastatic spread as a consequence of changes in protein expression and/or kinase activity (Summy and Gallick 2003; Johnson and Gallick 2007; Li 2008). Indeed, overexpression of Src kinases has been detected in several human malignancies, including carcinomas of the breast, lung, colon, esophagus, skin, pancreas, cervix as well as gastric tissues (Mazurenko et al. 1992; Ottenhoff-Kalff et al. 1992; Verbeek et al. 1996; Lutz et al. 1998; Jallal et al. 2007; Zhang et al. 2007). Bosutinib is capable of inhibiting Src kinase at nM concentrations; accordingly, an IC50 of 1.2 nM has been reported in an enzymatic assay. Inhibition of Src-dependent protein tyrosine phosphorylation can be detected at

		IC50 fold increase (WT = 1)				
		Imatinib	Bosutinib	Dasatinib	Nilotinib	Ponatinib
	Parental	10.8	38.3	568.3	38.4	570.0
	WT	1	1	1	1	1
P-Loop	M244V	0.9	0.9	2.0	1.2	3.2
	L248R	14.6	22.9	12.5	30.2	6.2
	L248V	3.5	3.5	5.1	2.8	3.4
	G250E	6.9	4.3	4.4	4.6	6.0
	Q252H	1.4	0.8	3.1	2.6	6.1
	Y253F	3.6	1.0	1.6	3.2	3.7
	Y253H	8.7	0.6	2.6	36.8	2.6
	E255K	6.0	9.5	5.6	6.7	8.4
	E255V	17.0	5.5	3.4	10.3	12.9
C-Helix	D276G	2.2	0.6	1.4	2.0	2.1
	E279K	3.6	1.0	1.6	2.0	3.0
	E292L	0.7	1.1	1.3	1.8	2.0
ATP-binding region (drug contact sites)	V299L	1.5	26.1	8.7	1.3	0.6
	T315A	1.7	6.0	58.9	2.7	0.4
	T315I	17.5	45.4	75.0	39.4	3.0
	T315V	12.2	29.3	738.8	57.0	2.1
	F317L	2.6	2.4	4.5	2.2	0.7
	F317R	2.3	33.5	114.8	2.3	4.9
	F317V	0.4	11.5	21.3	0.5	2.3
SH2-contact	M343T	1.2	1.1	0.9	0.8	0.9
	M351T	1.8	0.7	0.9	0.4	1.2
Substrate binding region (drug contact sites)	F359I	6.0	2.9	3.0	16.3	2.9
	F359V	2.9	0.9	1.5	5.2	4.4
A-Loop	L384M	1.3	0.5	2.2	2.3	2.2
	H396P	2.4	0.4	1.1	2.4	1.4
	H396R	3.9	0.8	1.6	3.1	5.9
C-terminal lobe	F486S	8.1	2.3	3.0	1.9	2.1
	L248R + F359I	11.7	39.3	13.7	96.2	17.7
Sensitive		≤ 2				
Moderately resistant		2.01 - 4				
Resistant		4.01 – 10				
Highly resistant		> 10				

Source: (12)

Fig. 9.1 Resistance profile of bosutinib, imatinib, nilotinib, dasatinib, and ponatinib. *Source* Redaelli et al. (2012)

comparable or lower concentrations (Boschelli et al. 2001). In addition, bosutinib successfully inhibited the growth of Src-transformed fibroblasts and Src overex-pressing HT29 colon tumors subcutaneously transplanted into athymic nu/nu mice (Compound 31a) (Boschelli et al. 2001).

2 Preclinical Data

2.1 Malignancies

2.1.1 BCR-ABL-Dependent Cancer Models

The anti-proliferative activity of bosutinib has been demonstrated in different BCR-ABL expressing leukemia cell lines. In line with its higher clinical efficacy compared to imatinib (Cortes et al. 2017), the in vitro efficacy of bosutinib is superior to IM with IC50 values ranging from 1 to 20 nM when compared to imatinib with 51–221 nM, respectively (Golas et al. 2003; Puttini et al. 2006). In addition, bosutinib successfully inhibits the growth of imatinib-resistant human cell lines, such as Lama84R, KCL22R, and K562R (Golas et al. 2003). In line with these findings, inhibition of proliferation of murine pro-B Ba/F3 cells, stably transformed by p210 BCR-ABL WT or four imatinib-resistant BCR-ABL point mutants (D276G, Y253F, E255K, and T315I), is more pronounced by bosutinib than by imatinib. However, the T315I BCR-ABL mutant requires excessively high concentrations of bosutinib to be sufficiently inhibited [i.e., one to two orders of magnitude higher when compared with wt BCR-ABL cells (Puttini et al. 2006)]. This is in line with the clinical observation that T315I mutated leukemias cannot be sufficiently be treated by bosutinib. According to these in vitro observations, in vivo experiments demonstrated that 75 mg/kg twice daily or 150 mg/kg once daily bosutinib therapy induces complete regression of human K562 xenografts for up to 40 days (Golas et al. 2003). Remarkably, while imatinib is unable to eradicate KU812 human tumor xenografts with a relapse rate of 30%, bosutinib treatment initiated at day 8 and 15 after leukemic cell injection induces complete disease eradication curing the animals for up to 210 days (Puttini et al. 2006). In mice s.c. injected with Ba/F3 BCR-ABL + xenografts containing WT or mutant BCR-ABL (E255K, Y253F, and D276G) and treated with bosutinib 1 day after tumor cell injection, the dual Src/ABL kinase inhibitor decreased tumor growth and prolonged event-free survival. However, animals with delayed start of bosutinib treatment, relapse of the disease cannot be prevented in the majority of mice. Furthermore, according to the above described in vitro data of almost complete resistance of the T315I mutation, bosutinib does not influence the growth of highly IM-resistant T315I xenografts (Puttini et al. 2006).

2.1.2 Breast Cancer

There is a high medical need to improve breast cancer therapy, particularly in the metastatic setting. Src activation has been implicated in both acquired and de novo trastuzumab-resistant cells (Zhang et al. 2011). Src regulation involved dephosphorylation by PTEN and increased Src activation conferred trastuzumab resistance in breast cancer cells and correlated with trastuzumab sensitivity in patients. Consequently, targeting Src in combination with trastuzumab re-sensitized multiple trastuzumab-resistant cells lines to trastuzumab and eliminated trastuzumab-resistant tumors in vivo, suggesting the potential clinical application of combining Src inhibitors with trastuzumab (Ocana et al. 2017). Bosutinib has been shown to cause reduced cell proliferation, migration, and invasion of breast cancer cell lines accompanied by an increase of cell-to-cell adhesions and a membrane localization of beta-catenin, a phosphoprotein that functions as both a structural component of the cell adhesion/actin cytoskeleton network and a signaling molecule when localized in the nucleus. Analysis of downstream effectors of Src reveals an inhibition of mitogen-activated protein kinase (MAPK) and Akt phosphorylation as well as a reduced phosphorylation of focal adhesion kinase (FAK), proline-rich tyrosine kinase 2 (Pyk2), and Crk-associated substrate (p130Cas). Thus, bosutinib inhibits signaling pathways involved in cell proliferation and malignant transformation as well as tumor cell motility and invasion (Jallal et al. 2007; Vultur et al. 2008). Accordingly, MDA-MB-231 cell in BALB/c nu/nu mice is significantly delayed by bosutinib therapy when compared to control animals. In addition, analysis of lung, liver, and spleen specimen has shown a significant reduction of metastatic spread in animals treated with the small molecule inhibitor at a well-tolerated dose.

2.1.3 Colorectal Cancer

Bosutinib decreases tumor growth in subcutaneous colorectal cancer xenograft models generated with different tumor cell lines (HT29, Colo205, HCT116, and DLD1) and causes substantial reduction of Src autophosphorylation at Tyr418 (Golas et al. 2005). In addition, it prevents Src-dependent activation of beta-catenin. However, protein levels of beta-catenin remain substantially unchanged by bosutinib, and a cytosolic/membranous retention of beta-catenin is promoted instead. The bosutinib-mediated relocalization of beta-catenin increases its binding affinity to E-cadherin and adhesion of colorectal cancer cells resulting in reduced cell motility (Coluccia et al. 2006). A decreased cell motion as well as the ability of bosutinib to reduce VEGF-mediated vascular permeability and tumor cell extravasation combined with the effect of Src inhibition in stromal cells may be responsible for the superior activity of bosutinib in vivo when compared with the attained effects in cell culture experiments.

2.1.4 Non-small Cell Lung Cell Cancer (NSCLC)

Immunohistochemical analyses of NSCLC biopsy samples reveal an up-regulation of Src kinase in 33% of the tumors. In NSCLC cell lines with elevated Src kinase activity, treatment with bosutinib induces apoptosis and causes a cleavage of caspase-3 and PARP (Zhang et al. 2007). However, monotherapy of bosutinib in solid cancer will probably not exert sufficient efficacy (Daud et al. 2012) and combination approaches have to be tested in the future to define the potential therapeutic value of additional Src inhibition as add-on to conventional cancer therapeutics.

2.2 Non-malignant Diseases

2.2.1 Polycystic Kidney Disease (PKD)

In polycystic kidney disease, the precise functions of the cystoprotein products remain unknown. Recent data suggest that multimeric cystoprotein complexes lead to aberrant signaling cascades involving c-Src kinases. In two different animal models, greater Src activity was found to correlate with disease progression in PKD. Inhibition of Src activity via bosutinib resulted in amelioration of renal cyst formation and biliary ductal abnormalities in both animal models (Sweeney et al. 2008), suggesting this strategy may provide therapeutic benefit in PKD (Sweeney et al. 2017).

2.2.2 Amyotrophic Lateral Sclerosis (ALS)

Amyotrophic lateral sclerosis (ALS) is a fatal neurological disease causing progressive motor neuron loss. No effective treatment option is available so far. A phenotypic drug screen using ALS motor neuron survival as readout identified the Src/c-ABL signaling pathway a most prominent hit. Motor neurons in this model were generated from induced pluripotent stem cells (iPSCs) derived from an ALS patient with a superoxide dismutase 1 (SOD1) mutation. Src/c-ABL inhibitors (including bosutinib) increased survival of ALS iPSC-derived motor neurons in vitro. Bosutinib boosted autophagy, reduced the amount of misfolded mutant SOD1 protein, and reduced altered expression of mitochondrial genes. Bosutinib also increased survival in vitro of ALS iPSC-derived motor neurons from patients with sporadic ALS or other forms of familial ALS caused by mutations in TAR DNA-binding protein (TDP-43) or repeat expansions in C9orf72. Finally, bosutinib treatment also extended survival of a mouse model of ALS with a SOD1 mutation, suggesting that inhibition of the Src/c-ABL by bosutinib is a potentially useful target for developing new drugs to treat ALS (Imamura et al. 2017).

3 Clinical Data

The initial approval of bosutinib in CML patients in 2013 was based on data published by Cortes et al. (2011) and Khoury et al. (2012) in their phase I/II trial, evaluating bosutinib in second-line and third-/fourth-line treatment upon intolerance or resistance to imatinib and/or intolerance or resistance to a second-generation TKI leading to the conditional approval of bosutinib for treatment in CML in chronic phase (CP), accelerated phase (AP), and blast crisis (BC) in Europe for patients after first-line therapy with first- or second-generation TKI for whom imatinib, nilotinib, or dasatinib are not considered appropriate treatment options. As mentioned before the approval in first-line CML treatment is still missing, however in addition to the failed first-line CML-CP BELA trial, another first-line trial with a limited starting dose of 400 mg/d was performed (the so-called BFORE trial) and recently published (Cortes et al. 2017). Based on this trial, widening of the approval of bosutinib in CML to first line is expected soon.

The phase I/II clinical trial, testing bosutinib in Philadelphia chromosome-positive leukemia, included 288 patients with imatinib resistance or intolerance between January 2006 and July 2008 where bosutinib was given as second-line treatment. Another 118 patients, which had been pretreated with at least two TKIs (imatinib *plus* one additional second-generation TKI), were recruited. Moreover, 134 patients in later disease phases (accelerated phase (AP) or blast crisis (BC) or Ph+ ALL) were formed the third cohort of this study. Bosutinib (500 mg) was established as current dosing regimen as 600 mg/d lead to dose-limiting toxicities (grade 3 rash, nausea, and vomiting).

Bosutinib has also been tested in several solid tumors and also in non-malignant diseases like polycystic kidney disease (PKD) not yet leading to any approval. The following chapter focuses on the clinical data available in all the different diseases.

3.1 Bosutinib in Treatment-Resistant/-Intolerant CML

3.1.1 Bosutinib as Second-Line Treatment

As mentioned before, the phase I/II trial on which approval of bosutinib was based on included three different cohorts of patients. In this trial, quality of life assessments has also been performed.

The second-line part included patients which were resistant or intolerant to imatinib. The definition of imatinib resistance in this trial (Cortes et al. 2011) applied if a patient did show no hematologic improvement within 4 weeks, no complete hematologic response (CHR) after 12 weeks, no cytogenetic response after 24 weeks, and/or no major cytogenetic response (MCR) after 12 months of therapy with an imatinib dose of at least 600 mg daily. Loss of a MyCR or any hematologic response defined an acquired resistance. Individuals have been considered to be intolerant to imatinib if toxicities grade 4 lasted longer than 7 days, if imatinib-related non-hematological toxicities grade 3 or higher occurred or persistent toxicities grade 2 not responding to adequate management and/or dose adjustments appeared. In addition, patients in whom dose reductions were necessary due to toxicities and who subsequently lost their response to treatment were considered imatinib-intolerant as well. Patients' characteristics are listed in Table 9.1. In total, 288 patients have been included in this part of the study with 69.4% exhibiting resistance and 20.6% intolerance to imatinib. Data on this trial were updated in 2014 by Gambacorti-Passerini et al. (2014) with a longer follow-up of at least 24 months. Response rates were reported as follows: 85% achieved/maintained CHR, 48% CCyR (59% with MyCR), and 35% presented with MMR. Probabilities of overall and progression-free survival were 91% and 81%. Age and cause of imatinib failure (intolerance or resistance) did not lead to

Table 9.1 Patient characteristics of chronic phase (CP) CML patients in the second-line setting

Characteristics	IM resistant (n = 200)	IM intolerant (n = 88)	Total (n = 288)
Median age: years (range)	51	54,5	53 (18–91)
Male sex	116	37	153
Median duration of disease in years (range)	4.0 (0.1–15.1)	2.8 (0.1–13.6)	3.6 (0.1–15.1)
Number of previous treatments			
1 (%)	128 (64)	65 (74)	193 (67)
2 (%)	72 (36)	23 (26)	95 (33)
Previous IFN (%)	69 (35)	23 (26)	92 (32)
Previous SCT (%)	6 (3)	2 (2)	8 (3)
BCR-ABL mutations			
Assessed patients	153	59	212
At least one mutation, n (%)	73 (48)	6 (10)	79 (37)

Source Gambacorti-Passerini et al. (2014a)

differential response rates. Brümmendorf et al. (2016) analyzed factors that impact long-term efficacy and safety in the context of the same trial. Prior cytogenetic response on imatinib, baseline MCyR, prior interferon therapy and duration from diagnosis to imatinib treatment initiation of less than 6 months without interferon intake before imatinib were identified as significant predictors of both MCyR and CCyR at 3 and 6 months.

3.1.2 Bosutinib After Failure of Second-Line Therapy

In the same study, 118 patients pretreated with imatinib and at least one other second-generation TKI had been recruited (Khoury et al. 2012). Bosutinib was administered in the 500 mg dose established in the phase I of the same trial. Among those, 118 patients who had previously been treated with IM 37 were dasatinib-resistant and 50 dasatinib intolerant. In addition, 27 were nilotinib resistant, and one patient was intolerant to nilotinib. Three patients had been treated with all three TKIs and failed. Median follow-up was 28.5 months (range 0.3–56.2), and median dose intensity was 478 mg/day (185–563 mg/day). MCyR rate was 32% among all patients with 24% (n = 26) achieving a CCyR; among them was one of the three patients being treated with all three TKIs before. Median time to MCyR among responders was 12.4 weeks (ranges 3.9–88.4 weeks). Molecular responses were assessed in 105 patients; among these, 16 (15%) achieved a MMR, including 12 (11%) with a CMR. Thirty-nine patients had known mutations at the beginning of treatment with bosutinib, and the results of these patients are summarized in Table 9.2.

In 2016, Cortes et al. (2016) published long-term data on this patient cohort proving data with a median follow-up of 32.7 months and a median treatment duration of 8.6 months. Table 9.3 summarizes the long-term probabilities and maintaining of response. Patient-reported outcome assessments in these third and

Table 9.2 Response by mutation status in CP CML after at least two lines of treatment

Mutation status	n	Cumulative response, n/n evaluable (%)	
		CHR	MCyR
No mutation	44	34/44 (77)	15/43 (Khoury et al. 2012)
Any mutation	39	26/39 (67)	11/35 (Sweeney et al. 2008)
>1 mutation	9	3/9 (33)	2/9 (22)
Mutation type			
P-loop	14	9/14 (64)	4/13 (Sweeney et al. 2008)
G250E	6	3/6	0/5
Y253H	6	5/6	4/6
E255 K	1	0/1	0/1
E255 V	1	1/1	0/1
Non-P-loop	29	18/29 (62)	9/26 (Khoury et al. 2012)
M244 V	3	3/3	2/3
V299L	2	1/2	0/2
Q300R	1	1/1	1/1
T315I	7	2/7	0/6
F317L	8	4/8	1/7
N336S	1	1/1	0/1
M351T	1	1/1	0/1
F359C	2	2/2	1/2
F359I	2	2/2	2/2
F359 V	2	0/2	1/2
L387F	1	1/1	0/1
H396R	1	0/1	0/1
E453A	1	1/1	0/0
C475 V	1	1/1	1/1
F486S	1	0/1	0/1

Source Khoury et al. (2012)

Table 9.3 Summary of the long-term response probabilities and rates in the third-/forth-line cohort (Cortes et al. 2016)

	Rate of %	Probability of maintaining at 4 years (%)
cCHR	74	63
MCyR	40	69
Incidence of PD on treatment/ death		24
4-year OS		78

further line patients as well as in the second-line patient cohort did show stabilization of health-related quality of life (QoL) during bosutinib treatment (Kantarjian et al. 2017).

3.1.3   Accelerated Phase (AP CML), Blast Phase (BP CML), and Ph+ ALL

Initially, data on patients with AP ($n = 77$) and BP CML ($n = 64$) and Ph+ ALL ($n = 24$) with an open-label continuous daily dosing schedule (bosutinib 500 mg/day) as part of the above-mentioned phase I/II trial were presented at the 2013 ASCO Annual Meeting (2013). All patients included were previously treated with imatinib *plus/minus* other TKIs and exhibited imatinib resistance or intolerance. In this analysis, patients were split into two different cohorts regarding their age (<65 years vs. ≥65 years). Hematologic and cytogenetic response data are shown in Table 9.4.

Long-term efficacy and safety of the whole patient group were analyzed and published in 2015 by Gambacorti-Passerini et al. (2015). Seventy-nine patients with AP, 64 with BP, and 24 patients with Ph+ ALL were treated with bosutinib and followed up for 28.4 (AP), 10.4 (BP), and 3.6 months (Ph+ ALL) (median). All patients had received prior imatinib treatment, and 9% had been treated with three prior TKIs. Median treatment duration was 10.2 months for AP patients, 2.8 months for BP patients, and 0.97 months for ALL patients. Responses were durable in approximately 50% of AP responders at 4 years with 57% maintaining baseline OHR, 40% attained/maintained MCyR by 4 years. For patients with blast crisis as approximately 25% responded at year 1, bosutinib seems to be a feasible treatment to bridge to allogeneic transplantation.

Attila et al. (2015) reported about a case with elderly acute lymphoblastic leukemia transformed from CML with suspected central nervous system involvement. This patient was pretreated with imatinib, dasatinib, and nilotinib as treatment for chronic phase CML, and after 7 years, the sickness transformed into acute B lymphoblastic leukemia occurring with simultaneous suspected central nervous system involvement. The patient was treated with bosutinib 500 mg/day (including

Table 9.4 Response to bosutinib treatment in AP/BC CML and Ph⁺ ALL

Response	ADV cohort	
	Aged ≥65 years (N = 30)	Aged <65 years (n = 135)
Hematologic response		
Evaluable patients, n	29	123
MHR, n (%)	8 (28)	38 (31)
CHR	4 (14)	31 (25)
2-year probability of maintaining a MHR	71%	54%
2-year probability of maintaining a CHR	75%	54%
Cytogenetic response		
Evaluable patients, n	26	117
MCyR, n (%)	8 (31)	45 (39)
CCyR	7 (27)	24 (29)
2-year probability of maintaining a MCyR	43%	34%

Source Brummendorf et al. (2013)

several treatment interruptions) and received cerebral radiotherapy and intrathecal chemotherapy with methotrexate and Ara-C. Maintenance therapy could only be performed including bosutinib as the patient could not stand further intrathecal treatment after six rounds of chemotherapy. At 14 months of follow-up, the patient still showed complete hematological and bone marrow response.

Whiteley et al. (2016) reported a significant improvement of several quality of life measurement tools in the AP/BC cohort during bosutinib treatment although the lack of comparison group handicaps the interpretation of these results.

3.2 Bosutinib in CML First-Line Treatment

In the BELA trial published 2012 by Cortes et al. (2012), bosutinib was evaluated in the first-line setting against imatinib in patients with chronic myeloid leukemia in chronic phase. The primary endpoint of this trial was the CCyR rate at 12 months which was the standard primary endpoint in first-line trials at that time, since the standardized molecular analysis was not available in all countries. 502 pts were randomized in a 1:1 manner to each arm, median duration of treatment in both study arms was 13.8 months, and median dose intensity was 489 mg/day for bosutinib and 400 mg/d for imatinib. In the IIT population, the CCyR rate at 12 months was similar in both treatment groups (70% for bosutinib vs. 68% for imatinib; $P = 0.601$). However, time to CCyR was significantly shorter with bosutinib (12.9 weeks vs. 24.6 weeks; $P < 0.001$) with higher rates for CCyR for bosutinib at months 3, 6, and 9. Molecular responses were also significantly higher in the bosutinib group, and in detail MMR rate at 12 months was 41% versus 27% ($P < 0.001$). Transformation to AP/BC CML on treatment occurred less frequently among the bosutinib-treated patients (4.2% vs. 10.4%).

Data from the BELA trial were updated in 2014 regarding safety aspects (Gambacorti-Passerini et al. 2014b) and efficacy in an update after 24 months of follow up (Brummendorf et al. 2015). The safety update stated clearly the low risk of long-term safety issues and the low amount of cardiovascular events comparable to imatinib treatment. Brümmendorf et al. reported durable responses from the 24-month follow-up of this BELA trial. Between the 12 and the 24 month update no new case of transformation to advanced stages of the disease occurred.

However, the BELA trial did not lead to approval of bosutinib in first-line CML treatment due to the missed primary endpoint; that is why after analysis of efficacy and safety data of individual dose levels of bosutinib, the so-called BFORE was established testing a reduced daily dose of 400 mg bosutinib again in first-line treatment compared to imatinib standard dose which closed recruitment in 2015 (NCT02130557). This hypothesis was supported by as well as based on the experience gained from other second-generation TKIs that first-line treatment requires lower doses of TKI as compared to second and later line treatments. At the end of 2016, the positive study results were announced meaning that bosutinib was superior to imatinib in first-line treatment regarding the MMR rate (and also again, regarding CCyR rate) at 12 months of treatment.

In this trial, patients with newly diagnosed chronic phase CML received 400 mg of bosutinib once daily ($n = 268$) or imatinib ($n = 268$) (Cortes et al. 2017). The median dose intensity was 392 mg per day for bosutinib and 400 mg per day for imatinib. The MMR rate at 12 months as mentioned before was significantly higher with bosutinib versus imatinib (47.2% vs. 36.9%; $P = 0.02$) as was the complete cytogenetic response (CCyR) rate by 12 months (77.2% vs. 66.4%; $P = 0.0075$). Bosutinib-treated patients achieved faster responses, and less patients discontinued treatment receiving bosutinib because of lack of efficacy in comparison with imatinib, whereas more patients discontinued treatment due to drug-related toxicity (12.7% for bosutinib and 8.7% for imatinib) (Cortes et al. 2017).

At this year's annual meeting of the American Society of Hematology, a comparison of both the first-line trials regarding exposure and response will be presented including 512 patients (Knight et al. 2017). The amount of side effects seemed to correlate with bosutinib exposure and furthermore the incidence of AEs associated with permanent discontinuation from bosutinib treatment was higher within the BELA trial (21.0% for a starting dose of 500 mg/day (BELA) vs. 14.2% for a starting dose of 400 mg/day (BFORE)). Time on treatment influenced efficacy with both bosutinib exposure and time on bosutinib treatment being significant predictors of MMR. The interpretation of this data might be that staying on treatment could be more important than receiving higher doses and may at least in part explain the suboptimal results achieved by bosutinib therapy in the BELA trial.

3.3 Bosutinib in Solid Tumors

Daud et al. (2012) published their phase I trial in patients with advanced solid tumor malignancies. This trial was conducted in two parts, a dose escalation part where 400 mg/day could be identified as recommended dose for phase II. In the second part, approximately 30 patients each with refractory colorectal, pancreas, or NSCLC were treated. A partial response (breast) and unconfirmed complete response (pancreas) were observed; 8 of 112 evaluable patients had stable disease for 22–101 weeks. However, the primary efficacy endpoints for part 2 were not met.

Campone et al. (2012) performed a phase II study which evaluated single-agent bosutinib in pretreated patients with locally advanced or metastatic breast cancer in 73 patients. The primary endpoint was the progression-free survival (PFS) rate at 16 weeks. For the intent-to-treat population, the PFS rate at 16 weeks was 39.6%. Unexpectedly, all responding patients ($n = 4$) were hormone receptor positive. The 2-year overall survival rate was 26.4%.

In 2014, Isakoff et al. (2014) published data of a phase I trial testing safety, efficacy, and maximum tolerated dose (MTD) of bosutinib in combination with capecitabine in several solid tumors. Thirty-two patients with locally advanced/metastatic cancer of the breast, pancreas and patients with cholangiocarcinoma, glioblastoma, or colorectal cancer received both drugs in eight different dose combinations with nine of them receiving MTD (300 mg bosutinib/day + capecitabine 1000 mg/m^2 bid). In 6% of the patients (2/31), dose-limiting toxicities occurred. Efficacy was limited as best overall confirmed PR or SD lasting longer than 24 was only observed in 6 and 13% of the patients, respectively. The safety profile was quite similar to the individual profiles of both drugs, and especially, regarding diarrhea most patients facing this side effect (91%) did only experience low-grade events (grade 1/2).

3.4 Bosutinib in Polycystic Kidney Disease (PKD)

Src kinase overactivation is one of the driving mechanisms in the pathogenesis of autosomal dominant polycystic kidney disease (ADPKD). As mentioned already above, this hypothesis leads to the preclinical and clinical testing of bosutinib in this disease. Tesar et al. (2017) published data from a multicentre phase II trial where 172 patients with ADPKD were randomized 1:1:1 to receive either bosutinib 200 mg/day, bosutinib 400 mg/day, or placebo. Bosutinib 200 mg/day and pooled bosutinib treatment showed a significant reduction (66%/82%) in the rate of kidney enlargement. Annualized eGFR decline was similar in all three arms. Toxicity findings were similar to the side effect profiles established in the hematologic trials.

4 Toxicity

While the general toxicity profile of bosutinib was very similar in hematological trials and studies in solid tumors, there were some expected differences in hematological adverse events.

In an update of the BELA trial (Brummendorf et al. 2015), comparing bosutinib versus imatinib for newly diagnosed patients with CML in CP, grade 1 or 2 side effects like diarrhea occurred in 58%, nausea in 31%, vomiting in 31%, rash in 22%, headache in 12%, and arthralgia in 7% of the patients. The most common cardiovascular AEs were hypertension (6% vs. 4%) and palpitations (2% vs. 2%). Cardiac failure occurred in one (<1%) bosutinib-treated patient and two (1%) imatinib-treated patients. There was no report of peripheral arterial occlusive disease. The most common grade 3/4 treatment-emergent AE was diarrhea (bosutinib, 12%; imatinib, 1%). In the bosutinib arm diarrhea of all grades typically occurred during the first month of treatment and was treated with anti-diarrheal medication. In some patients, temporary interruption was needed to control the side effects. But in most of the cases, it was self-limiting and transient. Hematological adverse events (neutropenia, thrombocytopenia, and anemia) of grade 3 and 4 were lower in the bosutinib arm (10% compared to imatinib 24%). Non-hematological adverse events like elevation of liver enzymes or bilirubin occurred more often in the bosutinib cohort. Side effects could be controlled with concurrent medication and dose modification. None of these effects led to hospitalization or to permanent hepatic injury.

Even in heavily pretreated patients with advanced CML (AP, BP) (Gambacorti-Passerini et al. 2015), the most common AEs were gastrointestinal (96%; 83%), primarily diarrhea (85%; 64%), which was typically low grade (maximum grade 1/2: 81%; 59%) and transient. Serious AEs were pneumonia and pyrexia.

Cortes et al. (2017) analyzed patients receiving bosutinib in first and in later lines regarding renal function. Long-term bosutinib treatment was associated with a reversible decline in renal function; this aspect seems to be similar to long-term imatinib treatment regarding frequency and characteristics. Patients at risk for renal side effects should be monitored closely.

In contrast to the hematological malignancies, myelosuppression in solid tumor studies was minimal. This could be explained by the fact that hematologic toxicity of TKI treatment in CML is not only a reflection of inhibition of normal hematopoiesis but at least in part mediated by suppression of the leukemic population itself by the TKI.

In part one of the solid cancer trial (Daud et al. 2012), dose-limiting toxicities of grade 3 diarrhea (two patients) and grade 3 rash occurred with bosutinib 600 mg/day and the maximum tolerable dose was defined as 500 mg/day. However, the majority of patients treated with 500 mg/day had grade 2 or greater gastrointestinal toxicity. The most common bosutinib-related adverse events were nausea (60% patients), diarrhea (47%), vomiting (40%), fatigue (38%), and anorexia (36%).

In a phase I study of advanced solid tumor patients treated with bosutinib in combination with capecitabine (Isakoff et al. 2014), the most frequent treatment-related adverse events (AEs) were diarrhea, nausea, vomiting, palmar-plantar erythrodysesthesia (PPE), fatigue; most frequent grade 3/4 AEs: PPE, fatigue, and increased alanine/aspartate aminotransferase. Although diarrhea was common, 91% of affected patients experienced maximum grade 1/2 toxicity that resolved. Among breast cancer patients, the main toxic effects were diarrhea (66%), nausea (55%), and vomiting (47%). Grade 3–4 liver aminotransferase elevation occurred in 14 (19%) patients.

5 Drug Interactions

Strong inhibitors of CYP3A4 should be avoided during treatment with bosutinib because of significant increase in bosutinib plasma levels. In this context antifungal treatment with azoles needs to get special attention and should be given with caution (Steegmann et al. 2012, 2016; Ono et al. 2017). Furthermore, some HIV-1 proteasome inhibitors and NNRT inhibitors need to be administered very carefully. In addition to that, grapefruit juice needs to be avoided (Steegmann et al. 2012, 2016; Ono et al. 2017). A full list of CYP3A inhibitors can be found at: http://medicine.iupui.edu/clinpharm/ddis/table.aspx.

Of course, concomitant use of CYP3A4 inducers should be avoided as well. Especially, treatment with rifampicin or anti-epileptic drugs as carbamazepine and phenytoin or the use of St. John´s Worth should not be used as bosutinib plasma levels might be decreased significantly (Steegmann et al. 2012, 2016; Hsyu et al. 2017). A full list of CYP3A4 inducers can be found at: http://medicine.iupui.edu/clinpharm/ddis/table.aspx.

Beside CYP3A4 interactions, special attention needs to be paid in case of usage of any drug with QTc prolongation potential (Steegmann et al. 2012, 2016). If concomitant medication cannot be avoided regularly ECG controls need to be performed. A full list of agents that prolong the QT interval can be found at: https://crediblemeds.org/pdftemp/pdf/CombinedList.pdf.

Resorption of bosutinib is pH dependent; therefore, if medication with proton pump inhibitors is necessary, they should be taken several hours before or after bosutinib medication (Steegmann et al. 2012, 2016; Abbas et al. 2013). Other interactions might be caused by bosutinib and substrates of P-glycoprotein. One in vitro study suggests that plasma levels of P-gp substrates such as digoxin, tacrolimus, some chemotherapeutic agents, and dexamethasone may be increased by bosutinib (Steegmann et al. 2012, 2016; Hsyu et al. 2017).

6 Biomarkers for Response

In CML, BCR-ABL transcript monitoring is essential with any TKI treatment. According to international guidelines (i.e., ELN guidelines (Baccarani et al. 2013), NCCN Guidelines 2.2018), BCR-ABL (expressed as % of housekeeping control gene transcripts) measuring should be performed every 3 months. The goal is to achieve an optimal response, as reflected by CCyR after 6 months and/or a BCR-ABL transcript level of less than 1%, and a reduction in BCR-ABL to equal or less than 0.1% after 12 months of treatment. Early achievement of molecular remission becomes increasingly important; with a decrease in BCR-ABL transcripts to below 10% after three months of treatment is associated with improved 5-year survival as compared to patients who do not achieve this goal (Hanfstein et al. 2012). An even better individual biomarker for response is the slope of the BCR-ABL transcript decline during therapy (Hanfstein et al. 2014; Branford et al. 2014).

In the BELA trial, which tested the efficacy and safety of bosutinib versus imatinib in the first-line setting in patients with newly diagnosed CP CML (Cortes et al. 2012), the rate of molecular response was generally higher at all time points for bosutinib. Bosutinib was also associated with deeper cytogenetic and molecular responses compared with imatinib. For both bosutinib and imatinib, reduction in BCR-ABL/ABL ratio to ≤ 1 or $\leq 10\%$ at months 3, 6, and 9 was associated with higher rates of CCyR and MMR by 12 and 24 months. Overall, these results suggest that early reduction in BCR-ABL/ABL ratio during bosutinib or imatinib therapy is linked to a higher likelihood of experiencing better long-term outcome.

However, the trial failed to show superiority of bosutinib in achieving its primary endpoint, CCyR at 12 months as outlined before (Cortes et al. 2012).

In the second randomized phase III trial (BFORE trial), the superiority of bosutinib over imatinib was validated in patients with CML in chronic phase (Cortes et al. 2017). This trial showed significant improvement of molecular responses in the bosutinib- versus imatinib-treated group, and CCyR by 12 months was also significantly higher in the bosutinib group. It remains to be seen whether these early molecular responses biomarker will translate into superior long-term event-free or even overall survival.

Generally, it is very important to perform these biomarker measurements according to international standards in a well-experienced laboratory following their recommendations for national standardization for quality assurance (Cross et al. 2012, 2015, 2016). Due to the established converting factor to the international scale, follow-up monitoring not necessarily needs to be performed in the same laboratory but in certified laboratories in order to guarantee comparable results.

7 Summary and Perspectives

In conclusion, bosutinib is a novel dual Src/ABL kinase inhibitor with high activity against imatinib-resistant CML as well as solid tumors overexpressing the Src kinase. Its profile of activity is specific with a limited number of molecular targets outside the ABL and Src kinase family. When compared with other second-generation tyrosine kinase inhibitors and with imatinib, bosutinib shows a distinct and very favorable long-term toxicity profile and therefore might be of advantage for a certain cohort of patients based on their pretreatment, toxicities, and/or preexisting comorbidities. Indeed, presumably PDGFR- and/or KIT-mediated side effects such as inhibition of normal hematopoiesis typically observed with other TKIs used in BCR-ABL-positive leukemias (Bartolovic et al. 2004) occur less frequent in patients treated with bosutinib. Furthermore, until now bosutinib treatment seems to be favorable regarding a low rate of long-term toxicity. However, the high rate of gastrointestinal side effects is still a problem that needs to be addressed. A lot of effort has been put in the side management of those events including prophylactic medication and guidelines for patient and physicians how to behave in case of GI toxicity. Furthermore, initial dose reduction has been and is currently tested in different trials with first results showing that time on treatment with bosutinib is important but initial dose decrease can avoid early treatment discontinuation due to side effects. The so-called BODO trial (NCT03205267) is currently recruiting patients and is testing the concept of toxicity-guided intra-individual dose escalation upon starting with a lower dose of bosutinib (300 mg/day) and will hopefully improve GI tolerability by defining the individual maximum tolerable dose while efficacy is preserved due to a more continuous treatment.

References

Abbas R, Leister C, Sonnichsen D (2013) A clinical study to examine the potential effect of lansoprazole on the pharmacokinetics of bosutinib when administered concomitantly to healthy subjects. Clin Drug Investig 33(8):589–595

Atilla E, Ataca P, Ozyurek E, Erden I, Gurman G (2015) Successful bosutinib experience in an elderly acute lymphoblastic leukemia patient with suspected central nervous system involvement transformed from chronic myeloid leukemia. Case Rep Hematol 2015:689423

Baccarani M, Deininger MW, Rosti G, Hochhaus A, Soverini S, Apperley JF et al (2013) European LeukemiaNet recommendations for the management of chronic myeloid leukemia: 2013. Blood 122(6):872–884

Bartolovic K, Balabanov S, Hartmann U, Komor M, Boehmler AM, Buhring HJ et al (2004) Inhibitory effect of imatinib on normal progenitor cells in vitro. Blood 103(2):523–529

Boschelli DH, Ye F, Wang YD, Dutia M, Johnson SL, Wu B et al (2001) Optimization of 4-phenylamino-3-quinolinecarbonitriles as potent inhibitors of Src kinase activity. J Med Chem 44(23):3965–3977

Branford S, Yeung DT, Parker WT, Roberts ND, Purins L, Braley JA et al (2014) Prognosis for patients with CML and >10% BCR-ABL1 after 3 months of imatinib depends on the rate of BCR-ABL1 decline. Blood 124(4):511–518

Brummendorf TH, Gambacorti-Passerini C, Cortes J (2013) Efficacy and Safety of bosutinib for Philadelphia chromosome-positive leukaemia in older versus younger patients. J Clin Oncol (official journal of the American Society of Clinical Oncology), suppl. (Abstract 6511)

Brummendorf TH, Cortes JE, de Souza CA, Guilhot F, Duvillie L, Pavlov D et al (2015) Bosutinib versus imatinib in newly diagnosed chronic-phase chronic myeloid leukaemia: results from the 24-month follow-up of the BELA trial. Br J Haematol 168(1):69–81

Brummendorf TH, Cortes JE, Khoury HJ, Kantarjian HM, Kim DW, Schafhausen P et al (2016) Factors influencing long-term efficacy and tolerability of bosutinib in chronic phase chronic myeloid leukaemia resistant or intolerant to imatinib. Br J Haematol 172(1):97–110

Campone M, Bondarenko I, Brincat S, Hotko Y, Munster PN, Chmielowska E et al (2012) Phase II study of single-agent bosutinib, a Src/Abl tyrosine kinase inhibitor, in patients with locally advanced or metastatic breast cancer pretreated with chemotherapy. Ann Oncol 23 (3):610–617

Coluccia AM, Benati D, Dekhil H, De Filippo A, Lan C, Gambacorti-Passerini C (2006) SKI-606 decreases growth and motility of colorectal cancer cells by preventing pp60(c-Src)-dependent tyrosine phosphorylation of beta-catenin and its nuclear signaling. Cancer Res 66(4):2279–2286

Cortes JE, Kantarjian HM, Brummendorf TH, Kim DW, Turkina AG, Shen ZX et al (2011) Safety and efficacy of bosutinib (SKI-606) in chronic phase Philadelphia chromosome-positive chronic myeloid leukemia patients with resistance or intolerance to imatinib. Blood 118 (17):4567–4576

Cortes JE, Kim DW, Kantarjian HM, Brummendorf TH, Dyagil I, Griskevicius L et al (2012) Bosutinib versus imatinib in newly diagnosed chronic-phase chronic myeloid leukemia: results from the BELA trial. J Clin Oncol 30(28):3486–3492

Cortes JE, Khoury HJ, Kantarjian HM, Lipton JH, Kim DW, Schafhausen P et al (2016) Long-term bosutinib for chronic phase chronic myeloid leukemia after failure of imatinib plus dasatinib and/or nilotinib. Am J Hematol 91(12):1206–1214

Cortes JE, Gambacorti-Passerini C, Deininger MW, Mauro MJ, Chuah C, Kim DW et al (2017) Bosutinib versus imatinib for newly diagnosed chronic myeloid leukemia: results from the randomized BFORE trial. J Clin Oncol, JCO2017747162

Cortes JE, Gambacorti-Passerini C, Kim DW, Kantarjian HM, Lipton JH, Lahoti A et al (2017) Effects of bosutinib treatment on renal function in patients with philadelphia chromosome-positive leukemias. Clin Lymphoma Myeloma Leuk 17(10):684–695 e6

Cross NC, White HE, Muller MC, Saglio G, Hochhaus A (2012) Standardized definitions of molecular response in chronic myeloid leukemia. Leukemia 26(10):2172–2175

Cross NC, White HE, Colomer D, Ehrencrona H, Foroni L, Gottardi E et al (2015) Laboratory recommendations for scoring deep molecular responses following treatment for chronic myeloid leukemia. Leukemia 29(5):999–1003

Cross NC, White HE, Ernst T, Welden L, Dietz C, Saglio G et al (2016) Development and evaluation of a secondary reference panel for BCR-ABL1 quantification on the International Scale. Leukemia 30(9):1844–1852

Daud AI, Krishnamurthi SS, Saleh MN, Gitlitz BJ, Borad MJ, Gold PJ et al (2012) Phase I study of bosutinib, a src/abl tyrosine kinase inhibitor, administered to patients with advanced solid tumors. Clin Cancer Res 18(4):1092–1100

Gambacorti-Passerini C, Brummendorf TH, Kim DW, Turkina AG, Masszi T, Assouline S et al (2014a) Bosutinib efficacy and safety in chronic phase chronic myeloid leukemia after imatinib resistance or intolerance: minimum 24-month follow-up. Am J Hematol 89(7):732–742

Gambacorti-Passerini C, Cortes JE, Lipton JH, Dmoszynska A, Wong RS, Rossiev V et al (2014b) Safety of bosutinib versus imatinib in the phase 3 BELA trial in newly diagnosed chronic phase chronic myeloid leukemia. Am J Hematol 89(10):947–953

Gambacorti-Passerini C, Kantarjian HM, Kim DW, Khoury HJ, Turkina AG, Brummendorf TH et al (2015) Long-term efficacy and safety of bosutinib in patients with advanced leukemia following resistance/intolerance to imatinib and other tyrosine kinase inhibitors. Am J Hematol 90(9):755–768

Golas JM, Arndt K, Etienne C, Lucas J, Nardin D, Gibbons J et al (2003) SKI-606, a 4-anilino-3-quinolinecarbonitrile dual inhibitor of Src and Abl kinases, is a potent antiproliferative agent against chronic myelogenous leukemia cells in culture and causes regression of K562 xenografts in nude mice. Cancer Res 63(2):375–381

Golas JM, Lucas J, Etienne C, Golas J, Discafani C, Sridharan L et al (2005) SKI-606, a Src/Abl inhibitor with in vivo activity in colon tumor xenograft models. Cancer Res 65(12):5358–5364

Greuber EK, Smith-Pearson P, Wang J, Pendergast AM (2013) Role of ABL family kinases in cancer: from leukaemia to solid tumours. Nat Rev Cancer 13(8):559–571

Hanfstein B, Muller MC, Hehlmann R, Erben P, Lauseker M, Fabarius A et al (2012) Early molecular and cytogenetic response is predictive for long-term progression-free and overall survival in chronic myeloid leukemia (CML). Leukemia 26(9):2096–2102

Hanfstein B, Shlyakhto V, Lauseker M, Hehlmann R, Saussele S, Dietz C et al (2014) Velocity of early BCR-ABL transcript elimination as an optimized predictor of outcome in chronic myeloid leukemia (CML) patients in chronic phase on treatment with imatinib. Leukemia 28 (10):1988–1992

Hegedus C, Ozvegy-Laczka C, Apati A, Magocsi M, Nemet K, Orfi L et al (2009) Interaction of nilotinib, dasatinib and bosutinib with ABCB1 and ABCG2: implications for altered anti-cancer effects and pharmacological properties. Br J Pharmacol 158(4):1153–1164

Heisterkamp N, Stam K, Groffen J, de Klein A, Grosveld G (1985) Structural organization of the bcr gene and its role in the Ph' translocation. Nature 315(6022):758–761

Hsyu PH, Pignataro DS, Matschke K (2017) Effect of aprepitant, a moderate CYP3A4 inhibitor, on bosutinib exposure in healthy subjects. Eur J Clin Pharmacol 73(1):49–56

Imamura K, Izumi Y, Watanabe A, Tsukita K, Woltjen K, Yamamoto T et al (2017) The Src/c-Abl pathway is a potential therapeutic target in amyotrophic lateral sclerosis. Sci Transl Med 9(391)

Isakoff SJ, Wang D, Campone M, Calles A, Leip E, Turnbull K et al (2014) Bosutinib plus capecitabine for selected advanced solid tumours: results of a phase 1 dose-escalation study. Br J Cancer 111(11):2058–2066

Jallal H, Valentino ML, Chen G, Boschelli F, Ali S, Rabbani SA (2007) A Src/Abl kinase inhibitor, SKI-606, blocks breast cancer invasion, growth, and metastasis in vitro and in vivo. Cancer Res 67(4):1580–1588

Johnson FM, Gallick GE (2007) SRC family nonreceptor tyrosine kinases as molecular targets for cancer therapy. Anticancer Agents Med Chem 7(6):651–659

Kantarjian HM, Mamolo CM, Gambacorti-Passerini C, Cortes JE, Brummendorf TH, Su Y et al (2017) Long-term patient-reported outcomes from an open-label safety and efficacy study of bosutinib in Philadelphia chromosome-positive chronic myeloid leukemia patients resistant or intolerant to prior therapy. Cancer

Khoury HJ, Cortes JE, Kantarjian HM, Gambacorti-Passerini C, Baccarani M, Kim DW et al (2012) Bosutinib is active in chronic phase chronic myeloid leukemia after imatinib and dasatinib and/or nilotinib therapy failure. Blood 119(15):3403–3412

Knight B, Garrett M, Cortes JE, Deininger MW (2017) Optimizing dose of bosutinib to minimize adverse events while maintaining efficacy in patients with newly diagnosed chronic myelogenous leukemia. In: ASH 59th annual meeting, Atlanta, GA

Laneuville P (1995) Abl tyrosine protein kinase. Semin Immunol 7(4):255–266

Levinson NM, Boxer SG (2012) Structural and spectroscopic analysis of the kinase inhibitor bosutinib and an isomer of bosutinib binding to the Abl tyrosine kinase domain. PLoS ONE 7 (4):e29828

Li S (2008) Src-family kinases in the development and therapy of Philadelphia chromosome-positive chronic myeloid leukemia and acute lymphoblastic leukemia. Leuk Lymphoma 49(1):19–26

Lutz MP, Esser IB, Flossmann-Kast BB, Vogelmann R, Luhrs H, Friess H et al (1998) Overexpression and activation of the tyrosine kinase Src in human pancreatic carcinoma. Biochem Biophys Res Commun 243(2):503–508

Mazurenko NN, Kogan EA, Zborovskaya IB, Kisseljov FL (1992) Expression of pp60c-src in human small cell and non-small cell lung carcinomas. Eur J Cancer 28(2–3):372–377

Nowell PC, Hungerford DA (1961) Chromosome studies in human leukemia. II. Chronic granulocytic leukemia. J Natl Cancer Inst 27:1013–1035

Ocana A, Gil-Martin M, Martin M, Rojo F, Antolin S, Guerrero A, et al (2017) A phase I study of the SRC kinase inhibitor dasatinib with trastuzumab and paclitaxel as first line therapy for patients with HER2-overexpressing advanced breast cancer. GEICAM/2010-04 study. Oncotarget 8(42):73144–73153

Ono C, Hsyu PH, Abbas R, Loi CM, Yamazaki S (2017) Application of physiologically based pharmacokinetic modeling to the understanding of bosutinib pharmacokinetics: prediction of drug-drug and drug-disease interactions. Drug Metab Dispos 45(4):390–398

Ottenhoff-Kalff AE, Rijksen G, van Beurden EA, Hennipman A, Michels AA, Staal GE (1992) Characterization of protein tyrosine kinases from human breast cancer: involvement of the c-src oncogene product. Cancer Res 52(17):4773–4778

Patel AB, O'Hare T, Deininger MW (2017) Mechanisms of resistance to ABL kinase inhibition in chronic myeloid leukemia and the development of next generation ABL kinase inhibitors. Hematol Oncol Clin North Am 31(4):589–612

Pendergast AM (1996) Nuclear tyrosine kinases: from Abl to WEE1. Curr Opin Cell Biol 8 (2):174–181

Puttini M, Coluccia AM, Boschelli F, Cleris L, Marchesi E, Donella-Deana A et al (2006) In vitro and in vivo activity of SKI-606, a novel Src-Abl inhibitor, against imatinib-resistant Bcr-Abl + neoplastic cells. Cancer Res 66(23):11314–11322

Redaelli S, Mologni L, Rostagno R, Piazza R, Magistroni V, Ceccon M et al (2012) Three novel patient-derived BCR/ABL mutants show different sensitivity to second and third generation tyrosine kinase inhibitors. Am J Hematol 87(11):E125–E128

Ren R (2005) Mechanisms of BCR-ABL in the pathogenesis of chronic myelogenous leukaemia. Nat Rev Cancer 5(3):172–183

Steegmann JL, Cervantes F, le Coutre P, Porkka K, Saglio G (2012) Off-target effects of BCR-ABL1 inhibitors and their potential long-term implications in patients with chronic myeloid leukemia. Leuk Lymphoma 53(12):2351–2361

Steegmann JL, Baccarani M, Breccia M, Casado LF, Garcia-Gutierrez V, Hochhaus A et al (2016) European LeukemiaNet recommendations for the management and avoidance of adverse events of treatment in chronic myeloid leukaemia. Leukemia 30(8):1648–1671

Summy JM, Gallick GE (2003) Src family kinases in tumor progression and metastasis. Cancer Metastasis Rev 22(4):337–358

Sweeney WE Jr, von Vigier RO, Frost P, Avner ED (2008) Src inhibition ameliorates polycystic kidney disease. J Am Soc Nephrol 19(7):1331–1341

Sweeney WE, Frost P, Avner ED (2017) Tesevatinib ameliorates progression of polycystic kidney disease in rodent models of autosomal recessive polycystic kidney disease. World J Nephrol 6 (4):188–200

Tesar V, Ciechanowski K, Pei Y, Barash I, Shannon M, Li R et al (2017) Bosutinib versus placebo for autosomal dominant polycystic kidney disease. J Am Soc Nephrol 28(11):3404–3413

Thomas SM, Brugge JS (1997) Cellular functions regulated by Src family kinases. Annu Rev Cell Dev Biol 13:513–609

Verbeek BS, Vroom TM, Adriaansen-Slot SS, Ottenhoff-Kalff AE, Geertzema JG, Hennipman A et al (1996) c-Src protein expression is increased in human breast cancer. An immunohistochemical and biochemical analysis. J Pathol 180(4):383–388

Vultur A, Buettner R, Kowolik C, Liang W, Smith D, Boschelli F et al (2008) SKI-606 (bosutinib), a novel Src kinase inhibitor, suppresses migration and invasion of human breast cancer cells. Mol Cancer Ther 7(5):1185–1194

Whiteley J, Reisman A, Shapiro M, Cortes J, Cella D (2016) Health-related quality of life during bosutinib (SKI-606) therapy in patients with advanced chronic myeloid leukemia after imatinib failure. Curr Med Res Opin 32(8):1325–1334

Zhang J, Kalyankrishna S, Wislez M, Thilaganathan N, Saigal B, Wei W et al (2007) SRC-family kinases are activated in non-small cell lung cancer and promote the survival of epidermal growth factor receptor-dependent cell lines. Am J Pathol 170(1):366–376

Zhang S, Huang WC, Li P, Guo H, Poh SB, Brady SW et al (2011) Combating trastuzumab resistance by targeting SRC, a common node downstream of multiple resistance pathways. Nat Med 17(4):461–469

Ponatinib: A Third-Generation Inhibitor for the Treatment of CML

Julius Wehrle and Nikolas von Bubnoff

Contents

Abstract

The establishment of imatinib as the standard therapy for CML marked the beginning of a new era of treatment. Due to occurring intolerance and resistance against the drug, the development of new inhibitors was promoted. This led to the second-generation inhibitors dasatinib, nilotinib, and bosutinib. Despite all achieved improvements, first- and second-generation inhibitors are ineffective against the BCR-ABL T315I "gatekeeper" mutation. In order to overcome this issue and to further improve the inhibitory effect, the third-generation inhibitor ponatinib was developed. Various clinical trials have been launched to study the effect of ponatinib in the clinical setting. Based on positive phase 1 and phase 2 trials, ponatinib was approved for the second-line treatment of CML and Ph⁺ ALL in December 2012 in the USA and in July 2013 in the European Union. The safety data of these trials particularly revealed a dose-dependent, increased risk for serious

J. Wehrle · N. von Bubnoff (✉)
Department of Medicine I, Medical Center, University of Freiburg, Freiburg, Germany
e-mail: nikolas.bubnoff@uniklinik-freiburg.de

N. von Bubnoff
German Cancer Consortium (DKTK) and German Cancer Research Center (DKFZ),
Heidelberg, Germany

© Springer International Publishing AG, part of Springer Nature 2018
U. M. Martens (ed.), *Small Molecules in Hematology*, Recent Results
in Cancer Research 211, https://doi.org/10.1007/978-3-319-91439-8_5

arterial occlusive events under treatment with ponatinib. Further trials investigate optimized dosing schemes to reduce side effects while maintaining clinical activity in CML and evaluate potential activity of the drug in other malignancies. In conclusion, ponatinib has proved to be a powerful BCR-ABL inhibitor, which exhibits clinical activity both in BCR-ABL wild-type and mutant CML, including the pan-resistant T315I mutation. Ponatinib should be used catiously with respect to increased cardiovascular risk. Despite previous TKI failure, chronic-phase CML patients can achieve sustained remissions using this drug, offering an important addition to therapeutic options in the treatment for CML.

Keywords
Ponatinib · CML · Tyrosine Kinase Inhibitor (TKI)

1 Resistance to Treatment in CML

The establishment of imatinib as the standard therapy for CML in 2001 (Druker et al. 2001) fundamentally changed the clinical course of this disease. For many patients, CML became a chronic disorder and patients experiencing major molecular response (MMR) might not face a loss in life expectancy (Jain et al. 2013). However, this favorable prognosis is not true for all patients. Around 20–30% of patients treated with imatinib do not respond adequately to treatment (primary resistance) or relapse after initial response to imatinib (secondary resistance) (Druker et al. 2006; de Lavallade et al. 2008).

Resistance against imatinib or newer Abl inhibitors is caused by various mechanisms that can occur in combination, especially in advanced stages of disease (von Bubnoff et al. 2005; Lahaye et al. 2005; Nicolini et al. 2007). Patient-related causes for primary as well as secondary resistance are mainly non-compliance with the treatment regime (Darkow et al. 2007). However, inadequate serum levels can arise despite proper compliance from individual differences in the activity of imatinib-metabolizing enzymes such as CYP3A4. In addition, these enzymes can be induced by co-medication and nutritional habits (Floyd et al. 2003).

At the cellular level, the ability of the malignant clone to transport drug out of the cell or to hinder drug influx can result in drug resistance. For example, the proteins ABCB1 and MDR-1 are considered responsible for the increased efflux of imatinib from CML cells (Kuwazuru et al. 1990; Mahon et al. 2003; Thomas et al. 2004).

Just as the BCR-ABL fusion protein represents the causative event for CML, it is also the main reason for the development of resistance (Shah and Sawyers 2003). Mutations of this fusion gene result in changes in critical amino acids, such that inhibitors become ineffective (von Bubnoff et al. 2002; Branford et al. 2003). More than 90 different mutations of BCR-ABL in CML have been described in recent years (Soverini et al. 2011). However, the majority of observed mutations occur at specific positions. One study found 14 mutations in 95% of cases (Zhou et al. 2011), while another analysis described 20 mutations in 88% of cases

(Branford et al. 2009). Hence, these common mutations are clinically most relevant and have directed the development of second- and third-generation inhibitors.

2 Second-Generation Inhibitors

After the approval of imatinib in 2002, second-generation BCR-ABL kinase inhibitors were developed. The need for these novel inhibitors became evident both from patients presenting with primary imatinib intolerance, or developing intolerance during treatment, and from primary or secondary imatinib resistance, many of them being the consequence of secondary mutations in BCR-ABL, which confer imatinib resistance.

Based on the positive results of phase 2 trials, the second-generation inhibitors dasatinib and nilotinib were approved as second-line therapy in imatinib-resistant or imatinib-intolerant CML and Ph$^+$ ALL (Kantarjian et al. 2007; Talpaz et al. 2006). In March 2013, bosutinib was also approved for second-line treatment. Recently, phase 3 trials (DAISION for dasatinib; ENESTnd for nilotinib) reported earlier and deeper remissions compared to imatinib in newly diagnosed, chronic-phase CML patients, as well as lower rates of progression to accelerated phase or blast crisis along with good tolerability of the drugs (Kantarjian et al. 2010, 2011; Saglio et al. 2010). These trials consequently led to the approval of both second-generation inhibitors, dasatinib and nilotinib, for the first-line treatment of CML. Although all second-generation inhibitors proved to be effective against a variety of known secondary BCR-ABL mutations, each of these inhibitors still faces a distinct spectrum of vulnerable mutations (Zhou et al. 2011; Branford et al. 2009; Bradeen et al. 2006; von Bubnoff et al. 2006) (Table 1).

Most notably, despite their differences, all first- and second-generation inhibitors are ineffective against the BCR-ABL T315I mutation. The exchange of threonine at position 315 for the more bulky isoleucine leads to a steric hindrance, inhibiting binding of all these inhibitors. Unable to bind the kinase, most Abl inhibitors lose their ability to block BCR-ABL kinase activity. Twenty percent of patients who are imatinib-resistant because of a BCR-ABL mutation harbor the T315I "gatekeeper" mutation (O'Hare et al. 2007).

3 Ponatinib: A Third-Generation Inhibitor

The small molecule ponatinib was developed specifically to overcome resistance based on the T315I mutation. The integration of a linear carbon–carbon triple bond into the structure of the molecule to link two functional groups avoids the blocking effect of the isoleucine in the context of the T315I mutation (Fig. 1). Furthermore,

Table 1 Resistance of BCR-ABL mutations against first-, second-, and third-generation inhibitors

	imatinib	dasatinib	nilotinib	bosutinib	ponatinib
WT	1,0	1,0	1,0	1,0	1,0
M244V	0,9	2,0	1,2	0,9	3,2
L248R	14,6	12,5	30,2	22,9	6,2
L248V	3,5	5,1	2,8	3,5	3,4
G250E	6,9	4,4	4,6	4,3	6,0
Q252H	1,4	3,1	2,6	0,8	6,1
Y253F	3,6	1,6	3,2	1,0	3,7
Y253H	8,7	2,6	36,8	0,6	2,6
E255K	6,0	5,6	6,7	9,5	8,4
E255V	17,0	3,4	10,3	5,5	12,9
D276G	2,2	1,4	2,0	0,6	2,1
E279K	3,6	1,6	2,0	1,0	3,0
E292L	0,7	1,3	1,8	1,1	2,0
V299L	1,5	8,7	1,3	26,1	0,6
T315A	1,7	58,9	2,7	6,0	0,4
T315I	17,5	75,0	39,4	45,4	3,0
T315V	12,2	738,8	57,0	29,3	2,1
F317L	2,6	4,5	2,2	2,4	0,7
F317R	2,3	114,0	2,3	33,5	4,9
F317V	0,4	21,3	0,5	11,5	2,3
M343T	1,2	0,9	0,8	1,1	0,9
M351T	1,8	0,9	0,4	0,7	1,2
F359I	6,0	3,0	16,3	2,9	2,9
F359V	2,9	1,5	5,2	0,9	4,4
L384M	1,3	2,2	2,3	0,5	2,2
H396P	2,4	1,1	2,4	0,4	1,4
H396R	3,9	1,6	3,1	0,8	5,9
F486S	8,1	3,0	1,9	2,3	2,1
L248R & F359I	1,2	13,7	96,2	39,3	17,7
Generation:	1st gen	2nd gen			3th gen.

Relative activity ($IC50^{MUT}/IC50^{WT}$) of imatinib, dasatinib, nilotinib, bosutinib, and ponatinib in the context of the respective mutation relative to the effectiveness against BCR-ABL^{WT}. Color code: *green* <2/sensitive; *yellow* 2, 1–4/moderately resistant; *orange* 4, 1–10/resistant; *red* >10/highly resistant. Note that ponatinib is the only inhibitor displaying activity against the common "gatekeeper" T315I mutation. Modified from Redaelli et al. (2012)

sites for interaction between the inhibitor and the kinase were optimized and are distributed over a wide range of protein residues. This increases the affinity and thereby reduces the required serum drug level. In addition, increased binding affinity ensures effectiveness of the inhibitor, even in those cases where one of the drug-binding site is lost, due to a mutation (Zhou et al. 2011).

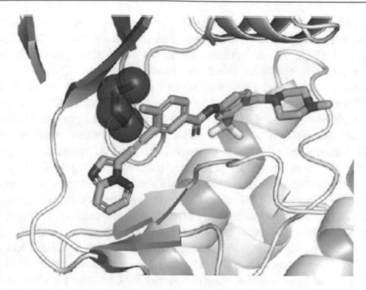

Fig. 1 Illustration of ponatinib in complex with the BCR-ABL protein. The *red spheres* represent the bulky side *chain* introduced by the T315I mutation. With kind permission of ARIAD Pharmaceuticals, Inc.

Initial preclinical studies of ponatinib—formerly referred to as AP24534—revealed the activity of the drug as a pan-BCR-ABL inhibitor in biochemical assays, in cell lines as well as in mouse models. In contrast to the previously approved first- and second-generation inhibitors, the activity profile of the new inhibitor included the T315I mutation. In addition, so-called compound mutants, defined by the co-occurrence of several concurrent mutations within the BCR-ABL fusion protein, were inhibited at a higher concentration by ponatinib (O'Hare et al. 2009).

In 2012, the first phase 1 trial for ponatinib in previously therapy-refractory patients was published (Cortes et al. 2012). This study included 60 CML and 5 Ph$^+$ ALL patients. The CML cases included 43 patients in chronic phase (CP), 9 in accelerated phase (AP), and 8 in blast phase (BP) and represented a highly pretreated collective ($59/60 \geq 2$ TKIs; $41/60 \geq 3$ TKIs). Ponatinib was given once daily at doses ranging from 2 to 60 mg. Among the CP-CML patients, 98% achieved a complete hematologic remission (CHR), 72% achieved a major cytogenetic response (MCyR), and 44% achieved a major molecular response (MMR). Given the refractory nature of CML in these patients and the high degree of pretreatment, these numbers were quite remarkable.

It should be highlighted that 12 of the 43 CP patients (28%) carried the T315I mutation and therefore were refractory to first- or second-generation inhibitors. Under ponatinib therapy, 100% of these T315I patients achieved a major hematologic response (MHR), 92% achieved a MCyR, and 67% achieved a MMR. Of the 13 refractory CML cases, which lacked any BCR-ABL mutation, rates for CHR, MCyR, and MMR of 100, 62, and 15%, respectively, were observed. Patients with advanced CML (AP, BP) were analyzed together with the Ph$^+$ ALL cohort in this study and responded to ponatinib as well. A MHR was achieved in 36%, MCyR in 32%, and MMR in 9% of patients. Thus, the novel third-generation inhibitor showed a clinically significant effect even in advanced-phase CML.

In order to further investigate the primary response rates to ponatinib (45 mg once daily) and its safety, a phase 2 trial (PACE trial) was launched. In total 449 patients in all phases of CML (CP, AP, and BP) and Ph$^+$ ALL, resistant or intolerant to dasatinib or nilotinib or with a known T315I mutation, were enrolled. In CP-CML patients ($n = 267$), the primary endpoint (MCyR at 12 months) was achieved in 56% of cases. In particular, patients carrying a T315I mutation responded better than those who were included because of resistance or intolerance (70% vs. 51%). In the CP-CML cohort, progression-free survival (PFS) and overall survival (OS) after twelve months were 80 and 94%, respectively. Furthermore, the study revealed that the response rates for MCyR, CCyR, and MMR of those patients decreased depending on the number of previously applied TKIs (Cortes et al. 2013). The primary endpoint (MHR after 12 months) was achieved in 55% of the AP CML and in 31% of the group containing BP CML and Ph$^+$. Altogether, the results of the PACE trial confirm the efficacy of ponatinib in second-generation TKI-resistant or TKI-intolerant CML and Ph$^+$ ALL patients at a dose of 45 mg daily. Importantly, the results confirm the efficacy of this new inhibitor against the "gatekeeper" T315I mutation. As the final data collection was scheduled for the end of 2017, an update of those results is expected in the near future.

Based on the two above-mentioned trials, ponatinib was approved for the second-line treatment of CML and Ph$^+$ ALL in December 2012 in the USA and in July 2013 in the European Union. The approval in the EU covers patients in all phases of CML.

- Who are resistant to dasatinib or nilotinib.
- Who are intolerant to dasatinib or nilotinib and for whom subsequent treatment with imatinib is not clinically appropriate.
- Who carry the T315I mutation.

The same terms apply to the approval for the use in Ph$^+$ ALL except that nilotinib is not considered here.

A phase 3 trial (EPIC trial) opened in July 2012 strived to compare ponatinib (45 mg daily) with imatinib (400 mg daily) in first-line therapy of newly diagnosed CML in CP. This trial aimed to enroll 528 patients, but was terminated due to safety concerns in October 2013 after the inclusion of 307 patients. This decision was based on the safety results of the aforementioned trails, showing an increased concurrency of serious arterial occlusive events. Due to the premature termination of the trail, the interpretation of the trial results is limited. Based on the preliminary data, patients treated with ponatinib in first line seem to achieve an MMR earlier and in a higher proportion of patients. The analysis of the adverse events showed increased frequency of arterial occlusive events.

In the PACE and EPIC trial, the following non-hematologic adverse reactions were reported in descending order of frequency (any grade, PACE/EPIC): rash (34%/31%), dry skin (32%/17%), abdominal pain (22%/27%), headaches (19%/32%), increased lipase (18%/32%), fatigue (17%/20%), constipation (16%/27%), myalgia (16%/25%), nausea (16%/21%), arthralgia (13%/18%), increased alanine aminotransferase (10%/18%), pancreatitis (6%/n.a.), and hypertension (7%/13%). Hematologic adverse effects have been observed more frequently compared to other Abl kinase inhibitors (thrombocytopenia > neutropenia > anemia). Focusing on the serious adverse events of grades 3 and 4, the increase in lipase (10%/12% of CP-CML patients) and hematologic adverse effects (thrombocytopenia 41%/6%, neutropenia 16%/3%, anemia 10%/n.a.) should receive special attention (Cortes et al. 2013; Lipton et al. 2016). Furthermore, the occurrence of arterial thrombotic events in the PACE trial (5.1% cardiovascular serious adverse events, 2.4% cerebrovascular serious adverse events, and 2.0% peripheral vascular serious adverse events) has to be highlighted (Cortes et al. 2013).

In order to improve the safety information about ponatinib with particular focus on the arterial thrombotic events, the available data of patients treated with ponatinib in the respective clinical trials (phase 1 trial, 81 patients; phase 2 PACE trial, 449 patients; phase 3 EPIC trial 153 patients) were recently analyzed retrospectively. A total of 671 patients were included in the multivariate analysis. The strongest independent predictors for the arterial thrombotic events were history of ischemic disease, dose intensity of ponatinib, and age. According to this analysis, a 15-mg/d decrease in ponatinib dose intensity results in a 33% reduction in the risk of an arterial occlusive event (Dorer et al. 2016). In the PACE phase 2 trial, 68% of the patients required dose reductions to 30 or 15 mg once daily during the course of therapy. The follow-up of these patients showed that the efficacy was retained at lower doses in most cases (Cortes et al. 2015). Along with this information, the current prescribing information recommends to consider dose reduction to 30 or 15 mg in patients achieving major cytogenetic response after patient's individual risk assessment taking into account cardiovascular risk factors, individual tolerability, time to cytogenetic response, and molecular response (status: 11/2016 FDA; 09/2017 EMA).

Based on the experience regarding the improved response rates achieved by ponatinib as well as the dose-related risk for adverse events (pancreatitis, arterial occlusive events, rash), further studies were initiated.

First, a phase 2 trial (OPTIC trial/NCT02467270) assays the activity and risk of three different starting doses of ponatinib (45/30/15 mg) in CP-CML patients who received at least two different TKI before. To address the safety concerns especially in higher doses of ponatinib, the drug will be reduced to 15 mg daily upon an achievement of MCyR. This trial aims to enroll 450 patients.

Second, a phase 3 trial (OPTIC-2L trial/NCT02627677) compares two doses of ponatinib (30 mg/15 mg once daily) and nilotinib 400 mg twice daily in CP-CML following resistance to imatinib. Again, a dose reduction of ponatinib (30–15 mg; 15–10 mg) is implemented in the study protocol after reaching MMR. A total of 600 patients will be included and randomized according to a 1:2:1 scheme.

Furthermore, a single-armed phase 2 trial (OPUS trial/NCT02398825) examines the activity and risk profile of 30 mg ponatinib, which will as well be adjusted to 15 mg daily once an MMR has been achieved.

In addition to the use of ponatinib in CML and Ph⁺ ALL, other diseases could potentially benefit from the treatment with this drug as well. Preclinical studies reported that ponatinib inhibits not only BCR-ABL but also RET, FLT3, KIT, SRC, as well as members of receptor kinase families VEGFR, FGFR, and PDGFR (O'Hare et al. 2009). Following these findings, in vitro as well as in vivo studies / mouse xenograft models investigated the effect of ponatinib in AML as well as breast cancer cell lines and carcinoma of the endometrium, bladder, stomach, colon, lung, and medullary thyroid. In these neoplasms, ponatinib was shown to inhibit proliferation and additionally to induce apoptosis in FLT3-ITD-driven AML. The activity of ponatinib in these preclinical studies constitutes the rational to examine ponatinib in a variety of additional cancer entities (Falco et al. 2013; Gozgit et al. 2011, 2012; Zirm et al. 2012). Respective clinical trials on FLT3-ITD positive AML, non-small cell lung cancer (NSCLC), glioblastoma, thyroid cancer, and others are currently evaluating the significance of ponatinib in those disease entities.

In conclusion, ponatinib constitutes a powerful BCR-ABL inhibitor and has been approved for the treatment of CML patients resistant or intolerant to imatinib, dasatinib, or nilotinib. It displays clinical activity both in wild-type and in BCR-ABL mutant CML, including activity against the T315I mutation. Ponatinib induces high rates of remission. On the other hand, it causes an increased risk for serious adverse events, especially arterial thrombotic events. Current clinical trials investigate optimized dosing schemes in order to reduce the occurrence of these adverse events while maintaining its clinical activity. Despite previous TKI failure, chronic-phase CML patients can achieve sustained remissions using the novel drug. For patients with advanced CML or Ph⁺ ALL, ponatinib therapy can successfully bridge the time to allogeneic stem cell transplantation.

References

Bradeen HA et al (2006) Comparison of imatinib mesylate, dasatinib (BMS-354825), and nilotinib (AMN107) in an N-ethyl-N-nitrosourea (ENU)-based mutagenesis screen: high efficacy of drug combinations. Blood 108(7):2332–2338

Branford S, Rudzki Z, Walsh S, Parkinson I, Grigg A, Szer J et al (2003) Detection of BCR-ABL mutations in patients with CML treated with imatinib is virtually always accompanied by clinical resistance, and mutations in the ATP phosphate-binding loop (P-loop) are associated with a poor prognosis. Blood 102(1):276–283

Branford S, Melo JV, Hughes TP (2009) Selecting optimal second-line tyrosine kinase inhibitor therapy for chronic myeloid leukemia patients after imatinib failure: does the BCR-ABL mutation status really matter? Blood 114(27):5426–5435

Cortes JE, Kantarjian H, Shah NP, Bixby D, Mauro MJ, Flinn I et al (2012) Ponatinib in refractory Philadelphia chromosome-positive leukemias. N Engl J Med 367(22):2075–2088

Cortes JE et al (2013) A phase 2 trial of ponatinib in Philadelphia chromosome–positive leukemias. N Engl J Med 369:1783–1796

Cortes J, Kim DW, Pinilla-Ibarz J, le Coutre PD, Paquette R, Chuah C et al (2015) Ponatinib efficacy and safety in heavily pretreated leukemia patients: 3-year results of the PACE trial [abstract P234]. Haematologica 100:64

Darkow T, Henk HJ, Thomas SK, Feng W, Baladi J-F, Goldberg GA et al (2007) Treatment interruptions and non-adherence with imatinib and associated healthcare costs: a retrospective analysis among managed care patients with chronic myelogenous leukaemia. Pharmacoeconomics 25(6):481–496

de Lavallade H, Apperley JF, Khorashad JS, Milojkovic D, Reid AG, Bua M et al (2008) Imatinib for newly diagnosed patients with chronic myeloid leukemia: incidence of sustained responses in an intention-to-treat analysis. J Clin Oncol 26(20):3358–3363

Dorer DJ, Knickerbocker RK, Baccarani M, Cortes JE, Hochhaus A, Talpaz M, Haluska FG (2016) Impact of dose intensity of ponatinib on selected adverse events: multivariate analyses from a pooled population of clinical trial patients. Leuk Res 48:84–91

Druker BJ, Talpaz M, Resta DJ, Peng B, Buchdunger E, Ford JM et al (2001) Efficacy and safety of a specific inhibitor of the BCR-ABL tyrosine kinase in chronic myeloid leukemia. N Engl J Med 344(14):1031–1037

Druker BJ, Guilhot F, O'Brien SG, Gathmann I, Kantarjian H, Gattermann N et al (2006) Five-year follow-up of patients receiving imatinib for chronic myeloid leukemia. N Engl J Med 355(23):2408–2417

Falco VD, Buonocore P, Muthu M, Torregrossa L, Basolo F, Billaud M et al (2013) Ponatinib (AP24534) is a novel potent inhibitor of oncogenic RET mutants associated with thyroid cancer. J Clin Endocrinol Metab (Internet). 22 Mar 2013 (cited 29 Apr 2013). Available from http://jcem.endojournals.org/content/early/2013/03/21/jc.2012-2672

Floyd MD, Gervasini G, Masica AL, Mayo G, George AL Jr, Bhat K et al (2003) Genotype-phenotype associations for common CYP3A4 and CYP3A5 variants in the basal and induced metabolism of midazolam in European- and African-American men and women. Pharmacogenetics 13(10):595–606

Gozgit JM, Wong MJ, Wardwell S, Tyner JW, Loriaux MM, Mohemmad QK et al (2011) Potent activity of ponatinib (AP24534) in models of FLT3-driven acute myeloid leukemia and other hematologic malignancies. Mol Cancer Ther 10(6):1028–1035

Gozgit JM, Wong MJ, Moran L, Wardwell S, Mohemmad QK, Narasimhan NI et al (2012) Ponatinib (AP24534), a multitargeted Pan-FGFR inhibitor with activity in multiple FGFR-amplified or mutated cancer models. Mol Cancer Ther 11(3):690–699

Jain P, Kantarjian H, Cortes J (2013) Chronic myeloid leukemia: overview of new agents and comparative analysis. Curr Treat Options Oncol 14(2):127–143

Kantarjian HM, Giles F, Gattermann N, Bhalla K, Alimena G, Palandri F et al (2007) Nilotinib (formerly AMN107), a highly selective BCR-ABL tyrosine kinase inhibitor, is effective in patients with Philadelphia chromosome–positive chronic myelogenous leukemia in chronic phase following imatinib resistance and intolerance. Blood 110(10):3540–3546

Kantarjian H, Shah NP, Hochhaus A, Cortes J, Shah S, Ayala M et al (2010) Dasatinib versus imatinib in newly diagnosed chronic-phase chronic myeloid leukemia. N Engl J Med 362 (24):2260–2270

Kantarjian HM, Hochhaus A, Saglio G, De Souza C, Flinn IW, Stenke L et al (2011) Nilotinib versus imatinib for the treatment of patients with newly diagnosed chronic phase, Philadelphia chromosome-positive, chronic myeloid leukaemia: 24-month minimum follow-up of the phase 3 randomised ENESTnd trial. Lancet Oncol 12(9):841–851

Kuwazuru Y, Yoshimura A, Hanada S, Ichikawa M, Saito T, Uozumi K et al (1990) Expression of the multidrug transporter, P-glycoprotein, in chronic myelogenous leukaemia cells in blast crisis. Br J Haematol 74(1):24–29

Lahaye T, Riehm B, Berger U, Paschka P, Müller MC, Kreil S et al (2005) Response and resistance in 300 patients with BCR-ABL–positive leukemias treated with imatinib in a single center. Cancer 103(8):1659–1669

Lipton JH, Chuah C, Guerci-Bresler A, Rosti G, Simpson D, Assouline S et al (2016) Ponatinib versus imatinib for newly diagnosed chronic myeloid leukaemia: an international, randomised, open-label, phase 3 trial. Lancet Oncol 17(5):612–21

Mahon F-X, Belloc F, Lagarde V, Chollet C, Moreau-Gaudry F, Reiffers J et al (2003) MDR1 gene overexpression confers resistance to imatinib mesylate in leukemia cell line models. Blood 101(6):2368–2373

Nicolini FE, Chabane K, Tigaud I, Michallet M, Magaud J-P, Hayette S (2007) BCR-ABL mutant kinetics in CML patients treated with dasatinib. Leuk Res 31(6):865–868

O'Hare T, Eide CA, Deininger MWN (2007) Bcr-Abl kinase domain mutations, drug resistance, and the road to a cure for chronic myeloid leukemia. Blood 110(7):2242–2249

O'Hare T, Shakespeare WC, Zhu X, Eide CA, Rivera VM, Wang F et al (2009) AP24534, a pan-BCR-ABL inhibitor for chronic myeloid leukemia, potently inhibits the T315I mutant and overcomes mutation-based resistance. Cancer Cell 16(5):401–412

Redaelli S, Mologni L, Rostagno R, Piazza R, Magistroni V, Ceccon M et al (2012) Three novel patient-derived BCR-ABL mutants show different sensitivity to second and third generation tyrosine kinase inhibitors. Am J Hematol 87(11):E125–E128

Saglio G, Kim D-W, Issaragrisil S, le Coutre P, Etienne G, Lobo C et al (2010) Nilotinib versus imatinib for newly diagnosed chronic myeloid leukemia. N Engl J Med 362(24):2251–2259

Shah NP, Sawyers CL (2003) Mechanisms of resistance to STI571 in Philadelphia chromosome-associated leukemias. Oncogene 22(47):7389–7395

Soverini S, Hochhaus A, Nicolini FE, Gruber F, Lange T, Saglio G et al (2011) BCR-ABL kinase domain mutation analysis in chronic myeloid leukemia patients treated with tyrosine kinase inhibitors: recommendations from an expert panel on behalf of European LeukemiaNet. Blood 118(5):1208–1215

Talpaz M, Shah NP, Kantarjian H, Donato N, Nicoll J, Paquette R et al (2006) Dasatinib in imatinib-resistant Philadelphia chromosome-positive leukemias. N Engl J Med 354(24):2531–2541

Thomas J, Wang L, Clark RE, Pirmohamed M (2004) Active transport of imatinib into and out of cells: implications for drug resistance. Blood 104(12):3739–3745

von Bubnoff N et al (2002) BCR-ABL gene mutations in relation to clinical resistance of Philadelphia-chromosome-positive leukaemia to STI571: a prospective study. Lancet 359 (9305):487–491

von Bubnoff N, Veach DR, van der Kuip H, Aulitzky WE, Sänger J, Seipel P et al (2005) A cell-based screen for resistance of Bcr-Abl-positive leukemia identifies the mutation pattern for PD166326, an alternative Abl kinase inhibitor. Blood 105(4):1652–1659

von Bubnoff N et al (2006) Bcr-Abl resistance screening predicts a limited spectrum of point mutations to be associated with clinical resistance to the Abl kinase inhibitor nilotinib (AMN107). Blood 108(4):1328–1333

Zhou T, Commodore L, Huang W-S, Wang Y, Thomas M, Keats J et al (2011) Structural mechanism of the pan-BCR-ABL inhibitor ponatinib (AP24534): lessons for overcoming kinase inhibitor resistance. Chem Biol Drug Des 77(1):1–11

Zirm E, Spies-Weisshart B, Heidel F, Schnetzke U, Böhmer F-D, Hochhaus A et al (2012) Ponatinib may overcome resistance of FLT3-ITD harbouring additional point mutations, notably the previously refractory F691I mutation. Br J Haematol 157(4):483–492

Ruxolitinib

Stefanie Ajayi, Heiko Becker, Heike Reinhardt,
Monika Engelhardt, Robert Zeiser,
Nikolas von Bubnoff and Ralph Wäsch

Contents

Stefanie Ajayi and Heiko Becker: These authors contributed equally.

S. Ajayi · H. Becker · H. Reinhardt · M. Engelhardt · R. Zeiser · N. von Bubnoff · R. Wäsch (✉)
Department of Hematology and Oncology, University of Freiburg Medical Center,
Hugstetter Str. 55, 79106 Freiburg, Germany
e-mail: ralph.waesch@uniklinik-freiburg.de

S. Ajayi · H. Becker · H. Reinhardt · M. Engelhardt · R. Zeiser · N. von Bubnoff · R. Wäsch
Comprehensive Cancer Center Freiburg (CCCF), Hugstetter Str. 55,
79106 Freiburg, Germany

© Springer International Publishing AG, part of Springer Nature 2018
U. M. Martens (ed.), *Small Molecules in Hematology*, Recent Results
in Cancer Research 211, https://doi.org/10.1007/978-3-319-91439-8_6

Abstract

Ruxolitinib, formerly known as INCB018424 or INC424, is a potent and selective oral inhibitor of Janus kinase (JAK) 1 and JAK2. Ruxolitinib has been approved for the treatment of myelofibrosis (MF) by the US Food and Drug Administration (FDA) in 2011 and by the European Medicines Agency (EMA) in 2012, followed by the approval for the treatment of hydroxyurea (HU)-resistant or -intolerant polycythemia vera (PV) in 2014. Both MF and PV are myeloproliferative neoplasms (MPNs) which are characterized by the aberrant activation of the JAK–STAT pathway. Clinically, MF features bone marrow fibrosis, splenomegaly, abnormal blood counts, and poor quality-of-life through associated symptoms. PV is characterized by the overproduction of primarily red blood cells (RBC), risk of thrombotic complications, and development of secondary MF. Ruxolitinib treatment results in a meaningful reduction in spleen size and symptom burden in the majority of MF patients and may also have a favorable effect on survival. In PV, ruxolitinib effectively controls the hematocrit and reduces splenomegaly. Since recently, ruxolitinib is also under investigation for the treatment of graft-versus-host disease (GvHD) after allogeneic hematopoietic stem cell transplantation (HSCT). Toxicities of ruxolitinib include myelosuppression, which results in dose-limiting thrombocytopenia and anemia, and viral reactivations. The metabolization of ruxolitinib through CYP3A4 needs to be considered particularly if co-administered with potent CYP3A4 inhibitors. Several further JAK inhibitors are currently under investigation for MPNs or other immuno-inflammatory diseases.

Keywords

Ruxolitinib · Polycythemia vera · Myelofibrosis · Graft-versus-host disease

1 Introduction

Ruxolitinib is licensed for the treatment of myelofibrosis (MF) and polycythemia vera (PV). Both diseases belong to the group of myeloproliferative neoplasms (MPNs). MF is associated with a continuous decrease in hematopoietic function of the bone marrow due to progressive fibrosis. This leads to extramedullary hematopoiesis with enlargement of liver and spleen in an attempt to compensate the marrow fibrosis and progressive pancytopenia at later stages of the disease. The disease is accompanied by general symptoms such as fatigue, night sweats, fever, and weight loss. The only curative approach to MF is allogeneic hematopoietic stem cell transplantation (HSCT). Ruxolitinib currently constitutes the best available medical treatment to temporarily improve symptoms and quality-of-life in many MF patients. Whether or not ruxolitinib is able to prolong the survival of MF patients continues to be a controversial issue. Alternative palliative therapies for MF are hydroxyurea (HU) and corticosteroids. PV is characterized by neoplastic proliferation of erythroid cells and secondary MF. Ruxolitinib can mitigate the red cell proliferation and splenomegaly and is approved as second-line therapy in PV patients with resistance to or intolerance of HU.

2 Structure, Mechanism of Action, and Pharmacokinetics

The Janus kinase (JAK) family consists of four intracellular, nonreceptor tyrosine kinases: JAK1, JAK2, JAK3, and tyrosine-protein kinase 2 (TYK2). JAKs are constitutively bound to cytokine receptors. Upon binding of a ligand to the receptor, JAKs phosphorylate and activate downstream targets such as signal transducers and activators of transcription (STAT) (Mertens and Darnell 2007). Thus, JAKs have a crucial role in regulation and homeostasis in hematopoiesis and immunity. In 2005, an activating mutation in the JAK2 pseudokinase, i.e., V617F, was identified in a high proportion of patients with myeloproliferative neoplasms, and expression of the mutant JAK2 in a murine model resulted in an MPN-like disease (James et al. 2005; Quintás-Cardama et al. 2010). These findings drove the development of drugs to target wild-type and/or mutant JAK2. Ruxolitinib is the first of these drugs that has been approved for treatment.

Ruxolitinib was formerly known as INCB018424 or INC424. The chemical name is (*R*)-3-(4-(7*H*-pyrrolo[2,3-*d*]pyrimidin-4-yl)-1*H*-pyrazol-1-yl)-3-cyclopentylpropanenitrile phosphate, and its molecular weight is 306.37 g/mol (Fig. 1).

Ruxolitinib is an oral, reversible class I inhibitor and competes with ATP in the catalytic site of the JAK tyrosine kinases. Accordingly, ruxolitinib is not specific for the JAK2 V617F mutation. Its efficacy in myelofibrosis has been primarily attributed to attenuation of the inflammatory state caused by constitutive JAK–STAT activation and a nonspecific myelosuppression. Peak plasma concentrations of ruxolitinib are achieved within one hour after administration and decline in a monophasic or biphasic manner with a mean terminal half-life of 2.3 h (Shilling et al. 2010).

Fig. 1 Chemical structure of ruxolitinib

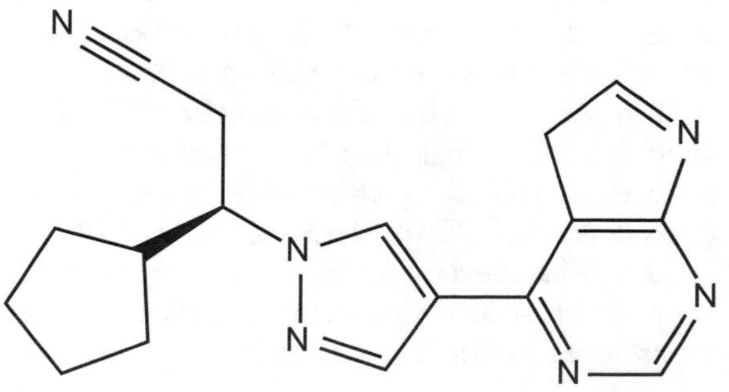

3 Preclinical Data

Ruxolitinib selectively inhibited JAK1 and JAK2 with IC_{50} values of 3.3 and 2.8 nM, respectively. The IC_{50} was approximately sixfold higher for TYK2 and 140-fold higher for JAK3 (Quintás-Cardama et al. 2010). Ruxolitinib also suppressed the proliferation of JAK2 V617-positive Ba/F3 cells with an IC_{50} of 127 nM as well as the cytokine-independent colony formation of erythroid progenitors from patients with JAK2 V617F-positive polycythemia vera with an IC_{50} of 67 nM (Quintás-Cardama et al. 2010). In Balb/c mice injected with JAK2 V617F-positive Ba/F3 cells, ruxolitinib reduced splenomegaly, decreased levels of circulating interleukin 6 and tumor necrosis factor alpha, and prolonged survival (Quintás-Cardama et al. 2010).

4 Clinical Data

4.1 Ruxolitinib in the Treatment of MF

The Food and Drug Administration (FDA) in the USA approved ruxolitinib for the treatment of MF in 2011 and the European Medicines Agency (EMA) in 2012. MF can occur as primary MF (PMF), post-essential thrombocythemia MF (PETMF), or post-PV MF (PPVMF). It is characterized by progressive bone marrow fibrosis, splenomegaly, abnormal blood counts as well as constitutional symptoms (fever, weight loss, and night sweats) and other debilitating symptoms, such as fatigue, bone pain, early satiety, abdominal pain, and pruritus. Abnormal levels of proinflammatory cytokines and the activation of the JAK–STAT pathway are characteristic for myelofibrosis. JAK2 V617F mutations are found in approximately half of the patients, most of the remaining patients harbor mutations in the calreticulin gene (CALR) or, less frequently, in the gene of the thrombopoietin receptor (MPL). The median survival of patients after the diagnosis of MF depends on the presence of risk factors and varies according to the International Prognostic Scoring System (IPSS) between 2 years for patients with high risk and 11 years for those with low-risk features (Cervantes et al. 2009). Major causes of death are leukemic transformation or progressive marrow fibrosis with pancytopenia (Cervantes et al. 2009). Except for allogeneic HSCT, the current therapeutic approaches are palliative and confer a temporary benefit.

In a phase 1/2 trial, which included 153 adult patients with MF (93% IPSS intermediate-2 or high risk), thrombocytopenia was found to be the dose-limiting toxic effect, and 25 mg twice daily was defined as the maximum tolerated dose (Verstovsek et al. 2010). Sixty-one (44%) of 140 patients with splenomegaly had a $\geq 50\%$ reduction in palpable splenomegaly in the first 3 months of treatment. Response rates were highest among patients who received 15 mg twice daily (response rate 52%) or 25 mg twice daily (response rate 49%). Considering also those with a less pronounced effect on splenomegaly, $\geq 70\%$ of patients with 10, 15, or 25 mg twice daily had $\geq 25\%$ reduction in palpable spleen size in the first 2 months of treatment. Response rates were similar among patients with or without JAK2 V617F mutation. In accordance, the suppression of STAT3 phosphorylation was observed regardless of the presence of JAK2 V617F. In addition to the reduction in the spleen size, the majority of patients with 10, 15, or 25 mg twice daily had a $\geq 50\%$ improvement of myelofibrosis-related symptoms. With regard to the blood counts, the mean white blood cell count decreased from 29.8×10^9 to 16.0×10^9/L, and patients with elevated platelet counts at baseline (mean 728×10^9/L) had reduced platelet counts (336×10^9/L) at 3 months of treatment. In the long-term follow-up of 107 patients included in the phase 1/2 trial, the median duration of a meaningful spleen size reduction was approximately 2 years from the onset of the response (Verstovsek et al. 2012a).

Subsequent to the phase 1/2 trial, two phase 3 studies (COMFORT-I and COMFORT-II) were initiated. In both trials, patients had PMF, PETMF, or PPVMF with palpable splenomegaly of at least 5 cm below the costal margin and an IPSS intermediate-2 or high risk. The starting dose depended on the baseline platelet count and was 15 mg twice daily for platelets of 100×10^9/L–200×10^9/L and 20 mg twice daily for platelets of more than 200×10^9/L. During the study, the dosing was reduced based on neutropenia or thrombocytopenia or escalated (to a maximum of 25 mg twice daily) to increase efficacy. While COMFORT-I was a double-blind, placebo-controlled trial including 155 patients in the ruxolitinib group and 154 in the placebo group, COMFORT-II was an open-label trial testing ruxolitinib in 146 patients against best available therapy (BAT, mostly HU or glucocorticoids) in 73 patients.

The primary efficacy endpoint was the proportion of patients achieving a $\geq 35\%$ reduction in spleen volume at 24 weeks (COMFORT-I) or 48 weeks (COMFORT-II), as assessed by MRI or CT scan. The respective endpoint was reached by 42% in the ruxolitinib and 1% in the placebo group in COMFORT-I (Verstovsek et al. 2012b) and by 28% in the ruxolitinib group compared with 0% in the BAT group in COMFORT-II (Harrison et al. 2012). The median time to the first observation of $\geq 35\%$ reduction in spleen volume was 12 weeks in the ruxolitinib group in COMFORT-II. Overall, almost every patient who received ruxolitinib had some degree of spleen size reduction.

A secondary endpoint in COMFORT-I was the proportion of patients with a $\geq 50\%$ reduction in the total symptom score at 24 weeks measured by the modified Myelofibrosis Symptom Assessment Form. This endpoint was reached by 46% of the ruxolitinib-treated patients and 5% of the patients receiving placebo in COMFORT-I (Verstovsek et al. 2012b). In contrast, only 4% of the ruxolitinib group had significant worsening of symptoms (>50% increase in total symptom score), compared with 33% in the placebo group (Mesa et al. 2013). Comparable results regarding quality-of-life and symptoms were obtained in COMFORT-II (Harrison et al. 2012).

Notably, ruxolitinib was effective in reducing spleen size and symptom burden regardless of age groups (≤ 65 and >65 years), MF subtype, IPSS risk, pretreatment spleen size, pretreatment platelet count, and JAK2 V617F status (Verstovsek et al. 2013). Although there were no significant differences according to the JAK2 V617F status, JAK2 V617F-positive patients had a mean reduction in the spleen volume of 35% and in the symptom burden of 53%, whereas those negative for JAK2 V617F had reductions of 24 and 28%, respectively, (Verstovsek et al. 2012b).

Ruxolitinib-treated patients also had a survival benefit compared with those receiving placebo in COMFORT-I (HR 0.5, 95%-CI 0.25–0.98, $P = 0.04$). In COMFORT-II, overall survival (OS) was similar between the ruxolitinib and BAT group after 48 weeks. No survival difference was observed between intermediate-2 and high-risk patients when treated with ruxolitinib (Verstovsek et al. 2012a). The finding of a survival benefit in one cohort of the phase 1/2 trial (Verstovsek et al. 2012a), but not another (Tefferi et al. 2011) was reasoned to be due to the lower discontinuation rates and a higher mean ruxolitinib dose in the cohort with the survival advantage by ruxolitinib (Verstovsek et al. 2012a). Disease progression or loss or lack of response was the reason for treatment discontinuation in 40% of the patients in the report by Tefferi et al. (2011), whereas progressive disease was the cause for discontinuation in 11% in the cohort studied by Verstovsek et al. (2012a).

Subsequent analyzes of these trials with longer periods of follow-up underlined the benefits conferred by ruxolitinib therapy. In the final, five-year update of the COMFORT-I trial, 28% of ruxolitinib-randomized patients and 25% of the patients who crossed over from placebo to ruxolitinib, were still on treatment, while no patients remained in the placebo arm. Among the patients, who were randomized to ruxolitinib, 59% achieved a $\geq 35\%$ reduction in spleen volume, with a median duration of response of 168 weeks (Verstovsek et al. 2017). The median OS in the ruxolitinib arm was not reached, while among patients randomized to placebo the median OS was 4.2 years (HR 0.69; 95%-CI 0.50-0.96; $P = 0.025$). Similarly, in the COMFORT-II trial, there was a 33% reduction in risk of death with ruxolitinib compared with BAT (HR 0.67; 95%-CI 0.44-1.02; $P = 0.06$). The OS benefit conferred by ruxolitinib remained significant after correction for crossover (HR 0.44, 95%-CI 0.18-1.04; $P = 0.06$) (Harrison et al. 2016). The exact reasons for the survival benefits remain to be determined, but may be related to spleen size reduction and alleviation of cytokine-driven symptoms and specific patient groups being included in these studies.

While the COMFORT-studies only included patients with IPSS intermediate-2 or high-risk MF, the phase 3b expanded access JUMP trial also comprised 163 intermediate-1 risk patients. The safety and efficacy profile in these patients was similar to that of the intermediate-2—and high-risk patients enrolled in the JUMP or COMFORT trials (Al-Ali et al. 2016). Accordant findings were reported from a retrospective analysis that included 25 IPSS low-risk and 83 IPSS intermediate-1 risk patients (Davis et al. 2015).

4.2 Ruxolitinib in the Treatment of PV

In 2014, ruxolitinib was granted approval for the treatment of HU-resistant or - intolerant PV patients. PV is a MPN characterized by the hyperproliferation of primarily red cells, which is often accompanied by increased white blood cell and platelet counts. Major complications of PV are the progression to MF (i.e., PPVMF) and, in particular, the increased rate of thromboembolic events, including cardio-vascular diseases.

The approval of ruxolitinib for the treatment of PV was based on two phase 3 trials (RESPONSE and RESPONSE-2) for patients with PV and HU resistance or intolerance. In RESPONSE-2, hematocrit control was achieved in 62% of 74 ruxolitinib-treated patients compared with 19% of the patients who received BAT. No cases of grade 3–4 anemia or thrombocytopenia occurred with ruxolitinib (Passamonti et al. 2017). The RESPONSE trial, which had been conducted before the RESPONSE-2 trial, was restricted to PV patients with splenomegaly. Here, in addition to the hematocrit control, 38% of patients in the ruxolitinib arm had a reduction of the spleen volume by $\geq 35\%$, compared with 1% in the BAT-arm (Vannucchi et al. 2015). Thromboembolic events occurred in one patient receiving ruxolitinib and in six patients receiving best available therapy.

4.3 Ruxolitinib in Combination Therapy

The combination of ruxolitinib with other agents is an attractive option for future MPN treatment. However, when searching for combination partners one needs to bear in mind the myelosuppressive effects of ruxolitinib.

The combination of ruxolitinib with immunomodulatory agents such as poma-lidomide or thalidomide is currently being investigated (Verstovsek and Bose 2017). In preliminary results from the POMINC trial (NCT01644110), which enrolls anemic patients with intermediate-2 or high-risk MF according to the dynamic IPSS (DIPSS) and investigates the combination of ruxolitinib with pomalidomide, 3 of 37 patients had an hemoglobin increase ≥ 2 mg/dL and/or reached RBC transfusion independence (Stegelmann et al. 2016).

Sotatercept is a first-in-class activin receptor type IIA fusion protein acting as a ligand trap that may relieve stromal inhibition of erythropoiesis (Iancu-Rubin et al. 2013). In an ongoing trial (NCT01712308) in MF patients with anemia, sotatercept is investigated as monotherapy at different dose levels and in combination with ruxolitinib. In preliminary results, sotatercept treatment is associated with a promising overall response rate (ORR) and RBC transfusion independence in some patients (Verstovsek and Bose 2017).

Aberrations in the DNA methylation are frequent in MPNs and may impact gene expression (McPherson et al. 2017). However, DNA methyltransferase (DNMT) inhibitors, such as azacytidine or decitabine, showed limited single-agent activity in MF. The addition of ruxolitinib to a DNMT inhibitor may have synergistic effects on gene expression. Preliminary results on such combinations are promising and point out that these regimens may be particularly beneficial for patients with advanced MF disease stages (Daver et al. 2016; Rampal et al. 2016).

4.4 Ruxolitinib as Salvage Treatment for Graft-versus-Host Disease (GvHD)

Corticosteroid-refractory GvHD causes high morbidity and mortality despite of the improvements in allogeneic HSCT over the past decades (Zeiser and Blazar 2017a, b). Preclinical evidence indicated the potent anti-inflammatory properties of JAK 1/2 inhibitors (Spoerl et al. 2014). Zeiser et al. (2015) performed a retrospective,

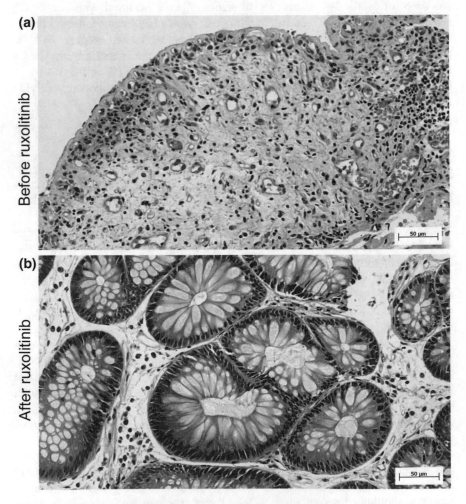

Fig. 2 Treatment of steroid-refractory acute graft-versus-host disease (aGvHD). **a** Grade IV aGvHD of the gut before treatment with ruxolitinib and **b** grade I after treatment with ruxolitinib

multicenter survey of 95 patients, who received ruxolitinib as salvage therapy for corticosteroid-refractory GvHD (the median number of previous GvHD-therapies was three). Despite this heavily pretreated population, the ORR was 81.5% in acute GvHD (including 46.3% complete responses (CR)) (Fig. 2) and 85.4% in chronic GvHD (78% of the patients achieved a partial response (PR)). Responses were durable and the rate of GvHD-relapse was low (acute GvHD: 6.8%, chronic GvHD: 5.7%). Several prospective trials in patients with acute or chronic GvHD are currently following up these initial observations, for example, RIG (NCT02396628), REACH2 (NCT02913261), or REACH3 (NCT03112603).

5 Toxicity

In phase 3 clinical trials in MF patients, the nonhematologic toxic effects were largely similar between the ruxolitinib and the placebo or BAT group (Verstovsek et al. 2012b; Harrison et al. 2012). In the COMFORT-I trial bruising, dizziness, and headache (mostly grade 1 or 2) were more frequently associated with ruxolitinib compared to placebo. Whereas in COMFORT-II, diarrhea (predominantly grade 1 or 2) was the only adverse event with a $\geq 10\%$ higher occurrence in the ruxolitinib than in the BAT group.

With regard to hematologic effects in MF patients, thrombocytopenia and anemia occurred more frequently in patients receiving ruxolitinib than in those receiving placebo or BAT (Verstovsek et al. 2012b; Harrison et al. 2012). Although anemia and thrombocytopenia were the most common adverse events under ruxolitinib, these were usually manageable with dose modifications, treatment interruption, or transfusion and rarely led to discontinuation of therapy. In COMFORT-II, mandatory dose reductions due to thrombocytopenia were required in 41% of patients receiving ruxolitinib. Overall, dose reductions or treatment interruptions due to adverse events were expectedly more frequent in the ruxolitinib (63%) than in the BAT group (15%) in COMFORT-II. It had already been observed in the preceding phase 1/2 trial that patients with a 25 mg twice daily dose more often experienced thrombocytopenia and new onset of anemia than those with 15 mg twice daily (Verstovsek et al. 2010).

In the RESPONSE trials conducted among patients with PV, the hematologic side effects were less pronounced; grade 3 or 4 anemia or thrombocytopenia occurred in less than 2 and 5% of patients, respectively, (Vannucchi et al. 2015; Passamonti et al. 2017).

Due to the hematological side effects, it is recommended to adapt the starting dose of ruxolitinib to the baseline platelet counts (Jakavi 2017). Patients with severe renal impairment should start with a reduced dosage of ruxolitinib. If dialysis is required, the dosage should be given after dialysis (on days of dialysis). For patients with hepatic impairment, it is recommended to reduce the starting dose by 50%. After careful monitoring, subsequent doses may be increased if well tolerated. Ruxolitinib treatment should be interrupted if the platelet count drops below 50,000/mm^3 or the neutrophil count below 500/mm^3. The hematological side effects are generally reversible and well manageable by treatment reduction or interruption. An ongoing trial aims to further investigate the safety and efficacy of ruxolitinib in patients with MF and low platelet counts (NCT01348490, Talpaz et al. 2013).

Following interruption of ruxolitinib, disease-associated symptoms returned to pretreatment levels within approximately 1 week among MF patients (Verstovsek et al. 2012b). Among the adverse events that occurred after discontinuation, no pattern was observed that would suggest a withdrawal syndrome (Verstovsek et al. 2012b). However, as acknowledged in the FDA prescribing information, a patient's clinical course may worsen after discontinuation of ruxolitinib during acute illness (Tefferi et al. 2011; Tefferi and Pardanani 2011). Although such a ruxolitinib withdrawal syndrome due to a cytokine rebound remains to be established, the FDA recommends that a gradual tapering of ruxolitinib (e.g., by 5 mg twice daily each week) may be considered, when therapy is discontinued for reasons other than thrombocytopenia.

Importantly, ruxolitinib treatment has been associated with severe infections (including opportunistic infections) and viral (re-)activation, such as CMV, HBV, or VZV (Herpes zoster) (Caocci et al. 2014; Vannucchi et al. 2015; Zeiser et al. 2015; Verstovsek et al. 2017). Thus, ruxolitinib should only be used with caution in patients with pertinent risks, and all patients should be carefully monitored for opportunistic infections and viral re-activation under ruxolitinib treatment.

6 Drug Interactions

Ruxolitinib is primarily metabolized by cytochrome P450 3A4 (CYP3A4). Co-administration of ruxolitinib with the strong CYP3A4 inhibitor ketoconazole or the moderate CYP3A4 inhibitor erythromycin increased ruxolitinib plasma exposure by 91 and 27%, respectively, which was consistent with the level of inhibition of interleukin 6-stimulated STAT3 phosphorylation (Shi et al. 2012). Co-administration of the CYP3A4 inducer rifampicin decreased the plasma levels of ruxolitinib by 71%, but reduced the inhibition of STAT3 phosphorylation by only 10%. This discrepancy may be explained by the presence of active ruxolitinib metabolites (Shi et al. 2012). Hence, adjustments in ruxolitinib doses may not be required when co-administered with inducers or moderate inhibitors of CYP3A4; however ruxolitinib doses should be reduced by 50% if co-administered with strong CYP3A4 inhibitors (for example, azoles).

7 Biomarkers

MF patients receiving ruxolitinib had increased plasma levels of leptin and erythropoietin and reduced plasma levels of proinflammatory tumor necrosis factor alpha and interleukin 6 (Verstovsek et al. 2010, 2012b; Harrison et al. 2012).

The decrease in proinflammatory cytokines was associated with symptomatic improvements by ruxolitinib in the phase 1/2 trial among MF patients (Verstovsek et al. 2010).

While most patients with MF benefit from ruxolitinib, some patients are refractory, have an inferior response or develop secondary resistance. No difference in the response to ruxolitinib has been observed between MF patients with a JAK2 or CALR mutation (Guglielmelli et al. 2014). Patel et al. (2015) assessed the mutations status of 28 genes in 95 MF patients treated with ruxolitinib. Patients with ≥ 3 mutations had lower odds to achieve a 50% reduction of spleen size and shorter OS than those with fewer mutations. This finding warrants further studies to establish biomarkers that are predictive for the response of MPN patients to ruxolitinib.

8 Other JAK Inhibitors

Based on the key role of JAKs in cytokine signaling, JAK inhibitors are also being studied in the treatment of other MPNs, such as essential thrombocythemia, as well as other immuno-inflammatory diseases, such as rheumatoid arthritis, inflammatory bowel disease, and psoriasis. Tofacitinib, which mainly inhibits JAK3, has been approved for the treatment of rheumatoid arthritis in the USA.

Clinical trials with newer JAK inhibitors in MF patients were particularly aimed to identify treatments which are less myelosuppressive than ruxolitinib. In phase 3 SIMPLIFY-1 trial, momelotinib, a JAK1/2 inhibitor, was noninferior to ruxolitinib with regard to spleen response but not with regard to symptom control in MF patients who had previously not been treated with a JAK inhibitor; importantly, momelotinib treatment was by trend associated with a reduced transfusion requirement (Mesa et al. 2017a). In the SIMPLIFY-2 trial which enrolled MF patients previously treated with ruxolitinib, momelotinib was not superior to BAT for the reduction of spleen size by $\geq 35\%$ (Harrison et al. 2017).

Pacritinib, a JAK2 inhibitor, was investigated in two phase 3 trials in MF patients. In PERSIST-1, patients could be enrolled irrespective of pre-existing anemia or thrombocytopenia. Here, at week 24, 19% of the patients in the pacritinib group had achieved a $\geq 35\%$ reduction in spleen volume (Mesa et al. 2017b). In contrast to PERSIST-1, the PERSIST-2 trial allowed prior JAK2 inhibitor treatment and ruxolitinib as best available therapy. In preliminary results, pacritinib was more effective in the reduction of spleen volume than BAT (Mascarenhas et al. 2016). In 2016, the FDA placed full clinical hold on pacritinib studies following reports on patient deaths related to intracranial hemorrhage, cardiac failure, or cardiac arrest in the PERSIST-2 trial. The full clinical hold has been removed in 2017. A new trial (PAC203, NCT03165734) is ongoing in order to evaluate the safety and the dose—response relationship for efficacy of three pacritinib dosing regimens.

9 Summary and Perspectives

Ruxolitinib is a potent and selective oral inhibitor of JAK1 and JAK2, which induces clinically meaningful responses in terms of reduced splenomegaly and debilitating symptoms in the majority of patients with MF, while its favorable impact on survival and bone marrow fibrosis has yet to be firmly established. Overall ruxolitinib is a precious addition to the palliative substances currently used in the treatment of patients with MF, who are not candidates for a potentially curative allogeneic HSCT. In addition, ruxolitinib has become a valuable addition to the treatment options in patients with PV with HU resistance or intolerance.

As with other therapies, future research has to focus on biomarkers that can reliably predict patients with response to ruxolitinib treatment. Being able to restrict treatment to only responsive patients would avoid exposition of the remaining patients to side effects and drastically reduce overall therapy costs. In addition, current and future research aims to identify agents to combine with ruxolitinib in the treatment of MPNs and expand the usage of ruxolitinib to other immuno-inflammatory diseases, such as GvHD.

References

Al-Ali HK, Griesshammer M, le Coutre P et al (2016) Safety and efficacy of ruxolitinib in an open-label, multicenter, single-arm phase 3b expanded-access study in patients with myelofibrosis: a snapshot of 1144 patients in the JUMP trial. Haematologica 101(9): 1065–1073

Caocci G, Murgia F, Podda L et al (2014) Reactivation of hepatitis B virus infection following ruxolitinib treatment in a patient with myelofibrosis. Leukemia 28(1):225–227

Cervantes F, Dupriez B, Pereira A et al (2009) New prognostic scoring system for primary myelofibrosis based on a study of the International Working Group for Myelofibrosis Research and Treatment. Blood 113(13):2895–2901

Daver N, Cortes JE, Pemmaraju N et al (2016) Ruxolitinib (RUX) in combination with 5-azacytidine (AZA) as therapy for patients (pts) with myelofibrosis (MF). Blood 128(22):4246

Davis KL, Côté I, Kaye JA et al (2015) Real-world assessment of clinical outcomes in patients with lower-risk myelofibrosis receiving treatment with ruxolitinib. Adv Hematol 2015:848473

Guglielmelli P, Biamonte F, Rotunno G et al (2014) Impact of mutational status on outcomes in myelofibrosis patients treated with ruxolitinib in the COMFORT-II study. Blood 123 (14):2157–2160

Harrison CN, Kiladjian JJ, Al-Ali HK et al (2012) JAK inhibition with ruxolitinib versus best available therapy for myelofibrosis. N Engl J Med 366(9):787–798

Harrison CN, Vannucchi AM, Kiladjian JJ et al (2016) Long-term findings from COMFORT-II, a phase 3 study of ruxolitinib versus best available therapy for myelofibrosis. Leukemia 30 (8):1701–1707

Harrison CN, Vannucchi AM, Platzbecker U et al (2017) Momelotinib versus best available therapy in patients with myelofibrosis previously treated with ruxolitinib (SIMPLIFY 2): a randomised, open-label, phase 3 trial. Lancet Haematol. 20 Dec (epup ehead of print)

Iancu-Rubin C, Mosoyan G, Wang J, Kraus T, Sung V, Hoffman R (2013) Stromal cell-mediated inhibition of erythropoiesis can be attenuated by Sotatercept (ACE-011), an activin receptor type II ligand trap. Exp Hematol 41(2):155–166

Jakavi® (2017) Summary of product characteristics, Novartis http://www.fachinfo.de. Last revised Apr 2017

James C, Ugo V, Le Couédic JP et al (2005) A unique clonal JAK2 mutation leading to constitutive signalling causes polycythaemia vera. Nature 434(7037):1144–1148

Mascarenhas J, Hoffman R, Talpaz M et al (2016) Results of the persist-2 phase 3 study of pacritinib (PAC) versus best available therapy (BAT), including ruxolitinib (RUX), in patients (pts) with myelofibrosis (MF) and platelet counts <100,000/µl. Blood 128(22):LBA-5

McPherson S, McMullin MF, Mills K (2017) Epigenetics in myeloproliferative neoplasms. J Cell Mol Med 21(9):1660–1667

Mertens C, Darnell JE Jr (2007) SnapShot: JAK-STAT signaling. Cell 131(3):612

Mesa RA, Gotlib J, Gupta V et al (2013) Effect of ruxolitinib therapy on myelofibrosis-related symptoms and other patient-reported outcomes in COMFORT-I: a randomized, double-blind, placebo-controlled trial. J Clin Oncol 31(10):1285–1292

Mesa RA, Kiladjian JJ, Catalano JV et al (2017a) SIMPLIFY-1: a phase III randomized trial of momelotinib versus ruxolitinib in janus kinase inhibitor-naïve patients with myelofibrosis. J Clin Oncol 35(34):3844–3850

Mesa RA, Vannucchi AM, Mead A et al (2017b) Pacritinib versus best available therapy for the treatment of myelofibrosis irrespective of baseline cytopenias (PERSIST-1): an international, randomised, phase 3 trial. Lancet Haematol 4(5):e225–e236

Passamonti F, Griesshammer M, Palandri F et al (2017) Ruxolitinib for the treatment of inadequately controlled polycythaemia vera without splenomegaly (RESPONSE-2): a randomised, open-label, phase 3b study. Lancet Oncol 18(1):88–99

Patel KP, Newberry KJ, Luthra R et al (2015) Correlation of mutation profile and response in patients with myelofibrosis treated with ruxolitinib. Blood 126(6):790–797

Quintás-Cardama A, Vaddi K, Liu P et al (2010) Preclinical characterization of the selective JAK1/2 inhibitor INCB018424: therapeutic implications for the treatment of myeloproliferative neoplasms. Blood 115(15):3109–3117

Rampal RK, Mascarenhas JO, Kosiorek HE et al (2016) Safety and efficacy of combined ruxolitinib and decitabine in patients with blast-phase MPN and post-MPN AML: results of a phase I study (Myeloproliferative Disorders Research Consortium 109 trial). Blood 128 (22):1124

Shi JG, Chen X, Emm T et al (2012) The effect of CYP3A4 inhibition or induction on the pharmacokinetics and pharmacodynamics of orally administered ruxolitinib (INCB018424 phosphate) in healthy volunteers. J Clin Pharmacol 52(6):809–818

Shilling AD, Nedza FM, Emm T et al (2010) Metabolism, excretion, and pharmacokinetics of [14C] INCB018424, a selective Janus tyrosine kinase 1/2 inhibitor, in humans. Drug Metab Dispos 38(11):2023–2031

Spoerl S, Mathew NR, Bscheider M et al (2014) Activity of therapeutic JAK 1/2 blockade in graft-versus-host disease. Blood 123(24):3832–3842

Stegelmann F, Hebart H, Bangerter M et al (2016) Ruxolitinib plus pomalidomide in myelofibrosis: updated results from the Mpnsg-0212 Trial (NCT01644110). Blood 128 (22):1939

Talpaz M, Paquette R, Afrin L et al (2013) Interim analysis of safety and efficacy of ruxolitinib in patients with myelofibrosis and low platelet counts. J Hematol Oncol 6(1):81

Tefferi A, Pardanani A (2011) Serious adverse events during ruxolitinib treatment discontinuation in patients with myelofibrosis. Mayo Clin Proc 86(12):1188–1191

Tefferi A, Litzow MR, Pardanani A (2011) Long-term outcome of treatment with ruxolitinib in myelofibrosis. N Engl J Med 365(15):1455–1457

Vannucchi AM, Kiladjian JJ, Griesshammer M et al (2015) Ruxolitinib versus standard therapy for the treatment of polycythemia vera. N Engl J Med 372(5):426–435

Verstovsek S, Bose P (2017) JAK2 inhibitors for myeloproliferative neoplasms: what is next? Blood 130(2):115–125

Verstovsek S, Kantarjian H, Mesa RA et al (2010) Safety and efficacy of INCB018424, a JAK1 and JAK2 inhibitor, in myelofibrosis. N Engl J Med 363(12):1117–1127

Verstovsek S, Kantarjian HM, Estrov Z et al (2012a) Long-term outcomes of 107 patients with myelofibrosis receiving JAK1/JAK2 inhibitor ruxolitinib: survival advantage in comparison to matched historical controls. Blood 120(6):1202–1209

Verstovsek S, Mesa RA, Gotlib J et al (2012b) A double-blind, placebo-controlled trial of ruxolitinib for myelofibrosis. N Engl J Med 366(9):799–807

Verstovsek S, Mesa RA, Gotlib J et al (2013) The clinical benefit of ruxolitinib across patient subgroups: analysis of a placebo-controlled, phase III study in patients with myelofibrosis. Br J Haematol 161(4):508–516

Verstovsek S, Mesa RA, Gotlib J et al (2017) Long-term treatment with ruxolitinib for patients with myelofibrosis: 5-year update from the randomized, double-blind, placebo-controlled, phase 3 COMFORT-I trial. J Hematol Oncol. 10(1):55

Zeiser R, Blazar BR (2017a) Acute graft-versus-host disease—biologic process, prevention, and therapy. N Engl J Med 377(22):2167–2179

Zeiser R, Blazar BR (2017b) Pathophysiology of chronic graft-versus-host disease and therapeutic targets. N Engl J Med 377(26):2565–2579

Zeiser R, Burchert A, Lengerke C et al (2015) Ruxolitinib in corticosteroid-refractory graft-versus-host disease after allogeneic stem cell transplantation: a multicenter survey. Leukemia 29(10):2062–2068

Ibrutinib

Andriani Charalambous, Mark-Alexander Schwarzbich
and Mathias Witzens-Harig

Contents

Disclosure: The authors have nothing to disclose.

A. Charalambous
School of Medicine and Dentistry,
Queen Mary University of London, London, UK
e-mail: a.charalambous@smd15.qmul.ac.uk

M.-A. Schwarzbich (✉)
Barts Cancer Institute, Barts and The London School of Medicine and Dentistry,
Queen Mary University of London, Charterhouse Square, London EC1M 6BQ, UK
e-mail: M.Schwarzbich@qmul.ac.uk

M.-A. Schwarzbich · M. Witzens-Harig
Department of Haematology, Oncology and Rheumatology, Heidelberg University Hospital,
Heidelberg, Germany
e-mail: witzens.harig@yahoo.de

Abstract

Abnormal B-cell receptor (BCR) signalling is a key mechanism of disease progression in B-cell malignancy. Bruton's tyrosine kinase (BTK) has a pivotal role in BCR signalling. Ibrutinib (PCI-32765) is a small molecule which serves as a covalent irreversible inhibitor of BTK. It is characterized by high selectivity for BTK and high potency. Ibrutinib is currently approved by the FDA and EMA for use in chronic lymphocytic leukaemia in any line of treatment, for treatment of Waldenstrom macroglobulinemia in patients who have received previous treatments or are not suitable to receive immunochemotherapy as well as for second line treatment of mantle cell lymphoma and for patients with marginal zone lymphoma who have received at least one prior anti-CD20-based therapy. In addition, there is emerging clinical data on its efficacy in ABC subtype diffuse large B-cell lymphoma, multiple myeloma and primary central nervous system lymphoma. Ibrutinib has opened new options for treatment of those patients that have relapsed or have been refractory to more classical modes of treatment. Moreover, Ibrutinib has been shown to be effective in patients that have been known to have little sensitivity to classical immunochemotherapy. Having a favourable risk profile, the substance is, unlike conventional immunochemotherapy, also suitable for the less physical fit patients. Cases of primary and secondary resistance to Ibrutinib have emerged and there is an ongoing effort to identify their mechanism and develop strategies to overcome them. Beyond its direct effects on survival and apoptosis of malignant B-cells, there is increasing evidence that Ibrutinib is able to modulate the tumour microenvironment to overcome mechanisms of immune evasion. This has sparked interest in use of the substance beyond lymphoid malignancy. This chapter discusses structure, mechanism of action and toxicities of Ibrutinib and also presents important preclinical and clinical data as well as mechanisms of Ibrutinib resistance.

Combination strategies with immunotherapeutic strategies such as immune checkpoint blockade and CAR T-cell therapy may be synergistic and are currently under investigation.

Keywords

Ibrutinib · B-cell receptor · Chronic lymphocytic leukemia · Mantel cell lymphoma · Waldenstrom's Macroglobulinemia · Marginal zone lymphoma · Tumour microenvironment · Immunomodulation

1 Introduction

The concept of targeted therapies is becoming increasingly popular in a coordinated attempt to investigate and possibly eliminate cancer. Extensive study of tumorigenesis and in-depth analysis of the genomic, biochemical and immunological aspects of cancer cells have given rise to a paradigm shift in the treatment of malignancies. In an era where the limitations of conventional therapies are becoming increasingly apparent, targeted therapies, including small molecule inhibitors, are important additions to the armamentarium against malignancies.

Excessive and uncontrolled proliferation of cells comprises a significant hallmark of cancer. This is largely due to activating mutations in either receptor or non-receptor tyrosine kinases. Receptor tyrosine kinase domains of growth factor receptors (GFRs) are responsible for regulating cell proliferation, growth and differentiation upon ligand binding. Such mutations result in constitutive activation of the kinases and hence, of downstream signalling pathways that regulate the aforementioned cell functions, thus bringing about growth factor independent growth. Alternatively, mutations in non-receptor tyrosine kinases, a subgroup of cytoplasmic kinases, also play an important role in cell differentiation, growth, as well as in migration and apoptosis. Not surprisingly, the role of both receptor and non-receptor tyrosine kinases in malignant transformation has rendered them significant targets for anti-cancer therapy.

Bruton's tyrosine kinase is an example of a cytoplasmic tyrosine kinase and is a vital constituent of the B-cell receptor (BCR) signalling pathway, B-cell activation and development. In 1952, Ogden Bruton first discovered a case of B-cell developmental arrest and inability to mount an effective humoral immune response in a paediatric patient. The discovery of this condition later dubbed X-linked agammaglobulinemia (XLA) has laid the basis for the discovery of Bruton's tyrosine kinase (BTK) and of related gene defects. BTK and its role in BCR signalling have thus rendered BTK inhibition a possible therapeutic mode for a range of malignancies (Bruton 1952).

PCI-32765, better known as Ibrutinib, is a small molecule first designed by Celera Genomics as a selective inhibitor of Bruton's tyrosine kinase (BTK). The compound has been approved by the FDA and EMA for therapeutic use in chronic lymphocytic leukaemia (CLL), Waldenstrom macroglobulinemia (WM), mantle cell lymphoma (MCL) and marginal zone lymphoma (MZL). In addition to this, there is emerging data on clinical use in activated B-cell (ABC) subtype diffuse large B-cell lymphoma (DLBCL), multiple myeloma (MM), solid malignancies and primary central nervous system lymphoma (PCNSL). In August 2017, it was also licensed for use in the treatment of chronic graft versus host disease (GvHD).

2 Structure and Mechanism of Action

2.1 Bruton's Tyrosine Kinase and B-cell Receptor Signalling

In B-cell malignancies, antigen-dependent and independent BCR signalling is widely appreciated as one of the main mechanisms to promote disease progression (Chiorazzi et al. 2005; Davis et al. 2010; Stevenson et al. 2011; Minden et al. 2012; Woyach et al. 2012). The early placement of BTK in the BCR signalling cascade essentially means it is a cornerstone in the functions of the BCR.

BTK belongs to the Tec family of non-receptor tyrosine kinases. It consists of 659 amino acids, has a molecular weight of 77 kDa (Sideras et al. 1994) and is encoded by the *BTK* gene which is located in the long arm (q) of the X chromosome at position 22.1 (Broides et al. 2006). Tec family kinases consist of a pleckstrin homology (PH) domain, which binds phosphoinositides, hence contributing to phosphotyrosine-mediated and phospholipid-mediated signalling systems. BTK also contains a catalytic domain (SH1), two Src homology (SH) domains (SH2 and SH3) and a Tec homology (TH) domain, which is in turn composed of a BTK homology (BH) region and a polyproline region (PPR) (Mohamed et al. 2009). Each of the aforementioned domains interacts with a multitude of intracellular signalling mediators.

The BCR is a complex consisting of a membrane-bound immunoglobulin (Ig) coupled with heterodimers of the transmembrane proteins CD79a (Ig-alpha) and CD79b (Ig-beta) joined together by disulphide bridges. Physiologically, engagement of the Ig by antigen results in receptor aggregation, which subsequently activates the Src family kinases Lyn, Blk, Fyn, Syk and BTK. Phosphorylation of the aforementioned kinases as well as phosphorylation of the immunoreceptor-based activation motifs (ITAMs) found in the cytoplasmic tail of CD79a/b occurs (Woyach et al. 2012). The phosphorylated BCR binds to either the Syk or Lyn protein tyrosine kinase, which consequently activates downstream signalling cascades. The B-cell linker protein (BLNK) acts as a scaffold for phospholipase C gamma 2 (PLCγ-2) and BTK to form a microsignalosome that initiates downstream calcium signalling. Hydrolysis of membrane PIP_2 results in the production of IP_3, and this activates the corresponding IP_3 receptors bringing about calcium egress from the endoplasmic reticulum (Hendriks et al. 2014; Seda and Mraz 2015). This promotes the influx of more Ca^{2+} through calcium release-activated channels (CRAC). The increased ionic calcium in the cytosol promotes activation of PKCβ which mediates the activation of transcription factors needed for B-cell proliferation and differentiation including NF-κB, NFAT as well

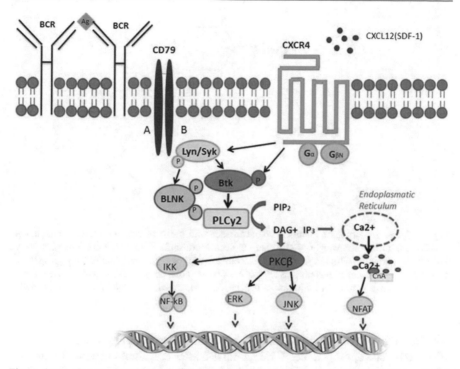

Fig. 1 BTK signalling pathways. *Abbreviations* PIP2—phosphatidylinositol 4,5-bisphosphate, DAG—diacylglycerol, IP3—inositol-1,4,5 trisphosphate, Ca^{2+}—calcium, CnA—calcineurin

as other protein kinases like ERK or JNK (Satterthwaite and Witte 2000; Scharenberg et al. 2007). These pathways normally achieve continuation of the cell cycle, as well as increased transcriptional activity, proliferation and survival. Through BTK inhibition, Ibrutinib abrogates or reduces the extent of the above processes. BTK is also involved in chemokine receptor signalling, namely in the activation of the chemokine receptors CXCR4 and CXCR5 by chemokines CXCL12 and CXCL13 which controls chemotaxis, adhesion and tissue-homing effects (Ortolano et al. 2006; de Gorter et al. 2007) (Fig. 1).

2.2 Ibrutinib Structure

For structure and chemical characteristics of Ibrutinib, refer to Fig. 2 (Pan et al. 2007; Honigberg et al. 2010).

2.3 Mode of Action and Pharmacokinetics

Ibrutinib and its active metabolite PCI-45227 bind covalently and irreversibly to cysteine residue 481 within the ATP binding domain of BTK. The inhibitory

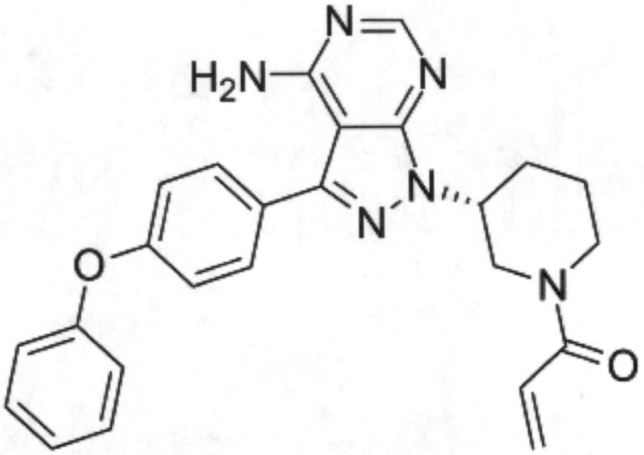

Fig. 2 Synonym, structure, chemical characteristics and mode of action of Ibrutinib. Synonym PCI-32765, molecular weight 440.50 Da, molecular formula C25H24N6O2, chemical name 1-[(3R)-3-[4-amino-3-(4-phenoxyphenyl)pyrazolo[3,4-d]pyrimidin-1-yl]piperidin-1-yl]prop-2-en-1-one, mode of action irreversible: BTK inhibitor binds covalently to cysteine-481 in the kinase domain. Highly potent BTK inhibition at IC50 = 0.5 nM, schedule 420–840 mg p.o. once daily

activity of the metabolite is 15 times lower than that of the drug. Occupancy of the BTK active site appears to be >95% within 4 h after oral administration. Ibrutinib is highly potent and selective for BTK, inhibiting the kinase activity with an IC50 0.5 nM (Honigberg et al. 2010). Ibrutinib has significant activity against other kinases, seven of which contain a cognate cysteine residue and hence are prone to irreversible inhibition. Reversible inhibition is also possible against a number of kinases, although clinical significance of this is questioned, taking into consideration the short in vivo half-life of the drug (2–3 h). The untoward effects of Ibrutinib have mainly been attributed to these off-target effects of the substance. The most prominent targets and corresponding IC50 values are listed in Table 1.

3 Preclinical Data

In 2007, a structure-based process for creating small molecules which serve as irreversible covalent inhibitors of BTK was first described by scientists at Celera Genomics (Pan et al. 2007). Of these molecules, the compound PCI-32765 was chosen for further preclinical development. Celera Genomics was at first trying to develop new compounds for treatment of rheumatoid arthritis. Therefore, the substance was initially tested in rheumatoid arthritis in vivo models. Later on the efficacy in lymphoma models was discovered (Honigberg et al. 2010; Chang et al. 2011; Di Paolo et al. 2011). Efficacy of Ibrutinib in B-cell lymphoma was first demonstrated by Honigberg et al. (2010) in spontaneous canine B-cell lymphoma. Orally administered substance induced a response in three out of eight dogs treated.

Table 1 IC50 and fold selectivity for enzymatic inhibition by Ibrutinib

Kinase	IC50 (nM)	BTK selectivity, fold
BTK	0.5	NA
BLK[a]	0.5	1
BMX[a]	0.8	1.6
CSK	2.3	4.6
FGR	2.3	4.6
BRK	3.3	6.6
HCK	3.7	7.4
EGFR[a]	5.6	11.2
YES	6.5	13
HER2[a]	9.4	18.8
ITK[a]	10.7	21.4
JAK3[a]	16.1	32.2
FRK	29.2	58.4
LCK	33.2	66.4
RET	36.5	73
FLT3	73	146
TEC[a]	78	156
ABL	86	172
FYN	96	192
RIPK2	152	304
c-SRC	171	342
LYN	200	400
PDGFRα	718	1436

[a]Kinases that contain a cysteine residue aligning with Cys-481 in BTK. Adapted from Honigberg et al. (2010)

3.1 Apoptosis and Survival in B-cell Malignancies

Herman et al. (2011) showed that Ibrutinib is able to induce apoptosis in CLL cells even in the presence of survival signals such as CD40L, BAFF, TNF-a, IL-4 and IL-6 albeit to a rather modest extent. Ponader et al. (2012) reported the inhibition of CLL cell survival and proliferation by Ibrutinib. In an adoptive transfer TCL1 mouse model of CLL, PCI-32765 also inhibited disease progression. Another study by Schwamb et al. (2012) reported Ibrutinib-mediated inhibition of BCR-dependent UDP-glucose ceramide glucosyltransferase expression which in turn sensitizes CLL cells to apoptosis. In addition, Sehgal et al. (2014) reported an increased sensitivity of lymphoma cell lines to FAS-induced apoptosis after Ibrutinib treatment due to a downregulation of EZH2, RBM5 and sFas. Dubovsky et al. (2013a, b) were able to demonstrate that Ibrutinib is able to inhibit BCR-induced activation of LCP1, a protein that has been implicated in crosslinking of F-actin filaments and hence providing a scaffold for critical signalling pathways in lymphocytes. This protein is highly overexpressed in CLL.

In DLCBL, Davis et al. (2010) demonstrated selective toxicity of Ibrutinib in DLCBL cell lines with chronically active BCR signalling. Yang et al. (2012) reported that the substance downregulates IRF4 and synergizes with Lenalidomide in killing activated B-cell like (ABC) subtype DLBCL cells. Dasmahapatra et al. (2013) showed that co-administration of Ibrutinib and Bortezomib increases apoptosis in DLCBL cells and MCL cells via AKT and nuclear factor (NF)-κB (NFKB1) inactivation, downregulation of MCl-1 (MCL1), Bcl-xL (BCL2L1), XIAP-enhanced DNA damage and endoplasmic reticulum (ER) stress, even in highly Bortezomib-resistant DLBCL and MCL cells.

Tai et al. (2012) showed that PCI-32765 inhibits RANKL/M-GCSG-induced phosphorylation of BTK and downstream PLC-gamma signalling in osteoclasts. Moreover, the substance also decreased chemokine and cytokine secretion by osteoclasts and bone marrow stromal cells, CLC12-induced migration of MM cells, IL6-induced growth of MM cells and in vivo MM cell growth as well as MM cell-induced osteolysis of implanted human bone chips in SCID mice. Rushworth et al. (2013) showed cytotoxic of Ibrutinib to MM cells and synergy with Bortezomib and Lenalidomide chemotherapies. This is mediated via inhibitory effects on the nuclear factor-κB (NF-κB) pathway resulting in downregulation of anti-apoptotic proteins Bcl-xL, FLIP(L) and survivin leading to apoptosis. Moreover, Murray et al. (2015) were able to demonstrate that Ibrutinib treatment resensitizes previously Bortezomib-resistant MM cells to further Bortezomib therapy.

3.2 B-cell Egress and Modulation of the Microenvironment

Ibrutinib treatment in CLL is associated with a phase of lymphocytosis in the first weeks of treatment that is not due to disease progression but rather redistribution of CLL B-cells to the bloodstream (Woyach et al. 2014a, b). Several studies have tried to address the mechanism of this phenomenon. De Rooij et al. (2012) demonstrated the inhibition of CLL cell chemotaxis and integrin-mediated CLL cell adhesion by Ibrutinib (Woyach et al. 2014a, b). Ponader et al. (2012) also showed reduced migration towards chemokines CXCL12 and CXCL13 (the ligands of CXCR4 and 5, respectively). PCI-32765 was also shown to downregulate secretion of BCR-dependent chemokines (CCL3, CCL4) by CLL cells, both in vitro and in vivo. A study on patient CLL cells after Ibrutinib treatment showed rapidly reduced capability of CLL cells to adhere to fibronectin, a moderate reduction of migration towards cytokines as well as a reduction of adhesion surface molecules CD49d, CD29 and CD44 (Herman et al. 2015). In addition, Chen et al. (2016a, b) showed reduced expression of CXCR4, CXCR5, CD49d and other homing-/adhesion-related surface molecules in a mouse model of CLL after Ibrutinib treatment.

As the direct cytotoxic effect of Ibrutinib against CLL B-cells in vitro is rather modest (Herman et al. 2011), it has been speculated that this egress of malignant B-cells from their protective microenvironment rather than its direct effects on

B-cell survival and apoptosis may be responsible for the high clinical efficacy of the substance. A study by Wodarz et al. (2014) sought to correlate serial lymphocyte counts of CLL patients after Ibrutinib treatment with CT-based volumetric assessment of lymph node and spleen size to address this question. However, it was estimated that only 23.3% $\pm$ 17% of total tissue disease burden was redistributed to the peripheral blood suggesting that CLL cell death rather than egress from nodal compartments is responsible for the clinical efficacy of the substance. Further support for these findings comes from a study by Burger et al. (2017) using isotopic labelling of CLL B-cells with deuterated water to directly measure the effects of Ibrutinib in 30 CLL patients. CLL proliferation rate was reduced from 0.39% of the clone per day to 0.05% per day with treatment, while death rates of CLL cells increased from 0.18% per day prior to treatment to 1.5% per day.

It has been suggested that modulation of T-cell and myeloid cell function by Ibrutinib contributes to increased malignant cell death after Ibrutinib treatment. Indeed, Dubovsky et al. (2013a, b) were able to demonstrate that Ibrutinib has the potential to shift T-helper cell polarity away from Th2 towards Th1 by targeting ITK and could thereby correct malignancy-associated T-cell defects. Moreover, Kondo et al. (2017) have reported downregulation of PD-L1 on the surface of CLL B-cells in the peripheral blood of Ibrutinib-treated CLL patients as well as down-regulation of expression of PD-1 on the surface of CD4+ and CD8+ T-cells, both in a STAT3-dependent manner. Stiff et al. (2016) demonstrate expression of BTK in both human and murine myeloid-derived suppressor cells (MDSCs) and showed that Ibrutinib treatment is able to inhibit BTK phosphorylation in these cells resulting in impaired nitrous oxide production, cell migration, expression of 2,3-dioxygenase as well as impaired in vitro generation of human MDSCs. Ibrutinib treatment resulted in reduced numbers of MDSCs in both spleen and tumours of mouse models of mammary cancer and melanoma. A study by Ping et al. (2017) demonstrated decreased production of CXCL12, CXCL13, CCL19 and VEGF by human macrophages after Ibrutinib treatment. Moreover, adhesion, migration and invasion of co-cultured lymphoid cells were significantly impaired. Finally, Gunderson et al. (2016) reported that tumour growth in a model of pancreatic ductal adenocarcinoma (PDAC) was dependent on a crosstalk between B-cells and FcRγ(+) tumour-associated macrophages resulting in a Th2-permissive macrophage phenotype via BTK activation in a PI3Kγ-dependent manner. Ibrutinib treatment results in a shift towards a more Th1-permissive macrophage phenotype and fostered CD8+ T-cell cytotoxicity.

3.3   Ibrutinib and Solid Malignancy

Reports of modulation of the tumour microenvironment by Ibrutinib have sparked interest in the therapeutic potential of the substance beyond lymphoid malignancy. In addition to what has been discussed above, several preclinical studies have tried to address a potential role of Ibrutinib treatment in solid malignancies.

Grabinski and Ewald (2014) have analysed the effects of Ibrutinib on Her2+ breast cancer cells in vitro showing a potential of the substance to suppress phosphorylation of ErbB1, ErbB2 and ErbB3, thereby suppressing AKT and ERK signalling. This was confirmed by Chen et al. (2016a, b) who reported growth inhibition of Her2+ breast cancer cell lines in vitro after Ibrutinib treatment which coincided with downregulation of phosphorylation of Her2 and EGFR and inhibition of downstream AKT and ERK signalling. Moreover, xenograft studies with Her2+ cell lines demonstrated significant inhibition of growth.

In Pancreatic ductal adenocarcinoma (PDAC), it has been demonstrated that tumour growth could effectively be limited by Ibrutinib treatment in both transgenic and patient-derived xenograft models. Ibrutinib treatment led to decreased fibrosis, extended survival and improved response to Gemcitabine therapy (Masso-Valles et al. 2015).

Zucha et al. (2015) reported high levels of cisplatin resistance dependent on BTK and JAK2/STAT3 in spheroid-forming ovarian cancer cells which highly expressed cancer stem-like cell (CSC) markers and BTK. The group was able to demonstrate synergistic effects of concomitant Ibrutinib and cisplatin treatment.

Kokabee et al. (2015) reported on BTK expression in human prostate cell lines and tumour samples from prostate cancer patients. Treatment with Ibrutinib reduced cell survival and induced apoptosis.

Downregulation of BTK expression as well as Ibrutinib treatment has been demonstrated to reduce colony formation, migration and sphere formation in glioblastoma multiforme (GBM) cell lines. In xenograft mouse models, tumorigenesis was significantly reduced in BTK-silenced or Ibrutinib-treated animals compared to controls. Glioma tissue microarray analysis indicated significantly higher BTK staining in malignant tumours than less malignant tumours and normal brain tissue (Wei et al. 2016). In a study by Wang et al. (2017), Ibrutinib inhibited cellular proliferation and migration, and induced apoptosis and autophagy in GBM cell lines. Inhibition of autophagy by 3-methyladenine (3MA) or Atg7 targeting with small interfering RNA (si-Atg7) enhanced the anti-GBM effect of Ibrutinib in vitro and in vivo suggesting an induction of autophagy by Ibrutinib through Akt/mTOR signalling pathways.

4   Clinical Data

Ibrutinib is currently approved by the FDA and EMA for use in CLL in any line of treatment, for treatment of WM in patients who have received previous treatments or are not suitable to receive immunochemotherapy as well as for second line treatment of MCL and for patients with MZL who have received at least one prior anti-CD20-based therapy. Below, we will present the most important clinical studies on these entities as well as emerging clinical data on ABC subtype DLBCL, MM, solid malignancies and PCNSL. Table 2 summarizes the relevant clinical studies.

Table 2 Overview of relevant clinical studies on Ibrutinib treatment. HTN—arterial hypertension

Trial/regimen	n	Median age (range) in years	ORR (%)	CR (%)	PFS	OS benefit	Neutropenia ≥ grade 3 (%)	Thrombocytopenia ≥ grade 3 (%)	Atrial fibrillation (%)	HTN ≥ grade 3 (%)	Major bleeding events (%)	≥ grade 3 infection (%)
Single-agent Ibrutinib in R/R CLL												
Byrd et al. (2013)/ Ibrutinib	101	66 (37–82)	89	10	Median: 52-mo	N/A	18	10	6	20	10	51
RESONATE (Brown et al. 2014)/Ibrutinib	195	67 (30–86)	90	6	24-mo: 74%	Yes	18	6	7	6	1	24
Ibrutinib combination treatment in R/R CLL												
Burger et al. (2014)/ Ibrutinib–Rituximab	40	63 (35–82)	95	8	26-mo: 75%	N/A	6	Not reported	6	Not reported	0	13
Jaglowski et al. (2015)/ Ibrutinib–Obinutuzumab	71	64 (48–85)	83	2	12-mo: 88.9%	N/A	24	Not reported	8.5	Not reported	10	20
HELIOS (Chanan-Khan et al. 2016/Ibrutinib–Bendamustine–Rituximab	289	64 (31–86)	83	10	18-mo: 79%	Yes	54	15	7	Not reported	4	29
Single-agent Ibrutinib as first-line treatment in CLL												
Byrd et al. (2015)/ Ibrutinib	31	71 (65–84)	84	23	30-mo: 96%	N/A	3	3	6	23	Not reported	6
Resonate-2 (Burger et al. 2015a, b/Ibrutinib del (17p) excluded	136	73 (65–89)	86	4	24-mo: 89%	Yes	10	2	6	4	4	8
Davids et al. (2016)/ Ibrutinib–FCR	27	55 (43–65)	100	45	Median: not reached	N/A	15	19	4	Not reported	0	9
Ibrutinib in CLL with del(17p) and/or TP53 mutation												
Farooqui et al. (2015a, b and c)/Ibrutinib del(17p) and/or TP53 only	51	63 (33–82)	92	5	24-mo: 82%	N/A	24	10	2	Not reported	0	6
Resonate-17 (O'Brien et al. 2016a, b/Ibrutinib del(17p) only	144	64 (57–72)	83	8	24-mo: 53%	N/A	22	11	5	13	9	30

(continued)

Table 2 (continued)

Trial/regimen	n	Median age (range) in years	ORR (%)	CR (%)	PFS	OS benefit	Neutropenia ≥ grade 3 (%)	Thrombocytopenia ≥ grade 3 (%)	Atrial fibrillation (%)	HTN ≥ grade 3 (%)	Major bleeding events (%)	≥ grade 3 infection (%)
Ibrutinib in Waldenstrom macroglobulinemia												
Treon et al. (2015)/ Ibrutinib	63	63 (44–86)	91	73	24-mo: 69%	N/A	14	13	5	0	6	10
iNNOVATE (Dimopoulos et al. 2015)/ Ibrutinib in Rituximab-refractory WM	42	67 (47–90)	88	64	Not reported	N/A	13	6	0	23	0	10
Ibrutinib in mantle cell lymphoma												
Wang et al. (2013)/ Ibrutinib	111	68 (40–84)	68	21	Median: 13.9 months	N/A	17	13	11	Not reported	26	6
Dreyling et al. (2016)/ Ibrutinib versus Temsirolimus	280	67 (not reported)	72	19	Median: 14.6 months	Yes	13	9	4	Not reported	10	Not reported
Wang et al. (2016a, b)/ Ibrutinib–Rituximab	50	67 (45–86)	88	44	Not reported	N/A	4	4	14	2	6	14
Ibrutinib in marginal zone lymphoma												
Noy et al. (2017)/ Ibrutinib	63	66 (3092)	48	3	Median: 14.2 months	N/A	5	0	NR	5	2	19

4.1   Ibrutinib in Relapsed/Refractory (R/R) CLL

In an initial phase I/IIb trial on 85 R/R CLL patients by Byrd et al. (2013), 51 patients received 420 mg Ibrutinib p.o. once daily, while 34 patients received 840 mg once daily. The patient cohort was heavily pretreated with a median of 4 priory therapies, and many of the patients had an unfavourable risk profile with del (17p) in 33%, del(11q) in 36% and unmutated IGHV in 81% of patients. Patients were largely elderly with a median age of 66. After a median follow-up of 20.9 month, an overall response rate (ORR) of 71% was reported independent of the administered dose. In addition to that, 20% of patients in the 420 mg cohort and 15% of patients in the 840 mg cohort had a partial remission with lymphocytosis (PR-L) (Hallek et al. 2008). In CLL, PCI-32765 induces lymphocytosis in the first weeks of treatment. This phenomenon is directly related to the presence of the drug, asymptomatic and temporary. It is believed that this is due to redistribution of CLL cells from solid lymphoma manifestations into the bloodstream. It should not be confused with lymphocytosis due to disease progression (Woyach et al. 2014a, b). Long-term follow-up data on this trial was reported in 2015/2016 with an additional 16 subjects showing an ORR of 89% (10% complete remission (CR)) and an impressive median progression-free survival (PFS) of 52 months (Byrd et al. 2015; O'Brien et al. 2016a, b). Patients with del(17p) had a median PFS of 26 months, and those with del(11q) had a median PFS of 55 months (O'Brien et al. 2016a, b). The presence of complex karyotype was predictive of poorer outcome (median PFS 33 months vs. not reached). No differences depending on IGVH mutation status were reported. Interestingly, almost all patients with initial PR-L achieved deeper remission with longer follow-up and had comparable outcomes then those without lymphocytosis (O'Brien et al. 2016a, b).

In the phase III RESONATE trial, 391 patients with R/R CLL/SLL were randomized to either single-agent Ibrutinib or Ofatumumab treatment. 32% of patients had del(17p), 32% had del(11q) and 68% had unmutated IGVH. About half of patients had received at least three prior treatments. The median age of patients included was 67. With a median follow-up of 16 month, an ORR of 90% in the Ibrutinib group versus only 25% in the Ofatumumab group was reached ($p < 0.0001$). Also, PFS was significantly improved in the Ibrutinib versus Ofatumumab groups (median not reached vs. 8.1 months). Moreover, Ibrutinib significantly increased 18 months OS (85 vs. 78%). Ibrutinib-treated patients demonstrated no differences in PFS regardless of the presence of del(17p) (Brown et al. 2014; Byrd et al. 2014). Together, these two studies demonstrate durable responses in patients with R/R CLL treated with single-agent Ibrutinib regardless of pretreatments or the presence of cytogenetic abnormalities.

A number of studies have sought to combine Ibrutinib with other substances to further improve outcomes. Researchers at the MD Anderson Cancer Centre, Houston, Texas, USA, have investigated the combination with Rituximab in a single arm phase II trial involving 40 patients with R/R CLL/SLL in a high-risk setting defined as the presence of del(17p), TP-53 mutation, del(11q) or a progression-free interval of <36 months after initial chemoimmunotherapy. Patients included had a median age of 63.2, 80% had unmutated IGVH, and 10% had del (17p). The ORR was 95%, the PFS of 78% with a median follow-up of 18.8 months (Burger et al. 2014). The utility of adding Rituximab to Ibrutinib has been called into question given that the reported PFS is very close to what has been reported with use of single-agent Ibrutinib (Byrd et al. 2013). Moreover, other groups have reported decreased antibody dependent cell-mediated cytotoxicity (ADCC) of Rituximab in vivo (Kohrt et al. 2014) as well as downregulation of CD20 in CLL B-cells following Ibrutinib treatment (Pavlasova et al. 2016). Ongoing studies like NCT02007044 randomizing R/R CLL patients to either Ibrutinib treatment alone or combined Ibrutinib/Rituximab treatment should help to clarify this question. Ibrutinib has been reported to affect ADCC of Obinutuzumab less than that of Rituximab (Duong et al. 2015). This has led to the development of combination strategies of both substances. Jaglowski et al. (2015) have reported on a study addressing this question: R/R CLL/SLL patients were randomized to one of the three treatment groups—group 1: Ibrutinib lead-in followed by Obinutuzumab ($n = 27$), group 2: concurrent start ($n = 20$) or group 3: Obinutuzumab lead-in followed by Ibrutinib ($n = 24$). Forty-four percentage of patients had del(17p), and 31% had del(11q). ORR was reported to be 100, 79 and 71% in groups 1, 2 and 3, respectively. Estimated 12-month PFS was reported to be 89, 85 and 75%, respectively.

Other groups have sought to combine Ibrutinib with chemoimmunotherapy. The HELIOS trial reported on 578 R/R CLL/SLL patients without del(17p) or prior allogeneic stem cell transplantation treated with either Bendamustine and Rituximab (BR) and placebo or BR and Ibrutinib (Chanan-Khan et al. 2016). The median age of patients was 63 in the placebo group and 64 in the Ibrutinib group with a median of 2 prior therapies in both groups, and 80% of patients had unmutated IGVH. At a median follow-up of 17 month, Ibrutinib improved PFS compared to placebo (median not reached vs. 13.3 months). Median OS was not reached in either group. However, after adjusting for patients that crossed over from the placebo to the Ibrutinib arm, OS was significantly increased in the Ibrutinib group (HR = 0.577, $p = 0.033$). Based on this data, the benefit of combining Ibrutinib with classical immunochemotherapy has been questioned as the 24-month PFS in the Ibrutinib group was 72% in this trial—very close to 30-month PFS of 69% in long-term follow-up after single-agent Ibrutinib treatment (Byrd et al. 2015). Critics argue that while addition of BR to Ibrutinib does seem to increase outcomes, similar results may be achieved with less potential toxicity by single-agent Ibrutinib.

4.2 Ibrutinib as First-Line Treatment in CLL

The initial phase I/IIb trial by Byrd et al. (2015) included a cohort of 31 previously untreated CLL/SLL patient ≥ 65 years of age. In this cohort, an ORR of 84% and a 30-month PFS of 96% were achieved. Based on this successful early-phase data, the RESONATE-2 trial to analyse efficacy of first-line Ibrutinib treatment in treatment-naïve CLL/SLL patients ≥ 65 years of age was developed

(Burger et al. 2015). Two hundred and sixty-nine patients were randomized to either single-agent Ibrutinib until disease progression or unacceptable adverse events or bi-weekly Chlorambucil up to 12 months. The median age of patients was 73. Patients with del(17p) were ineligible, 45% of patients had unmutated IGVH, and 20% had del(11q). With a median follow-up of 18.4 months, the ORR was 86% in the Ibrutinib cohort and 35% in the Chlorambucil cohort. Moreover, Ibrutinib significantly increased 18-month PFS from just 52% in the Chlorambucil cohort to 90% in the Ibrutinib cohort. Long-term follow-up data was presented at the ASH meeting in 2016 (Barr et al. 2016): with a median follow-up of 28.6 months, 24-month PFS was 89% in the Ibrutinib group versus only 34% in the Chlorambucil group, while 24-month OS was 95% versus 84%, respectively. The findings of the RESONATE-2 study have been called into question due to the choice of Chlorambucil in the comparative arm. Critics believe that a choice of Chlorambucil/Obinutuzumab would have been more informative given the improved outcomes over Chlorambucil only in the CLL11 study (Goede et al. 2014). Furthermore, many patients included in the RESONATE-2 trial may have been eligible for chemoimmunotherapy with BR. Single agent Ibrutinib treatment, Ibrutinib-Rituximab and BR are currently compared in the ALLIANCE trial (NCT01886872) with pending results.

Several studies are currently underway to compare combinations of Ibrutinib and monoclonal antibodies to standard Fludarabine, Cyclophosphamide and Rituximab (FCR) treatment in younger patients with no reported results yet (NCT02048813, EudraCT 2013-001944-76).

Last but not least, preliminary data has been reported on a phase II study sponsored by the Dana–Faber Cancer Institute looking at the efficacy of Ibrutinib plus FCR in younger adults as frontline treatment in CLL (Davids et al. 2016). Of 35 enrolled patients, 27% had del(11q), 12% had del(17p) and 65% had unmutated IGVH. In this patient cohort, an ORR of 100% with 47% CR or CRi was achieved. The rate of CR with MRD bone marrow was 43% compared to only 20% in historic studies of FCR (Böttcher et al. 2012). With a median follow-up of 12.1 months, all patients were still alive at the date of presentation.

4.3   Ibrutinib in CLL Patients with del(17p) or TP53 Mutation

Del(17p) and/or TP53 mutations are well established to cause poor sensitivity to classical immunochemotherapy, poor outcomes and shorter survival (Döhner et al. 2000). A single arm phase II study from the National Institute of Health, Bethesda, Maryland, USA, hence tried to address the question of Ibrutinib efficacy in this patient subset specifically (Farooqui et al. 2015a, b and c). Fifty-one CLL patients with del(17p) or TP53 mutation, 35 of whom were treatment naïve, were treated with single-agent Ibrutinib. The median follow-up was 2 years. An ORR of 97% was achieved in the treatment-naïve cohort and 80% in the R/R CLL cohort. The estimated 24-month PFS was 82%. An update on the extend 36 months follow-up found no difference in ORR compared to a cohort of patients without del(17p) and

TP53 mutation ($n = 35$) (Farooqui et al. 2015a, b and c). Support for the notion of high Ibrutinib efficacy even in the presence of del(17p)/TP53 mutations also comes from the initial phase I/IIb trial by Byrd et al. (2015). The group reported a ORR of 79% in the cohort of R/R CLL patients with del(17p) and median PFS of 28 month, a stark improvement over historic data on del(17p) CLL (Hallek et al. 2010; Hillmen et al. 2007; Fischer et al. 2016). In the RESONATE trial, the presence or absence of del(17p) did not affect the outcome in Ibrutinib-treated patients (Byrd et al. 2014).

In addition to these findings, O'Brien et al. (2016a, b) reported outcomes of the phase II RESONATE-17 trial in 2016. One hundred and forty-four patients with del (17p) R/R CLL were treated using single-agent Ibrutinib. Sixteen percentage of patients had del(11q) in addition, 92% had TP53 mutation, and the median number of prior therapies was 2. With a median follow-up of 27.6 month, the estimated PFS was 63%. In conclusion, these data clearly demonstrate high efficacy of Ibrutinib in this patient cohort compared to historical trials in any line of treatment.

4.4 Ibrutinib in Waldenstrom Macroglobulinemia

A phase II trial analysed efficacy of single-agent Ibrutinib in 63 patients with R/R WM (Treon et al. 2015). The median age of patients was 63, the median number of prior therapies 2 and the median IgM level 3520 mg/dl. An ORR of 91% was achieved with 73% of responding subjects reaching a major response (CR or IgM reduction of $\geq 50\%$). The median PFS was not reached, and the estimated 24-month PFS was 69%. ORR was dependent on MYD88 and CXCR4 mutation status with an ORR of 100% in MYD88^{L265P} and wild-type CXCR4 cases, 85.7% among MYD88^{L265P} and CXCR4^{WHIM} cases and 71.4% in patients with both wild-type MYD88 and CXCR4. Based on this trial, Ibrutinib was approved for treatment of R/R WM patients.

In addition, there are ongoing studies to evaluate Ibrutinib in combination treatments: the iNNOVATE study is a phase III trial randomizing R/R WM patients to Ibrutinib–Rituximab or placebo–Rituximab (Dimopoulos et al. 2015)—results are pending, but preliminary data on a third arm including Rituximab-refractory WM patients treated with single-agent Ibrutinib was presented at the 2015 ASH meeting showing a very promising ORR of 88% (CR 64%) in 42 patients. However, the follow-up was short with only 8 months.

A study trying to establish efficacy as a frontline treatment is currently ongoing (NCT02604511).

4.5 Ibrutinib in Mantle Cell Lymphoma

A phase II registration study published in 2013 evaluated 111 R/R MCL patients treated with 560 mg Ibrutinib once daily as a single agent (Wang et al. 2013). The median age of patients was 68, the median number of prior therapies was 3, and

90% of patients had intermediate or high-risk MCL international prognostic index (MIPI) scores. An ORR of 68% (CR 21%) was achieved. After a median follow-up of 15.3 months, an estimated median PFS of 13.9 months was reached. Updated results after a median follow-up of 26.7 months showed durable response with a median PFS of 13 months (Wang et al. 2015). Based on this study, Ibrutinib was approved for the treatment of R/R MCL.

In addition, a phase III randomized study was conducted comparing single-agent Ibrutinib to single-agent Temsirolimus in 280 R/R MCL patients (Dreyling et al. 2016). The median age of enrolled patients was 68, the median number of prior therapies was 2, and 69% of patients had intermediate or high-risk MIPI scores. With a median follow-up of 20 months, a median PFS of 14.6 months in the Ibrutinib arm compared to 6.2 months in the Temsirolimus arm was reached. Moreover, Ibrutinib treatment was associated with a trend towards improved OS.

Combining Ibrutinib and Rituximab has also been evaluated for R/R MCL. In a trial by Wang et al. (2016a, b), 50 patients received 560 mg Ibrutinib once daily in 28-day cycles with 375 mg/m^2 Rituximab once weekly for 4 weeks during cycle 1, on the first day of cycles 3–8 and then every other cycle for the next 2 years. The median age of patients was 67 and the median number of prior therapies 3. After a median follow-up of 15.6 months, an ORR of 88% (44% CR) and a 15-month PFS of 69% were reached. The combination of Ibrutinib and Rituximab was also analysed as frontline treatment in young MCL patients in a phase II trial (Wang et al. 2016a, b): fifty patients were treated with Rituximab/Ibrutinib for up to 12 months until best response (phase I) followed by a shortened number of cycles of Rituximab, cyclophosphamide, vincristine, doxorubicin and dexamethasone (hyper-CVAD). The best ORR was 100% after phase I alone, and the overall CR rate was 73%. Responses are expected to deepen as the majority of PR patients had not complete phase I at the time of report.

Several trials to evaluate the combination of Ibrutinib and chemoimmunotherapy in MCL are currently in progress. An early-phase study evaluated the combination of BR and Ibrutinib in 17 R/R MCL patients yielding a promising 94% ORR (Maddocks et al. 2015a, b). A phase III randomized trial (SHINE) evaluating first-line BR with and without Ibrutinib is currently ongoing and results pending (NCT01776840). Preliminary results on the phase II PHILEMON trial have been reported in 2016: Ibrutinib/Lenalidomide was analysed in 50 R/R MCL patients with an ORR of 88% (CR 64%) (Jerkeman et al. 2016).

4.6 Ibrutinib in Marginal Zone Lymphoma

An open-label phase II study was conducted to evaluate the efficacy of Ibrutinib in R/R MZL with at least one prior anti-CD20-containing line of therapy (Noy et al. 2017). Sixty-three patients with a median age of 66 (30–92) were enrolled. The median number of prior therapies was 2. With a median follow-up of 19.4 months, an ORR of 48% and a median progression-free survival of 14.2 months were reached. Based on this study, Ibrutinib was licensed for use in R/R MZL with at least on prior anti-CD20-containing line of therapy. A phase III clinical trial (SELENE study) evaluating Ibrutinib versus placebo in addition to either BR or R-CHOP immunochemotherapy is currently ongoing with pending results (NCT01974440).

4.7 Ibrutinib in Activated B-cell (ABC) Subtype Diffuse Large B-cell Lymphoma (DLBCL)

ABC subtype has persistently increased BCR signalling and in some cases activating mutations of the BCR (Young et al. 2015). It has hence been speculated that ABC subtype may be amenable to Ibrutinib treatment. An early-phase trial evaluated Ibrutinib in 80 patients with R/R DLBCL showing better OR in the ABC subtype compared to GCB subtype patients (37% vs. 5%) (Wilson et al. 2015). In addition, a phase Ib study by Younes et al. (2014) evaluated the role of Ibrutinib in combination with R-CHOP for CD20-positive B-cell non-Hodgkin lymphoma. Thirty-three patients were enrolled. Of 18 patients who had DLBCL and received the recommended dose all achieved an objective response with 15 CRs (83%) and 3 PRs (17%). Several clinical trials to evaluate the role of Ibrutinib in the treatment of DLBCL are currently ongoing: A phase III trial assesses the combination of Ibrutinib with Rituximab, cyclophosphamide, doxorubicin, vincristine and prednisone (R-CHOP) in the frontline treatment of non-GCB DLBCL patients (NCT01855750), a phase II trial from Australia evaluates Ibrutinib in combination with dose-reduced CHOP in DLBCL patients ≥ 75 years of age (ALLG NHL29), and a phase II study trial of R/R non-GCB DLBCL patients who are ineligible to autologous stem cell transplantation evaluates single-agent Ibrutinib for this patient cohort (NCT02692248).

4.8 Ibrutinib in Multiple Myeloma

A phase II trial currently evaluates efficacy of Ibrutinib in a dose of 560 or 840 mg once daily alone or in combination with 40 mg dexamethasone once weekly in MM (Vij et al. 2014). The authors reported on preliminary results of 69 patients with a median age of 64, 20% of which had either del(17p) or TP53 mutation. The median number of prior therapies was 4. Sixty-two percentage of patients were refractory to their last line of therapy, and 44% were refractory to both an immunomodulatory agent and a proteasome inhibitory. Outcomes were rather modest, however, with 1 PR, 4 MRs and 5 sustained SDs as best outcome in the Ibrutinib 840 mg + dexamethasone cohort.

In addition, Ibrutinib is currently being evaluated in combination with Carfilzomib in an ongoing Phase1/2b study (NCT01962792).

4.9   Ibrutinib in Solid Malignancies

Reports of Ibrutinib's ability to modulate functions of T-cells and other components of the tumour microenvironment have generated interest in exploring Ibrutinib for the use in solid malignancies as well. Most available data on this subject is still in the preclinical stage.

A number of clinical trials have been initiated to elucidated Ibrutinib's efficacy in gastroesophageal cancer (NCT02884453), non-small cell lung cancer (NCT02321 540, NCT02950038 and NCT02403271), pancreatic adenocarcinoma (NCT02562 898, NCT02436668), renal cell carcinoma (NCT02899078), melanoma (NCT025 81930, NCT03021460) and prostate cancer (NCT02643667). Results of all these trials are currently pending.

4.10   Ibrutinib in Primary Central Nervous System Lymphoma

The high efficacy of Ibrutinib in other forms of lymphoma has sparked interest in the substance regarding PCNSL. An early-phase study investigating single-agent Ibrutinib in R/R PCNSL enrolled 13 patients with a median age of 69. The median number of treatments was 2, and eight patients had failed prior methotrexate-based salvage therapy. Of 13, 10 patients (77%) showed a clinical response (5 CR, 5 PR). The median PFS was 4.6 months, and the median overall survival was 15 months (Grommes et al. 2017).

5   Toxicity

Data from CLL and MCL trials suggests that in general Ibrutinib is well tolerated. This is attributed to the restricted expression of BTK on the B-cell lineage. Adverse events include nausea, fatigue, myalgias and muscle spasms, as well as pyrexia, skin rashes and headaches. The majority of these untoward effects are grade 1 or 2 adverse events, and they are usually self-limiting. In a 3-year follow-up study of CLL and SLL patients receiving Ibrutinib, adverse events led to discontinuation of treatment in 13% of the patients, while 17% of patients discontinued Ibrutinib treatment due to disease progression (Byrd et al. 2015).

Hypertension following Ibrutinib therapy is a common adverse event. The rate of treatment emergent hypertension has been described to be up to 23% in the long-term follow-up of initial studies (Burger et al. 2015; Byrd et al. 2015). A retrospective analysis of 153 CLL patients receiving single-agent Ibrutinib treatment found that the rate of patients on two or more anti-hypertension medications increased from 20% pre-Ibrutinib to 30% during Ibrutinib treatment. Median pre-Ibrutinib blood pressure was 127/70 mmHg. At 1, 3, 6, 9, 12 months, median blood pressures were 137/73, 141/75, 143/76, 140/75, 142/77, respectively (7 months to peak blood pressure) (Gashonia et al. 2017). The frequency of $\geq$

grade 3 arterial hypertension requiring medical intervention ranges from 2 to 23% (Byrd et al. 2015; Noy et al. 2017). While treatment-associated hypertension is generally amenable to treatment and does not usually require dose reduction or discontinuation of treatment, it is an important factor to manage, particularly as it is an important risk factor for atrial fibrillation and bleeding events—both of which are common and potential severe adverse events during Ibrutinib therapy.

Atrial arrhythmias, namely atrial fibrillation (AF), constitute one of the most serious adverse events of Ibrutinib treatment. Major complications of AF include stroke and other systemic thromboembolic events, as well as increased mortality. Although definite evidence regarding the aetiology of AF is lacking, it is believed that it relates to the phosphoinositide 3-kinase (PI3K)-Akt signalling pathway which mediates cardiac protection (McMullen et al. 2007). Therapeutic doses of the drug were associated with reduced PI3K expression and Akt activation in ventricular myocytes from rats (McMullen et al. 2014). The incidence of AF in clinical trials ranges from 6 to 16%, which suggests Ibrutinib may possibly increase the risk of atrial arrhythmias (Byrd et al. 2014; Burger et al. 2015; Farooqui et al. 2015a, b and c; Chanan-Khan et al. 2016; Dreyling et al. 2016; Thompson et al. 2016). This was most apparent in the RESONATE trial with 6% of Ibrutinib-treated patients developing AF as opposed to only 1% of patients in the Ofatumumab arm (Brown et al. 2014). In a meta-analysis, the pooled rate of atrial fibrillation was 3.3 (95% CI: 2.5, 4.1) per 100 person-years in Ibrutinib-treated patients, whereas the pooled rate was 0.84 (95% CI: 0.3 2, 1.6) per 100 person-years in non-Ibrutinib-treated patients (Leong et al. 2016). It should be noted, however, that the advanced age of most CLL patients constitutes an important risk factor for cardiac rhythm disorders in itself. Moreover, emerging data suggests that CLL/SLL patients are at an increased risk of developing AF at baseline (Benjamin et al. 1998; Barrientos et al. 2015). Further evidence is therefore required in order to delineate the association between Ibrutinib therapy and AF occurrence, as well as data regarding the incidence of the different subtypes of AF. Anti-arrhythmic drugs are useful in the management of AF, although more targeted treatment algorithms are required, due to the emergence of drug–drug interactions complicating the use of anti-arrhythmic agents in TKI-treated patients (Vrontikis et al. 2016; Asnani et al. 2017).

Bleeding is a common adverse event of Ibrutinib therapy and is observed in up to 50% of Ibrutinib-treated patients. The majority of these events are either grade 1 or 2 and usually require no treatment. Long-term follow-up studies of MCL and CLL patients who receive the drug report that 5% of the patients experience grade 3 or higher bleeding—mainly intracranial or gastrointestinal (Advani et al. 2013; Byrd et al. 2013; Asnani et al. 2017). In addition, in a phase 1b/2 clinical trial examining the safety and activity of Ibrutinib versus Ofatumumab in CLL patients, Jaglowski et al. (2015) found that bleeding of any grade was more common in patients in the Ibrutinib arm (44% vs. 12%). BTK is present on platelets and is known to play a role in GPVI- and GP1b-mediated platelet aggregation and adhesion on von Willebrand factor. BTK inhibition also results in qualitative platelet dysfunction, since it is associated with giant platelets and increased megakaryocytes in peripheral blood. Nevertheless, it is still questionable whether

BTK inhibition results in bleeding, since X-linked agammaglobulinemia patients do not have an increased risk of bleeding, despite the absence of functional BTK (Oda et al. 2000). Bleeding is mainly attributed to the drug's off-target effects, including TEC kinase inhibition, while thrombocytopenia also plays a significant role. Judicious use of anticoagulants, along with platelet transfusion following clearance of the drug can improve haemostasis (Levade et al. 2014; Kamel et al. 2015).

Haemototoxicity and cytopenias may also present as neutropenia, thrombocytopenia or anaemia. In a phase I study, 15% of patients experienced grade 3 or 4 neutropenia, which was accompanied by fever in a quarter of them. Anaemia was observed in 6% of the patients, which was treated with erythropoietin (EPO)-stimulating agents. Ibrutinib induced cytopenias are not usually associated with treatment discontinuation, mainly because they occur early during the treatment course and are short-lasting (Advani et al. 2013; Burger et al. 2015). Importantly, Ibrutinib is not associated with significant myelosuppression, and in some cases, it has been shown to promote marrow restoration. This constitutes a significant finding for patients with marrow-related cytopenias or for patients previously treated with chemotherapy.

Diarrhoea comprises one of the most common adverse events associated with Ibrutinib. Approximately 60% of the patients experience at least 1 episode of diarrhoea (Byrd et al. 2015). The majority of diarrhoea episodes across studies occurred within the first 4 weeks of treatment, and the majority were mild and self-limiting. Severe diarrhoea is rare and can be effectively treated using anti-motility agents. Dose reduction and treatment discontinuation are generally uncommon.

Infection is another common adverse event during Ibrutinib treatment. A recent retrospective analysis on 200 patients receiving Ibrutinib for various haematological malignancies found that 52% developed infection with pneumonia (30%) and upper airway infection (26%) being the leading courses (Barbosa et al. 2017). The majority of these infectious complications are self-limiting and are commonly observed early in the course of Ibrutinib treatment (Byrd et al. 2013, 2014; Burger et al. 2014; O'Brien et al. 2014; Brown et al. 2015). The frequency of pulmonary infections experienced by relapsed/refractory patients tended to be higher as opposed to treatment-naïve patients on long-term follow-up (Byrd et al. 2015). Supportive therapy with antibiotics and intravenous immunoglobulin infusions is often substantial to assist with recovery (Falchi et al. 2016). Other common infectious complications include skin infection (28%) and sinusitis (13%). Barbosa et al. (2017) found a hospitalization rate of 44%, and the median time to infection after starting Ibrutinib was 70 days. Cases of severe opportunistic infections like invasive aspergillosis (Arthurs et al. 2017) and disseminated cryptococcal infection (Okamoto et al. 2016) have recently emerged. While such events are rare, treating physicians should be aware of them and monitor patients carefully.

6 Drug Interactions

It is generally advised that Ibrutinib should be taken 30 min before or 2 h after meals. It has been proven that administration of Ibrutinib in fasted conditions yields 60% of plasma exposure (AUC_{last}) as opposed to the administration of the drug in the aforementioned time range. The drug is metabolized primarily by the cytochrome P450 enzyme CYP3A4 and to a lesser extent by CYP2D6. Increased intestinal blood flow as a result of food intake promotes increased passage of the drug from the intestine to the portal circulation. This reduces the first-pass effect induced by intestinal CYP3A4. Nevertheless, due to the drug's favourable safety profile, it is licensed in the USA and EU for use regardless of food intake (de Jong et al. 2015a, b).

Ibrutinib, being a CYP3A4/5 substrate, should not be administered with strong or moderate CYP3A inducers or inhibitors as these can decrease or increase drug exposure, respectively (Scheers et al. 2015; de Zwart et al. 2016). Concomitant treatment with Ketoconazole, a drug that strongly inhibits CYP3A, increased Cmax by 29-fold while AUC0-last by 24-fold (de Jong et al. 2015a, b). Although more data is required in order to delineate the effect of CYP3A inhibitors on toxicity, it is widely agreed that co-administration of strong inhibitors including Ketoconazole, Nelfinavir, Indinavir, Clarithromycin, Telithromycin, Cobicistat and Itraconazole or moderate inhibitors including Crizotinib, Ciprofloxacin, Erythromycin, Diltiazem, Ritonavir, Imatinib and Verapamil should be avoided. It is generally advised that Ibrutinib treatment should temporarily be withheld or the dose reduced in cases where administration of any of the aforementioned drugs is considered essential. Grapefruit, star fruit and Seville oranges should also be avoided, since they contain moderate CYP3A4 inhibitors. Mild CYP3A inhibitors, such as Azithromycin have been found to increase Ibrutinib exposure by a factor of less than twofold. No treatment cessation or dose adjustments are required in cases of co-administration of mild inhibitors, although patients should still be closely monitored for toxicity (de Zwart et al. 2016). Inducers of CYP3A4 can possibly reduce plasma concentrations of Ibrutinib if used concomitantly with the drug. Strong inducers, such as St. John's-wort, Carbamazepine and Phenytoin, should be avoided, since they can decrease the efficacy of Ibrutinib therapy (McNally et al. 2015). For an extensive list of drug interactions involving cytochrome P450 drug interactors, refer to http://medicine.iupui.edu/clinpharm/ddis/.

In vitro data suggests that Ibrutinib can inhibit OCT2, P-glycoprotein (P-gp) and breast cancer resistance protein (BCRP). It is possible that gastrointestinal BCRP and P-gp are prone to inhibition in patients receiving Ibrutinib. The drug could also result in systemic inhibition of BCRP, hence increasing the plasma exposure of drugs undergoing BCRP-mediated hepatic efflux, including Pitavastatin and Rosuvastatin, although in vivo proof of this is still required. It is generally advised that if P-gp or BCRP substrates need to be co-administered with Ibrutinib, they should be staggered by >6 h (Shao et al. 2014).

Additionally, agents that affect stomach pH, including proton pump inhibitors, could possibly decrease Ibrutinib exposure; the solubility of the drug is pH dependent and is significantly reduced as the pH increases. However, such drug interactions require further in vivo data (de Jong et al. 2016).

7 Biomarkers

Ibrutinib has proven to be one of the most effective agents in the treatment of numerous haematological malignancies, especially in the treatment of MCL and CLL. However, cases of primary and secondary resistance have emerged. It has generally been demonstrated that Ibrutinib resistance and relapse in haematological malignancies resulted in poor prognosis. Although a large proportion of patients do respond to Ibrutinib, emerging cases of resistance have underlined the need for clinical biomarkers to predict sensitivity or resistance to the drug.

7.1 Chronic Lymphocytic Leukaemia

Disease progression during Ibrutinib therapy has been reported to be associated with a dismal prognosis. Outcomes are especially poor among CLL patients who develop Richter's transformation (RT) where a median OS of merely 3 months has been reported (Jain et al. 2015; Maddocks et al. 2015a, b). Also, Ibrutinib failure due to RT tended to occur more quickly than due to progressive CLL (Maddocks et al. 2015a, b). Whether Ibrutinib treatment truly increases the risk of RT or merely permits high-risk patients to live long enough to develop RT is highly controversial.

Acquired resistance to Ibrutinib therapy has been attributed to a number of mutations. Woyach et al. (2014a, b) identified acquired cysteine to serine mutations at the Ibrutinib binding site at C481. Functional characterization of C481 mutations showed a significant reduction in the binding affinity of Ibrutinib for BTK, while it was also observed that there was a shift from irreversible BTK inhibition to reversible inhibition (Burger et al. 2016). Several PLCγ2 mutations have been identified, and these are assumed to be gain-of-function. PLCγ2 lies immediately downstream of the kinase, and hence mutant forms bypass the inactive BTK enabling distal BCR signalling to take place (Woyach et al. 2014a, b; Burger et al. 2016). Burger et al. (2016) have also reported recurrent 8p deletion resulting in haploinsufficiency of TRAIL-R and hence potentially resistance to Ibrutinib-induced apoptosis.

It is questionable whether these mutations leading to secondary Ibrutinib resistance are truly acquired during Ibrutinib therapy or are rather present at baseline already. Using droplet microfluidic technology, Burger et al. (2016) were able to show the presence of Ibrutinib-resistant subclones even before treatment initiation suggesting that Ibrutinib-resistant clones may be present at baseline. Mutated subclones have been detected in CLL patients up to 15 months before manifestation of clinical progression which could comprise a useful indicative marker of Ibrutinib resistance (Ahn et al. 2017).

Although there are no definitive upfront biomarkers to predict Ibrutinib sensitivity, Byrd et al. (2013) reported that patients with unmutated *IGHV* are more sensitive to Ibrutinib inhibition, while other studies involving Ibrutinib-containing therapies have similar findings. These findings have been supported further by a recent study by Guo et al. (2016a, b).

7.2 Mantle Cell Lymphoma

Although Ibrutinib has proven very effective for the treatment of R/R MCL, cases of both primary and secondary resistances have emerged and the mechanisms for these appear to be unrelated. Primary resistance is surprisingly not associated with BTK mutations, and BTK activity is not related to clinical response in MCL. Instead, the degree of ERK and/or AKT inhibition correlated with the extent of cell death, thus predicting Ibrutinib sensitivity. This suggests that resistance to the drug may not be entirely due to ineffective BTK inhibition, but could possibly involve PIK3-AKT activation sustaining distal BCR signalling (Chiron et al. 2014; Ma et al. 2014). Additionally, genomic studies have identified somatic mutations in TRAF2 and TRAF3, which negatively regulate the alternative NF-κB pathway. Activation of the alternative pathway possibly renders BTK inhibition an ineffective treatment for patients possessing these mutations (Rahal et al. 2014). A study on MCL cell lines by Mohgarty et al. (2016) identified several mutation of cell cycle regulatory protein D1 (CCND1) leading to increased protein stability as a primary resistance mechanism to Ibrutinib.

Secondary resistance in MCL has also been shown to involve BTK^{C481S} mutations similar to findings in CLL (Chiron et al. 2014). New data presented at the American Society of Haematology 58th Annual Meeting suggests that upregulation of genes coding for fatty acid synthase (FASN), septin 3 (SEPT3), isocitrate dehydrogenase subunit alpha (IDH3A) and phosphatidylinositol-3,4,5-trisphosphate 5-phosphatase 1 (INPP5) could possibly correlate to Ibrutinib resistance in R/R MCL (Guo et al. 2016a, b).

7.3 Waldenstrom Macroglobulinemia

It has been demonstrated that mutations in CXCR4 are associated with primary resistance to Ibrutinib. CXCR4 comprises a transmembrane chemokine receptor which undergoes internalization upon binding to CXCL12, resulting in AKT and ERK activation. Mutations frequently affect the C-terminal region of the receptor, and they are usually germline nonsense or frameshift mutations. CXCR4$^{WHIM-like}$ prevents receptor internalization and can also prolong G protein signalling, hence sustained ERK and AKT activity and achieving increased cell survival. Such mutations are therefore predictive of reduced Ibrutinib sensitivity (Cao et al. 2015).

Limited data is available on mutations leading to acquired Ibrutinib resistance in WM. Xu et al. (2017) reported C481 BTK mutations and PLCγ2 mutations similar to findings in CLL as well as CARD11 mutations.

7.4 DLBCL

Clinical data on Ibrutinib treatment of DLBCL has yet to mature and is not yet an established treatment modality—similarly no established biomarkers exist. Limited early-phase data suggests that within ABC subtype DLBCL response depends on mutational status of MYD88 and CD79A/B: in a trial of 80 DLBCL patients by Wilson et al. (2015), Ibrutinib-resistant ABC subtype DLBCL patients carried mutant MYD88 and WT CD79A/B, whereas all other genotypic combinations (CD79A/BWT + MYD88WT, CD79A/B mutant + MYD88WT and CD79A/B mutant + MYD88 mutant) were responsive to Ibrutinib therapy.

Preclinical data suggests that activity of Ibrutinib in ABC subtype DLBCL may be limited to cases with wild-type CARD11. However, not clinical data is available on the subject (Davis et al. 2010; Yang et al. 2012).

Takahashi et al. (2015) have demonstrated increased sensitivity of DLBCL cells secreting high levels of CCL3 and CLL4 to BCR pathway inhibition in vitro. Serum concentrations of these markers have hence been proposed as prognostic biomarker for BCR inhibition—more clinical data is necessary to substantiate this suggestion.

8 Summary and Perspective

Ibrutinib is a covalent and irreversible inhibitor of BTK that is characterized by high selectivity and potency. The substance has revolutionized treatment of B-cell malignancy, especially CLL and MCL, and continues to shape the way we think about and advance treatment of these conditions.

Ibrutinib has opened new options for treatment of those patients that have relapsed or have been refractory to more classical modes of treatment. Moreover, Ibrutinib has been shown to be effective in patients that have been known to have little sensitivity to classical immunochemotherapy as those with del(17p)/TP53 mutation in CLL. Having a favourable risk profile, the substance is, unlike conventional immunochemotherapy, also suitable for the less physical fit patients (i.e. elderly or having significant comorbidities). Particularly, the absence of significant myelosuppression compared to conventional cytostatics makes it a particularly useful tool in this subset of patients.

In CLL, Ibrutinib causes rapid redistribution of tissue-resident CLL cells into the bloodstream leading to resolution of lymphadenopathy and a temporary increase in lymphocytosis which, however, must not be confused with disease progression.

Beyond its direct effects on survival and apoptosis of malignant B-cells, the substance also seems to have immunomodulatory properties. There is increasing evidence that the substance has a potential to modulate the tumour microenvironment and overcome immunosuppressive features of tumour-associated lymphocytes and myeloid cells—this has sparked interest in therapeutic potential beyond lymphoid malignancy, and several studies addressing the efficacy of Ibrutinib in solid malignancy such as pancreatic adenocarcinoma are now underway.

Its immunomodulatory properties make Ibrutinib an interesting candidate for combination strategies involving immunotherapeutic treatment strategies which may have synergistic properties. First evidence pointing towards improved efficacy of combinations with immune checkpoint blockade (Sagiv-Barfi et al. 2015) and CAR T-cell therapy (Gill et al. 2017) has been described, and early clinical trials investigating the combination of anti-PD-L1 immune checkpoint blockade and Ibrutinib (NCT02733042, NCT02846623) have been initiated.

References

Advani RH, Buggy JJ, Sharman JP, Smith SM, Boyd TE, Grant B, Kolibaba KS, Furman RR, Rodriguez S, Chang BY (2013) Bruton tyrosine kinase inhibitor ibrutinib (PCI-32765) has significant activity in patients with relapsed/refractory B-cell malignancies. J Clin Oncol 31

Ahn IE, Underbayev C, Albitar A, Herman SEM, Tian X, Maric I, Arthur DC, Wake L, Pittaluga S, Yuan CM, Stetler-Stevenson M, Soto S, Valdez J, Nierman P, Lotter J, Xi L, Raffeld M, Farooqui M, Albitar M, Wiestner A (2017) Clonal evolution leading to ibrutinib resistance in chronic lymphocytic leukemia. Blood 129(11):1469–1479

Arthurs B, Wunderle K, Hsu M, Kim S (2017) Invasive aspergillosis related to ibrutinib therapy for chronic lymphocytic leukemia. Respir Med Case Rep 21:27–29

Asnani A, Manning A, Mansour M, Ruskin J, Hochberg EP, Ptaszek LM (2017) Management of atrial fibrillation in patients taking targeted cancer therapies. Cardio-Oncology 3(1):2

Barbosa CC, DeAngelis LM, Grommes C (2017) Ibrutinib associated infections: a retrospective study. J Clin Oncol 35(15_suppl):e19020–e19020

Barr P, Robak T, Owen CJ, Tedeschi A, Bairey O, Bartlett NL, Burger J, Hillmen P, Coutre S, Devereux S, Grosicki S, McCarthy H, Li J, Simpson D, Offner F, Moreno C, Zhou C, Styles L, James DF, Kipps TJ, Ghia P (2016) Updated efficacy and safety from the phase 3 resonate-2 study: ibrutinib as first-line treatment option in patients 65 years and older with chronic lymphocytic leukemia/small lymphocytic leukemia. Blood 128(22):234

Barrientos JC, Meyer N, Song X, Rai KR (2015) Characterization of atrial fibrillation and bleeding risk factors in patients with chronic lymphocytic leukemia (cll): a population-based retrospective cohort study of administrative medical claims data in the United States (US). Blood 126(23):3301

Benjamin EJ, Wolf PA, D'Agostino RB, Silbershatz H, Kannel WB, Levy D (1998) Impact of atrial fibrillation on the risk of death: the Framingham Heart Study. Circulation 98(10):946–952

Böttcher S, Ritgen M, Fischer K, Stilgenbauer S, Busch RM, Fingerle-Rowson G, Fink AM, Bühler A, Zenz T, Wenger MK, Mendila M, Wendtner C-M, Eichhorst BF, Döhner H, Hallek MJ, Kneba M (2012) Minimal residual disease quantification is an independent predictor of progression-free and overall survival in chronic lymphocytic leukemia: a multivariate analysis from the randomized GCLLSG CLL8 trial. J Clin Oncol 30(9):980–988

Broides A, Yang W, Conley ME (2006) Genotype/phenotype correlations in X-linked agammaglobulinemia. Clin Immunol 118(2–3):195–200

Brown JR, Hillmen P, O'Brien S, Barrientos JC, Reddy N, Coutre S, Tam C, Mulligan S, Jaeger U, Barr PM, Furman RR, Kipps TJ, Cymbalista F, Thornton P, Caligaris-Cappio F, Delgado J, Montillo M, DeVos S, Moreno C, Pagel J, Burger JA, Chung D, Lin J, Gau L, Chang B, McGreivy J, James DF, Byrd JC (2014) Updated efficacy including genetic and clinical subgroup analysis and overall safety in the phase 3 resonate trial of ibrutinib versus ofatumumab in previously treated chronic lymphocytic leukemia/small lymphocytic lymphoma. Blood 124(21):3331

Brown JR, Barrientos JC, Barr PM, Flinn IW, Burger JA, Tran A, Clow F, James DF, Graef T, Friedberg JW, Rai K, O'Brien S (2015) The Bruton tyrosine kinase inhibitor ibrutinib with chemoimmunotherapy in patients with chronic lymphocytic leukemia. Blood 125(19):2915–2922

Bruton OC (1952) Agammaglobulinemia. Pediatrics 9(6):722–728

Burger JA, Keating MJ, Wierda WG, Hartmann E, Hoellenriegel J, Rosin NY, de Weerdt I, Jeyakumar G, Ferrajoli A, Cardenas-Turanzas M, Lerner S, Jorgensen JL, Nogueras-González GM, Zacharian G, Huang X, Kantarjian H, Garg N, Rosenwald A, O'Brien S (2014) Safety and activity of ibrutinib plus rituximab for patients with high-risk chronic lymphocytic leukaemia: a single-arm, phase 2 study. Lancet Oncol 15(10):1090–1099

Burger JA, Tedeschi A, Barr PM, Robak T, Owen C, Ghia P, Bairey O, Hillmen P, Bartlett NL, Li J, Simpson D, Grosicki S, Devereux S, McCarthy H, Coutre S, Quach H, Gaidano G, Maslyak Z, Stevens DA, Janssens A, Offner F, Mayer J, O'Dwyer M, Hellmann A, Schuh A, Siddiqi T, Polliack A, Tam CS, Suri D, Cheng M, Clow F, Styles L, James DF, Kipps TJ (2015) Ibrutinib as initial therapy for patients with chronic lymphocytic leukemia. N Engl J Med 373(25):2425–2437

Burger JA, Landau DA, Taylor-Weiner A, Bozic I, Zhang H, Sarosiek K, Wang L, Stewart C, Fan J, Hoellenriegel J, Sivina M, Dubuc AM, Fraser C, Han Y, Li S, Livak KJ, Zou L, Wan Y, Konoplev S, Sougnez C, Brown JR, Abruzzo LV, Carter SL, Keating MJ, Davids MS, Wierda WG, Cibulskis K, Zenz T, Werner L, Cin PD, Kharchencko P, Neuberg D, Kantarjian H, Lander E, Gabriel S, O'Brien S, Letai A, Weitz DA, Nowak MA, Getz G, Wu CJ (2016) Clonal evolution in patients with chronic lymphocytic leukaemia developing resistance to BTK inhibition. Nat commun 7:11589

Burger JA, Li KW, Keating MJ, Sivina M, Amer AM, Garg N, Ferrajoli A, Huang X, Kantarjian H, Wierda WG, O'Brien S, Hellerstein MK, Turner SM, Emson CL, Chen SS, Yan XJ, Wodarz D, Chiorazzi N (2017) Leukemia cell proliferation and death in chronic lymphocytic leukemia patients on therapy with the BTK inhibitor ibrutinib. JCI Insight 2(2): e89904

Byrd JC, Furman RR, Coutre SE, Flinn IW, Burger JA, Blum KA, Grant B, Sharman JP, Coleman M, Wierda WG, Jones JA, Zhao W, Heerema NA, Johnson AJ, Sukbuntherng J, Chang BY, Clow F, Hedrick E, Buggy JJ, James DF, O'Brien S (2013) Targeting BTK with ibrutinib in relapsed chronic lymphocytic leukemia. N Engl J Med 369(1):32–42

Byrd JC, Brown JR, O'Brien S, Barrientos JC, Kay NE, Reddy NM, Coutre S, Tam CS, Mulligan SP, Jaeger U, Devereux S, Barr PM, Furman RR, Kipps TJ, Cymbalista F, Pocock C, Thornton P, Caligaris-Cappio F, Robak T, Delgado J, Schuster SJ, Montillo M, Schuh A, de Vos S, Gill D, Bloor A, Dearden C, Moreno C, Jones JJ, Chu AD, Fardis M, McGreivy J, Clow F, James DF, Hillmen P (2014) Ibrutinib versus ofatumumab in previously treated chronic lymphoid leukemia. N Engl J Med 371(3):213–223

Byrd JC, Furman RR, Coutre SE, Burger JA, Blum KA, Coleman M, Wierda WG, Jones JA, Zhao W, Heerema NA, Johnson AJ, Shaw Y, Bilotti E, Zhou C, James DF, O'Brien S (2015) Three-year follow-up of treatment-naïve and previously treated patients with CLL and SLL receiving single-agent ibrutinib. Blood 125(16):2497–2506

Cao Y, Hunter ZR, Liu X, Xu L, Yang G, Chen J, Tsakmaklis N, Kanan S, Castillo JJ, Treon SP (2015) CXCR4 WHIM-like frameshift and nonsense mutations promote ibrutinib resistance but do not supplant MYD88(L265P)-directed survival signalling in Waldenstrom macroglobulinaemia cells. Br J Haematol 168(5):701–707

Chanan-Khan A, Cramer P, Demirkan F, Fraser G, Silva RS, Grosicki S, Pristupa A, Janssens A, Mayer J, Bartlett NL, Dilhuydy M-S, Pylypenko H, Loscertales J, Avigdor A, Rule S, Villa D, Samoilova O, Panagiotidis P, Goy A, Mato A, Pavlovsky MA, Karlsson C, Mahler M, Salman M, Sun S, Phelps C, Balasubramanian S, Howes A, Hallek M (2016) Ibrutinib combined with bendamustine and rituximab compared with placebo, bendamustine, and rituximab for previously treated chronic lymphocytic leukaemia or small lymphocytic lymphoma (HELIOS): a randomised, double-blind, phase 3 study. Lancet Oncol 17(2):200–211

Chang BY, Huang MM, Francesco M, Chen J, Sokolove J, Magadala P, Robinson WH, Buggy JJ (2011) The Bruton tyrosine kinase inhibitor PCI-32765 ameliorates autoimmune arthritis by inhibition of multiple effector cells. Arthritis Res Ther 13(4):R115

Chen J, Kinoshita T, Sukbuntherng J, Chang BY, Elias L (2016a) Ibrutinib inhibits ERBB receptor tyrosine kinases and HER2-amplified breast cancer cell growth. Mol Cancer Ther 15(12):2835–2844

Chen SS, Chang BY, Chang S, Tong T, Ham S, Sherry B, Burger JA, Rai KR, Chiorazzi N (2016b) BTK inhibition results in impaired CXCR4 chemokine receptor surface expression, signaling and function in chronic lymphocytic leukemia. Leukemia 30(4):833–843

Chiorazzi N, Rai KR, Ferrarini M (2005) Chronic lymphocytic leukemia. N Engl J Med 352(8):804–815

Chiron D, Di Liberto M, Martin P, Huang X, Sharman J, Blecua P, Mathew S, Vijay P, Eng K, Ali S, Johnson A, Chang B, Ely S, Elemento O, Mason CE, Leonard JP, Chen-Kiang S (2014) Cell-cycle reprogramming for PI3K inhibition overrides a relapse-specific C481S BTK mutation revealed by longitudinal functional genomics in mantle cell lymphoma. Cancer Discov 4(9):1022–1035

Dasmahapatra G, Patel H, Dent P, Fisher RI, Friedberg J, Grant S (2013) The Bruton tyrosine kinase (BTK) inhibitor PCI-32765 synergistically increases proteasome inhibitor activity in diffuse large-B cell lymphoma (DLBCL) and mantle cell lymphoma (MCL) cells sensitive or resistant to bortezomib. Br J Haematol 161(1):43–56

Davids MS, Kim HT, Brander DM, Bsat J, Savell A, Francoeur K, Hellman J, Jacobson CA, Hochberg E, Takvorian R, Abramson JS, Fisher DC, Brown JR (2016) Initial results of a multicenter, phase II study of ibrutinib plus fcr (iFCR) as frontline therapy for younger CLL patients. Blood 128(22):3243

Davis RE, Ngo VN, Lenz G, Tolar P, Young RM, Romesser PB, Kohlhammer H, Lamy L, Zhao H, Yang Y, Xu W, Shaffer AL, Wright G, Xiao W, Powell J, Jiang JK, Thomas CJ, Rosenwald A, Ott G, Muller-Hermelink HK, Gascoyne RD, Connors JM, Johnson NA, Rimsza LM, Campo E, Jaffe ES, Wilson WH, Delabie J, Smeland EB, Fisher RI, Braziel RM, Tubbs RR, Cook JR, Weisenburger DD, Chan WC, Pierce SK, Staudt LM (2010) Chronic active B-cell-receptor signalling in diffuse large B-cell lymphoma. Nature 463(7277):88–92

de Gorter DJ, Beuling EA, Kersseboom R, Middendorp S, van Gils JM, Hendriks RW, Pals ST, Spaargaren M (2007) Bruton's tyrosine kinase and phospholipase Cgamma2 mediate chemokine-controlled B cell migration and homing. Immunity 26(1):93–104

de Jong J, Skee D, Murphy J, Sukbuntherng J, Hellemans P, Smit J, de Vries R, Jiao JJ, Snoeys J, Mannaert E (2015a) Effect of CYP3A perpetrators on ibrutinib exposure in healthy participants. Pharmacol Res Perspect 3(4):e00156

de Jong J, Sukbuntherng J, Skee D, Murphy J, O'Brien S, Byrd JC, James D, Hellemans P, Loury DJ, Jiao J, Chauhan V, Mannaert E (2015b) The effect of food on the pharmacokinetics of oral ibrutinib in healthy participants and patients with chronic lymphocytic leukemia. Cancer Chemother Pharmacol 75(5):907–916

de Jong J, Hellemans P, Jiao J, Sukbuntherng J, Ouellet D (2016) An open-label, sequential-design drug interaction study of the effects of omeprazole on the pharmacokinetics of ibrutinib in healthy adults. Blood 128(22):1588

de Rooij MFM, Kuil A, Geest CR, Eldering E, Chang BY, Buggy JJ, Pals ST, Spaargaren M (2012) The clinically active BTK inhibitor PCI-32765 targets B-cell receptor—and chemokine-controlled adhesion and migration in chronic lymphocytic leukemia. Blood 119 (11):2590–2594

de Zwart L, Snoeys J, De Jong J, Sukbuntherng J, Mannaert E, Monshouwer M (2016) Ibrutinib dosing strategies based on interaction potential of CYP3A4 perpetrators using physiologically based pharmacokinetic modeling. Clin Pharmacol Ther 100(5):548–557

Di Paolo JA, Huang T, Balazs M, Barbosa J, Barck KH, Bravo BJ, Carano RA, Darrow J, Davies DR, DeForge LE, Diehl L, Ferrando R, Gallion SL, Giannetti AM, Gribling P, Hurez V, Hymowitz SG, Jones R, Kropf JE, Lee WP, Maciejewski PM, Mitchell SA, Rong H, Staker BL, Whitney JA, Yeh S, Young WB, Yu C, Zhang J, Reif K, Currie KS (2011) Specific Btk inhibition suppresses B cell- and myeloid cell-mediated arthritis. Nat Chem Biol 7(1): 41–50

Dimopoulos MA, Trotman J, Tedeschi A, Matous JV, Macdonald D, Tam C, Tournilhac O, Ma S, Oriol A, Heffner LT, Shustik C, García-Sanz R, Cornell RF, Fernández de Larrea C, Castillo JJ, Granell M, Kyrtsonis M-C, Leblond V, Symeonidis A, Singh P, Li J, Graef T, Bilotti E, Treon S, Buske C (2015) Ibrutinib therapy in rituximab-refractory patients with Waldenström's macroglobulinemia: initial results from an international, multicenter, open-label phase 3 substudy (iNNOVATE). Blood 126(23):2745

Döhner H, Stilgenbauer S, Benner A, Leupolt E, Kröber A, Bullinger L, Döhner K, Bentz M, Lichter P (2000) Genomic aberrations and survival in chronic lymphocytic leukemia. N Engl J Med 343(26):1910–1916

Dreyling M, Jurczak W, Jerkeman M, Silva RS, Rusconi C, Trneny M, Offner F, Caballero D, Joao C, Witzens-Harig M, Hess G, Bence-Bruckler I, Cho SG, Bothos J, Goldberg JD, Enny C, Traina S, Balasubramanian S, Bandyopadhyay N, Sun S, Vermeulen J, Rizo A, Rule S (2016) Ibrutinib versus temsirolimus in patients with relapsed or refractory mantle-cell lymphoma: an international, randomised, open-label, phase 3 study. Lancet 387(10020):770–778

Dubovsky JA, Beckwith KA, Natarajan G, Woyach JA, Jaglowski S, Zhong Y, Hessler JD, Liu TM, Chang BY, Larkin KM, Stefanovski MR, Chappell DL, Frissora FW, Smith LL, Smucker KA, Flynn JM, Jones JA, Andritsos LA, Maddocks K, Lehman AM, Furman R, Sharman J, Mishra A, Caligiuri MA, Satoskar AR, Buggy JJ, Muthusamy N, Johnson AJ, Byrd JC (2013a) Ibrutinib is an irreversible molecular inhibitor of ITK driving a Th1-selective pressure in T lymphocytes. Blood 122(15):2539–2549

Dubovsky JA, Chappell DL, Harrington BK, Agrawal K, Andritsos LA, Flynn JM, Jones JA, Paulaitis ME, Bolon B, Johnson AJ, Byrd JC, Muthusamy N (2013b) Lymphocyte cytosolic protein 1 is a chronic lymphocytic leukemia membrane-associated antigen critical to niche homing. Blood 122(19):3308–3316

Duong MN, Matera EL, Mathe D, Evesque A, Valsesia-Wittmann S, Clemenceau B, Dumontet C (2015) Effect of kinase inhibitors on the therapeutic properties of monoclonal antibodies. MAbs 7(1):192–198

Falchi L, Baron JM, Orlikowski CA, Ferrajoli A (2016) BCR signaling inhibitors: an overview of toxicities associated with ibrutinib and idelalisib in patients with chronic lymphocytic leukemia. Mediterr J Hematol Infect Dis 8(1):e2016011

Farooqui M, Valdez J, Soto S, Bray A, Tian X, Wiestner A (2015a) Atrial fibrillation in CLL/SLL patients on ibrutinib. Blood 126(23):2933

Farooqui M, Valdez J, Soto S, Stetler-Stevenson M, Yuan CM, Thomas F, Tian X, Maric I, Wiestner A (2015b) Single agent ibrutinib in CLL/SLL patients with and without deletion 17p. Blood 126(23):2937

Farooqui MZH, Valdez J, Martyr S, Aue G, Saba N, Niemann CU, Herman SEM, Tian X, Marti G, Soto S, Hughes TE, Jones J, Lipsky A, Pittaluga S, Stetler-Stevenson M, Yuan C, Lee YS, Pedersen LB, Geisler CH, Calvo KR, Arthur DC, Maric I, Childs R, Young NS, Wiestner A (2015c) Ibrutinib for previously untreated and relapsed or refractory chronic lymphocytic leukaemia with TP53 aberrations: a phase 2, single-arm trial. Lancet Oncol 16(2): 169–176

Fischer K, Bahlo J, Fink AM, Goede V, Herling CD, Cramer P, Langerbeins P, von Tresckow J, Engelke A, Maurer C, Kovacs G, Herling M, Tausch E, Kreuzer K-A, Eichhorst B, Böttcher S, Seymour JF, Ghia P, Marlton P, Kneba M, Wendtner C-M, Döhner H, Stilgenbauer S, Hallek M (2016) Long-term remissions after FCR chemoimmunotherapy in previously untreated patients with CLL: updated results of the CLL8 trial. Blood 127(2):208–215

Gashonia LM, Carver JR, O'Quinn R, Clasen S, Hughes ME, Schuster SJ, Isaac K, Kennard K, Svoboda J, Daniel C, Tsai DE, Fanning MJ, Nasta S, Landsburg DJ, Nabhan C, Mato AR (2017) Persistence of ibrutinib-associated hypertension in CLL pts treated in a real-world experience. J Clin Oncol 35(15_suppl):7525–7525

Gill S, Frey NV, Hexner EO, Lacey SF, Melenhorst JJ, Byrd JC, Metzger S, Marcus T, Gladney W, Marcucci K, Hwang W-T, June CH, Porter DL (2017) CD19 CAR-T cells combined with ibrutinib to induce complete remission in CLL. J Clin Oncol 35(15_suppl): 7509–7509

Goede V, Fischer K, Busch R, Engelke A, Eichhorst B, Wendtner CM, Chagorova T, de la Serna J, Dilhuydy M-S, Illmer T, Opat S, Owen CJ, Samoylova O, Kreuzer K-A, Stilgenbauer S, Döhner H, Langerak AW, Ritgen M, Kneba M, Asikanius E, Humphrey K, Wenger M, Hallek M (2014) Obinutuzumab plus chlorambucil in patients with CLL and coexisting conditions. N Engl J Med 370(12):1101–1110

Grabinski N, Ewald F (2014) Ibrutinib (ImbruvicaTM) potently inhibits ErbB receptor phosphorylation and cell viability of ErbB2-positive breast cancer cells. Invest New Drugs 32(6):1096–1104

Grommes C, Pastore A, Palaskas N, Tang SS, Campos C, Schartz D, Codega P, Nichol D, Clark O, Hsieh WY, Rohle D, Rosenblum M, Viale A, Tabar VS, Brennan CW, Gavrilovic IT, Kaley TJ, Nolan CP, Omuro A, Pentsova E, Thomas AA, Tsyvkin E, Noy A, Palomba ML, Hamlin P, Sauter CS, Moskowitz CH, Wolfe J, Dogan A, Won M, Glass J, Peak S, Lallana EC, Hatzoglou V, Reiner AS, Gutin PH, Huse JT, Panageas KS, Graeber TG, Schultz N, DeAngelis LM, Mellinghoff IK (2017) Ibrutinib unmasks critical role of Bruton tyrosine kinase in primary CNS lymphoma. Cancer Discov 7(9):1018–1029

Gunderson AJ, Kaneda MM, Tsujikawa T, Nguyen AV, Affara NI, Ruffell B, Gorjestani S, Liudahl SM, Truitt M, Olson P, Kim G, Hanahan D, Tempero MA, Sheppard B, Irving B, Chang BY, Varner JA, Coussens LM (2016) Bruton tyrosine kinase-dependent immune cell cross-talk drives pancreas cancer. Cancer Discov 6(3):270–285

Guo A, Lu P, Galanina N, Nabhan C, Smith SM, Coleman M, Wang YL (2016a) Heightened BTK-dependent cell proliferation in unmutated chronic lymphocytic leukemia confers increased sensitivity to ibrutinib. Oncotarget 7(4):4598–4610

Guo H, Huang S, Liu Y, Li CJ, Wang J, Zhang V, Ahmed M, Lam LT, Zhang H, Nomie K, Zhang L, Wang M (2016b) Genetic and molecular characterization of ibrutinib-resistant mantle cell lymphoma: designing innovative therapeutic strategies. Blood 128(22):1838

Hallek M, Cheson BD, Catovsky D, Caligaris-Cappio F, Dighiero G, Döhner H, Hillmen P, Keating MJ, Montserrat E, Rai KR, Kipps TJ (2008) Guidelines for the diagnosis and treatment of chronic lymphocytic leukemia: a report from the International Workshop on Chronic Lymphocytic Leukemia updating the National Cancer Institute-Working Group 1996 guidelines. Blood 111(12):5446–5456

Hallek M, Fischer K, Fingerle-Rowson G, Fink AM, Busch R, Mayer J, Hensel M, Hopfinger G, Hess G, von Grünhagen U, Bergmann M, Catalano J, Zinzani PL, Caligaris-Cappio F, Seymour JF, Berrebi A, Jäger U, Cazin B, Trneny M, Westermann A, Wendtner CM, Eichhorst BF, Staib P, Bühler A, Winkler D, Zenz T, Böttcher S, Ritgen M, Mendila M, Kneba M, Döhner H, Stilgenbauer S (2010) Addition of rituximab to fludarabine and cyclophosphamide in patients with chronic lymphocytic leukaemia: a randomised, open-label, phase 3 trial. Lancet 376(9747):1164–1174

Hendriks RW, Yuvaraj S, Kil LP (2014) Targeting Bruton's tyrosine kinase in B cell malignancies. Nat Rev Cancer 14(4):219–232

Herman SEM, Gordon AL, Hertlein E, Ramanunni A, Zhang X, Jaglowski S, Flynn J, Jones J, Blum KA, Buggy JJ, Hamdy A, Johnson AJ, Byrd JC (2011) Bruton tyrosine kinase represents a promising therapeutic target for treatment of chronic lymphocytic leukemia and is effectively targeted by PCI-32765. Blood 117(23):6287–6296

Herman SE, Mustafa RZ, Jones J, Wong DH, Farooqui M, Wiestner A (2015) Treatment with ibrutinib inhibits BTK- and VLA-4-dependent adhesion of chronic lymphocytic leukemia cells in vivo. Clin Cancer Res 21(20):4642–4651

Hillmen P, Skotnicki AB, Robak T, Jaksic B, Dmoszynska A, Wu J, Sirard C, Mayer J (2007) Alemtuzumab compared with chlorambucil as first-line therapy for chronic lymphocytic leukemia. J Clin Oncol 25(35):5616–5623

Honigberg LA, Smith AM, Sirisawad M, Verner E, Loury D, Chang B, Li S, Pan Z, Thamm DH, Miller RA, Buggy JJ (2010) The Bruton tyrosine kinase inhibitor PCI-32765 blocks B-cell activation and is efficacious in models of autoimmune disease and B-cell malignancy. Proc Natl Acad Sci USA 107(29):13075–13080

Jaglowski SM, Jones JA, Nagar V, Flynn JM, Andritsos LA, Maddocks KJ, Woyach JA, Blum KA, Grever MR, Smucker K, Ruppert AS, Heerema NA, Lozanski G, Stefanos M, Munneke B, West J-S, Neuenburg JK, James DF, Hall N, Johnson AJ, Byrd JC (2015) Safety and activity of BTK inhibitor ibrutinib combined with ofatumumab in chronic lymphocytic leukemia: a phase 1b/2 study. Blood 126(7):842–850

Jain P, Keating M, Wierda W, Estrov Z, Ferrajoli A, Jain N, George B, James D, Kantarjian H, Burger J, O'Brien S (2015) Outcomes of patients with chronic lymphocytic leukemia after discontinuing ibrutinib. Blood 125(13):2062–2067

Jerkeman M, Hutchings M, Räty R, Wader KF, Laurell A, Kuitunen H, Toldbod H, Pedersen LB, Eskelund CW, Grønbæk K, Niemann CU, Geisler CH, Kolstad A (2016) Ibrutinib-lenalidomide-rituximab in patients with relapsed/refractory mantle cell lymphoma: first results from the Nordic Lymphoma Group MCL6 (PHILEMON) phase II trial. Blood 128 (22):148

Kamel S, Horton L, Ysebaert L, Levade M, Burbury K, Tan S, Cole-Sinclair M, Reynolds J, Filshie R, Schischka S, Khot A, Sandhu S, Keating MJ, Nandurkar H, Tam CS (2015) Ibrutinib inhibits collagen-mediated but not ADP-mediated platelet aggregation. Leukemia 29(4):783–787

Kohrt HE, Sagiv-Barfi I, Rafiq S, Herman SEM, Butchar JP, Cheney C, Zhang X, Buggy JJ, Muthusamy N, Levy R, Johnson AJ, Byrd JC (2014) Ibrutinib antagonizes rituximab-dependent NK cell–mediated cytotoxicity. Blood 123(12):1957–1960

Kokabee L, Wang X, Sevinsky CJ, Wang WL, Cheu L, Chittur SV, Karimipoor M, Tenniswood M, Conklin DS (2015) Bruton's tyrosine kinase is a potential therapeutic target in prostate cancer. Cancer Biol Ther 16(11):1604–1615

Kondo K, Shaim H, Thompson PA, Burger JA, Keating M, Estrov Z, Harris D, Kim E, Ferrajoli A, Daher M, Basar R, Muftuoglu M, Imahashi N, Alsuliman A, Sobieski C, Gokdemir E, Wierda W, Jain N, Liu E, Shpall EJ, Rezvani K (2017) Ibrutinib modulates the immunosuppressive CLL microenvironment through STAT3-mediated suppression of regulatory B-cell function and inhibition of the PD-1/PD-L1 pathway. Leukemia

Leong DP, Caron F, Hillis C, Duan A, Healey JS, Fraser G, Siegal D (2016) The risk of atrial fibrillation with ibrutinib use: a systematic review and meta-analysis. Blood

Levade M, David E, Garcia C, Laurent PA, Cadot S, Michallet AS, Bordet JC, Tam C, Sie P, Ysebaert L, Payrastre B (2014) Ibrutinib treatment affects collagen and von Willebrand factor-dependent platelet functions. Blood 124(26):3991–3995

Ma J, Lu P, Guo A, Cheng S, Zong H, Martin P, Coleman M, Wang YL (2014) Characterization of ibrutinib-sensitive and -resistant mantle lymphoma cells. Br J Haematol 166(6):849–861

Maddocks K, Christian B, Jaglowski S, Flynn J, Jones JA, Porcu P, Wei L, Jenkins C, Lozanski G, Byrd JC, Blum KA (2015a) A phase 1/1b study of rituximab, bendamustine, and ibrutinib in patients with untreated and relapsed/refractory non-hodgkin lymphoma. Blood 125(2):242–248

Maddocks KJ, Ruppert AS, Lozanski G, Heerema NA, Zhao W, Abruzzo L, Lozanski A, Davis M, Gordon A, Smith LL, Mantel R, Jones JA, Flynn JM, Jaglowski SM, Andritsos LA, Awan F, Blum KA, Grever MR, Johnson AJ, Byrd JC, Woyach JA (2015b) Etiology of ibrutinib therapy discontinuation and outcomes in patients with chronic lymphocytic leukemia. JAMA Oncol 1(1):80–87

Masso-Valles D, Jauset T, Serrano E, Sodir NM, Pedersen K, Affara NI, Whitfield JR, Beaulieu ME, Evan GI, Elias L, Arribas J, Soucek L (2015) Ibrutinib exerts potent antifibrotic and antitumor activities in mouse models of pancreatic adenocarcinoma. Cancer Res 75(8): 1675–1681

McMullen JR, Amirahmadi F, Woodcock EA, Schinke-Braun M, Bouwman RD, Hewitt KA, Mollica JP, Zhang L, Zhang Y, Shioi T, Buerger A, Izumo S, Jay PY, Jennings GL (2007) Protective effects of exercise and phosphoinositide 3-kinase(p110alpha) signaling in dilated and hypertrophic cardiomyopathy. Proc Natl Acad Sci USA 104(2):612–617

McMullen JR, Boey EJ, Ooi JY, Seymour JF, Keating MJ, Tam CS (2014) Ibrutinib increases the risk of atrial fibrillation, potentially through inhibition of cardiac PI3K-Akt signaling. Blood 124(25):3829–3830

McNally GA, Long JM, Brophy LR, Badillo MR (2015) Ibrutinib: implications for use in the treatment of mantle cell lymphoma and chronic lymphocytic leukemia. J Adv Pract Oncol 6(5):420–431

Minden MD-V, Übelhart R, Schneider D, Wossning T, Bach MP, Buchner M, Hofmann D, Surova E, Follo M, Köhler F, Wardemann H, Zirlik K, Veelken H, Jumaa H (2012) Chronic lymphocytic leukaemia is driven by antigen-independent cell-autonomous signalling. Nature 489:309

Mohamed AJ, Yu L, Backesjo CM, Vargas L, Faryal R, Aints A, Christensson B, Berglof A, Vihinen M, Nore BF, Smith CI (2009) Bruton's tyrosine kinase (Btk): function, regulation, and transformation with special emphasis on the PH domain. Immunol Rev 228(1):58–73

Mohanty A, Sandoval N, Das M, Pillai R, Chen L, Chen RW, Amin HM, Wang M, Marcucci G, Weisenburger DD, Rosen ST, Pham LV, Ngo VN (2016) CCND1 mutations increase protein stability and promote ibrutinib resistance in mantle cell lymphoma. Oncotarget 7(45):73558–73572

Murray MY, Zaitseva L, Auger MJ, Craig JI, MacEwan DJ, Rushworth SA, Bowles KM (2015) Ibrutinib inhibits BTK-driven NF-kappaB p65 activity to overcome bortezomib-resistance in multiple myeloma. Cell Cycle 14(14):2367–2375

Noy A, de Vos S, Thieblemont C, Martin P, Flowers CR, Morschhauser F, Collins GP, Ma S, Coleman M, Peles S, Smith S, Barrientos JC, Smith A, Munneke B, Dimery I, Beaupre DM, Chen R (2017) Targeting Bruton tyrosine kinase with ibrutinib in relapsed/refractory marginal zone lymphoma. Blood 129(16):2224–2232

O'Brien S, Furman RR, Coutre SE, Sharman JP, Burger JA, Blum KA, Grant B, Richards DA, Coleman M, Wierda WG (2014) Ibrutinib as initial therapy for elderly patients with chronic lymphocytic leukaemia or small lymphocytic lymphoma: an open-label, multicentre, phase 1b/2 trial. Lancet Oncol 15

O'Brien S, Jones JA, Coutre SE, Mato AR, Hillmen P, Tam C, Osterborg A, Siddiqi T, Thirman MJ, Furman RR, Ilhan O, Keating MJ, Call TG, Brown JR, Stevens-Brogan M, Li Y, Clow F, James DF, Chu AD, Hallek M, Stilgenbauer S (2016a) Ibrutinib for patients with relapsed or refractory chronic lymphocytic leukaemia with 17p deletion (RESONATE-17): a phase 2, open-label, multicentre study. Lancet Oncol 17(10):1409–1418

O'Brien SM, Furman RR, Coutre SE, Flinn IW, Burger J, Blum K, Sharman J, Wierda WG, Jones J, Zhao W, Heerema NA, Johnson AJ, Luan Y, James DF, Chu AD, Byrd JC (2016b) Five-year experience with single-agent ibrutinib in patients with previously untreated and relapsed/refractory chronic lymphocytic leukemia/small lymphocytic leukemia. Blood 128(22): 233

Oda A, Ikeda Y, Ochs HD, Druker BJ, Ozaki K, Handa M, Ariga T, Sakiyama Y, Witte ON, Wahl MI (2000) Rapid tyrosine phosphorylation and activation of Bruton's tyrosine/Tec kinases in platelets induced by collagen binding or CD32 cross-linking. Blood 95(5):1663–1670

Okamoto K, Proia LA, Demarais PL (2016) Disseminated cryptococcal disease in a patient with chronic lymphocytic leukemia on ibrutinib. Case Rep Infect Dis 2016:4642831

Ortolano S, Hwang IY, Han SB, Kehrl JH (2006) Roles for phosphoinositide 3-kinases, Bruton's tyrosine kinase, and Jun kinases in B lymphocyte chemotaxis and homing. Eur J Immunol 36 (5):1285–1295

Pan Z, Scheerens H, Li S-J, Schultz BE, Sprengeler PA, Burrill LC, Mendonca RV, Sweeney MD, Scott KCK, Grothaus PG, Jeffery DA, Spoerke JM, Honigberg LA, Young PR, Dalrymple SA, Palmer JT (2007) Discovery of selective irreversible inhibitors for Bruton's tyrosine kinase. ChemMedChem 2(1):58–61

Pavlasova G, Borsky M, Seda V, Cerna K, Osickova J, Doubek M, Mayer J, Calogero R, Trbusek M, Pospisilova S, Davids MS, Kipps TJ, Brown JR, Mraz M (2016) Ibrutinib inhibits CD20 upregulation on CLL B cells mediated by the CXCR4/SDF-1 axis. Blood 128(12):1609–1613

Ping L, Ding N, Shi Y, Feng L, Li J, Liu Y, Lin Y, Shi C, Wang X, Pan Z, Song Y, Zhu J (2017) The Bruton's tyrosine kinase inhibitor ibrutinib exerts immunomodulatory effects through regulation of tumor-infiltrating macrophages. Oncotarget 8(24):39218–39229

Ponader S, Chen S-S, Buggy JJ, Balakrishnan K, Gandhi V, Wierda WG, Keating MJ, O'Brien S, Chiorazzi N, Burger JA (2012) The Bruton tyrosine kinase inhibitor PCI-32765 thwarts chronic lymphocytic leukemia cell survival and tissue homing in vitro and in vivo. Blood 119(5):1182–1189

Rahal R, Frick M, Romero R, Korn JM, Kridel R, Chan FC, Meissner B, Bhang HE, Ruddy D, Kauffmann A, Farsidjani A, Derti A, Rakiec D, Naylor T, Pfister E, Kovats S, Kim S, Dietze K, Dorken B, Steidl C, Tzankov A, Hummel M, Monahan J, Morrissey MP, Fritsch C, Sellers WR, Cooke VG, Gascoyne RD, Lenz G, Stegmeier F (2014) Pharmacological and genomic profiling identifies NF-kappaB-targeted treatment strategies for mantle cell lymphoma. Nat Med 20(1):87–92

Rushworth SA, Bowles KM, Barrera LN, Murray MY, Zaitseva L, MacEwan DJ (2013) BTK inhibitor ibrutinib is cytotoxic to myeloma and potently enhances bortezomib and lenalidomide activities through NF-kappaB. Cell Signal 25(1):106–112

Sagiv-Barfi I, Kohrt HEK, Czerwinski DK, Ng PP, Chang BY, Levy R (2015) Therapeutic antitumor immunity by checkpoint blockade is enhanced by ibrutinib, an inhibitor of both BTK and ITK. Proc Natl Acad Sci 112(9):E966–E972

Satterthwaite AB, Witte ON (2000) The role of Bruton's tyrosine kinase in B-cell development and function: a genetic perspective. Immunol Rev 175:120–127

Scharenberg AM, Humphries LA, Rawlings DJ (2007) Calcium signalling and cell-fate choice in B cells. Nat Rev Immunol 7(10):778–789

Scheers E, Leclercq L, de Jong J, Bode N, Bockx M, Laenen A, Cuyckens F, Skee D, Murphy J, Sukbuntherng J, Mannens G (2015) Absorption, metabolism, and excretion of oral ^{14}C radiolabeled ibrutinib: an open-label, phase I, single-dose study in healthy men. Drug Metab Dispos 43(2):289–297

Schwamb J, Feldhaus V, Baumann M, Patz M, Brodesser S, Brinker R, Claasen J, Pallasch CP, Hallek M, Wendtner C-M, Frenzel LP (2012) B-cell receptor triggers drug sensitivity of primary CLL cells by controlling glucosylation of ceramides. Blood 120(19):3978–3985

Seda V, Mraz M (2015) B-cell receptor signalling and its crosstalk with other pathways in normal and malignant cells. Eur J Haematol 94(3):193–205

Sehgal L, Mathur R, Braun FK, Wise JF, Berkova Z, Neelapu S, Kwak LW, Samaniego F (2014) FAS-antisense 1 lncRNA and production of soluble versus membrane Fas in B-cell lymphoma. Leukemia 28(12):2376–2387

Shao J, Markowitz JS, Bei D, An G (2014) Enzyme-transporter-mediated drug interactions with small molecule tyrosine kinase inhibitors. J Pharm Sci 103(12):3810–3833

Sideras P, Muller S, Shiels H, Jin H, Khan WN, Nilsson L, Parkinson E, Thomas JD, Branden L, Larsson I et al (1994) Genomic organization of mouse and human Bruton's agammaglobulinemia tyrosine kinase (Btk) loci. J Immunol 153(12):5607–5617

Stevenson FK, Krysov S, Davies AJ, Steele AJ, Packham G (2011) B-cell receptor signaling in chronic lymphocytic leukemia. Blood 118(16):4313–4320

Stiff A, Trikha P, Wesolowski R, Kendra K, Hsu V, Uppati S, McMichael E, Duggan M, Campbell A, Keller K, Landi I, Zhong Y, Dubovsky J, Howard JH, Yu L, Harrington B, Old M, Reiff S, Mace T, Tridandapani S, Muthusamy N, Caligiuri MA, Byrd JC, Carson WE 3rd (2016) Myeloid-derived suppressor cells express Bruton's tyrosine kinase and can be depleted in tumor-bearing hosts by ibrutinib treatment. Cancer Res 76(8):2125–2136

Tai Y-T, Chang BY, Kong S-Y, Fulciniti M, Yang G, Calle Y, Hu Y, Lin J, Zhao J-J, Cagnetta A, Cea M, Sellitto MA, Zhong MY, Wang Q, Acharya C, Carrasco DR, Buggy JJ, Elias L, Treon SP, Matsui W, Richardson P, Munshi NC, Anderson KC (2012) Bruton tyrosine kinase inhibition is a novel therapeutic strategy targeting tumor in the bone marrow microenvironment in multiple myeloma. Blood 120(9):1877–1887

Takahashi K, Sivina M, Hoellenriegel J, Oki Y, Hagemeister FB, Fayad L, Romaguera JE, Fowler N, Fanale MA, Kwak LW, Samaniego F, Neelapu S, Xiao L, Huang X, Kantarjian H, Keating MJ, Wierda W, Fu K, Chan WC, Vose JM, O'Brien S, Davis RE, Burger JA (2015) CCL3 and CCL4 are biomarkers for B cell receptor pathway activation and prognostic serum markers in diffuse large B cell lymphoma. Br J Haematol 171(5):726–735

Thompson PA, Levy V, Tam CS, Al Nawakil C, Goudot FX, Quinquenel A, Ysebaert L, Michallet AS, Dilhuydy MS, Van Den Neste E, Dupuis J, Keating MJ, Meune C, Cymbalista F (2016) Atrial fibrillation in CLL patients treated with ibrutinib. An international retrospective study. Br J Haematol 175(3):462–466

Treon SP, Tripsas CK, Meid K, Warren D, Varma G, Green R, Argyropoulos KV, Yang G, Cao Y, Xu L, Patterson CJ, Rodig S, Zehnder JL, Aster JC, Harris NL, Kanan S, Ghobrial I, Castillo JJ, Laubach JP, Hunter ZR, Salman Z, Li J, Cheng M, Clow F, Graef T, Palomba ML, Advani RH (2015) Ibrutinib in previously treated Waldenström's macroglobulinemia. N Engl J Med 372(15):1430–1440

Vij R, Huff CA, Bensinger WI, Siegel DS, Jagannath S, Berdeja J, Lendvai N, Lebovic D, Anderson LD, Costello CL, Stockerl-Goldstein KE, Laubach JP, Elias L, Clow F, Fardis M, Graef T, Bilotti E, Richardson PG (2014) Ibrutinib, single agent or in combination with dexamethasone, in patients with relapsed or relapsed/refractory multiple myeloma (mm): preliminary phase 2 results. Blood 124(21):31

Vrontikis A, Carey J, Gilreath JA, Halwani A, Stephens DM, Sweetenham JW (2016) Proposed algorithm for managing ibrutinib-related atrial fibrillation. Oncology (Williston Park) 30 (11):970–974, 980-971, C973

Wang ML, Rule S, Martin P, Goy A, Auer R, Kahl BS, Jurczak W, Advani RH, Romaguera JE, Williams ME, Barrientos JC, Chmielowska E, Radford J, Stilgenbauer S, Dreyling M, Jedrzejczak WW, Johnson P, Spurgeon SE, Li L, Zhang L, Newberry K, Ou Z, Cheng N, Fang B, McGreivy J, Clow F, Buggy JJ, Chang BY, Beaupre DM, Kunkel LA, Blum KA (2013) Targeting BTK with ibrutinib in relapsed or refractory mantle-cell lymphoma. N Engl J Med 369(6):507–516

Wang ML, Blum KA, Martin P, Goy A, Auer R, Kahl BS, Jurczak W, Advani RH, Romaguera JE, Williams ME, Barrientos JC, Chmielowska E, Radford J, Stilgenbauer S, Dreyling M, Jedrzejczak WW, Johnson P, Spurgeon SE, Zhang L, Baher L, Cheng M, Lee D, Beaupre DM, Rule S (2015) Long-term follow-up of MCL patients treated with single-agent ibrutinib: updated safety and efficacy results. Blood 126(6):739–745

Wang M, Lee HJ, Thirumurthi S, Chuang HH, Hagemeister FB, Westin JR, Fayad LE, Samaniego F, Turturro F, Chen W, Oriabure O, Huang SY, Li S, Zhang L, Badillo M, Hartig KH, Ahmed M, Nomie K, Lam LT, Addison AA, Romaguera JE (2016a) Chemotherapy-free induction with ibrutinib-rituximab followed by shortened cycles of chemo-immunotherapy consolidation in young, newly diagnosed mantle cell lymphoma patients: a phase II clinical trial. Blood 128(22):147

Wang ML, Lee H, Chuang H, Wagner-Bartak N, Hagemeister F, Westin J, Fayad L, Samaniego F, Turturro F, Oki Y, Chen W, Badillo M, Nomie K, DeLa Rosa M, Zhao D, Lam L, Addison A, Zhang H, Young KH, Li S, Santos D, Medeiros LJ, Champlin R, Romaguera J, Zhang L (2016b) Ibrutinib in combination with rituximab in relapsed or refractory mantle cell lymphoma: a single-centre, open-label, phase 2 trial. Lancet Oncol 17(1):48–56

Wang J, Liu X, Hong Y, Wang S, Chen P, Gu A, Guo X, Zhao P (2017) Ibrutinib, a Bruton's tyrosine kinase inhibitor, exhibits antitumoral activity and induces autophagy in glioblastoma. J Exp Clin Cancer Res 36(1):96

Wei L, Su YK, Lin CM, Chao TY, Huang SP, Huynh TT, Jan HJ, Whang-Peng J, Chiou JF, Wu AT, Hsiao M (2016) Preclinical investigation of ibrutinib, a Bruton's kinase tyrosine (Btk) inhibitor, in suppressing glioma tumorigenesis and stem cell phenotypes. Oncotarget 7 (43):69961–69975

Wilson WH, Young RM, Schmitz R, Yang Y, Pittaluga S, Wright G, Lih C-J, Williams PM, Shaffer AL, Gerecitano J, de Vos S, Goy A, Kenkre VP, Barr PM, Blum KA, Shustov A, Advani R, Fowler NH, Vose JM, Elstrom RL, Habermann TM, Barrientos JC, McGreivy J, Fardis M, Chang BY, Clow F, Munneke B, Moussa D, Beaupre DM, Staudt LM (2015) Targeting B cell receptor signaling with ibrutinib in diffuse large B cell lymphoma. Nat Med 21 (8):922–926

Wodarz D, Garg N, Komarova NL, Benjamini O, Keating MJ, Wierda WG, Kantarjian H, James D, O'Brien S, Burger JA (2014) Kinetics of CLL cells in tissues and blood during therapy with the BTK inhibitor ibrutinib. Blood 123(26):4132–4135

Woyach JA, Johnson AJ, Byrd JC (2012) The B-cell receptor signaling pathway as a therapeutic target in CLL. Blood 120(6):1175–1184

Woyach JA, Furman RR, Liu T-M, Ozer HG, Zapatka M, Ruppert AS, Xue L, Li DH-H, Steggerda SM, Versele M, Dave SS, Zhang J, Yilmaz AS, Jaglowski SM, Blum KA, Lozanski A, Lozanski G, James DF, Barrientos JC, Lichter P, Stilgenbauer S, Buggy JJ, Chang BY, Johnson AJ, Byrd JC (2014a) Resistance mechanisms for the Bruton's tyrosine kinase inhibitor ibrutinib. N Engl J Med 370(24):2286–2294

Woyach JA, Smucker K, Smith LL, Lozanski A, Zhong Y, Ruppert AS, Lucas D, Williams K, Zhao W, Rassenti L, Ghia E, Kipps TJ, Mantel R, Jones J, Flynn J, Maddocks K, O'Brien S, Furman RR, James DF, Clow F, Lozanski G, Johnson AJ, Byrd JC (2014b) Prolonged lymphocytosis during ibrutinib therapy is associated with distinct molecular characteristics and does not indicate a suboptimal response to therapy. Blood 123(12):1810–1817

Xu L, Tsakmaklis N, Yang G, Chen JG, Liu X, Demos M, Kofides A, Patterson CJ, Meid K, Gustine J, Dubeau T, Palomba ML, Advani R, Castillo JJ, Furman RR, Hunter ZR, Treon SP (2017) Acquired mutations associated with ibrutinib resistance in Waldenström macroglobulinemia. Blood 129(18):2519–2525

Yang Y, Shaffer AL 3rd, Emre NC, Ceribelli M, Zhang M, Wright G, Xiao W, Powell J, Platig J, Kohlhammer H, Young RM, Zhao H, Yang Y, Xu W, Buggy JJ, Balasubramanian S, Mathews LA, Shinn P, Guha R, Ferrer M, Thomas C, Waldmann TA, Staudt LM (2012) Exploiting synthetic lethality for the therapy of ABC diffuse large B cell lymphoma. Cancer Cell 21(6):723–737

Younes A, Thieblemont C, Morschhauser F, Flinn I, Friedberg JW, Amorim S, Hivert B, Westin J, Vermeulen J, Bandyopadhyay N, de Vries R, Balasubramanian S, Hellemans P, Smit JW, Fourneau N, Oki Y (2014) Combination of ibrutinib with rituximab, cyclophosphamide, doxorubicin, vincristine, and prednisone (R-CHOP) for treatment-naive patients with CD20-positive B-cell non-Hodgkin lymphoma: a non-randomised, phase 1b study. Lancet Oncol 15(9):1019–1026

Young RM, Shaffer AL 3rd, Phelan JD, Staudt LM (2015) B-cell receptor signaling in diffuse large B-cell lymphoma. Semin Hematol 52(2):77–85

Zucha MA, Wu AT, Lee WH, Wang LS, Lin WW, Yuan CC, Yeh CT (2015) Bruton's tyrosine kinase (Btk) inhibitor ibrutinib suppresses stem-like traits in ovarian cancer. Oncotarget 6(15): 13255–13268

Pomalidomide

Monika Engelhardt, Stefanie Ajayi, Heike Reinhardt,
Stefan Jürgen Müller, Sandra Maria Dold and Ralph Wäsch

Contents

Abstract

Pomalidomide (originally CC-4047 or 3-amino-thalidomide) is a derivative of thalidomide that is antiangiogenic and also acts as immunomodulatory. Pomalidomide, the recent immunomodulatory agent (IMiD), has shown substantial

M. Engelhardt (✉) · S. Ajayi · H. Reinhardt · S. J. Müller · S. M. Dold · R. Wäsch
Hematology and Oncology, University of Freiburg, Hugstetter Str. 55, 79106 Freiburg, Germany
e-mail: monika.engelhardt@uniklinik-freiburg.de

M. Engelhardt · S. Ajayi · R. Wäsch
Comprehensive Cancer Center Freiburg (CCCF), Hugstetter Str. 55, 79106 Freiburg, Germany

© Springer International Publishing AG, part of Springer Nature 2018
U. M. Martens (ed.), *Small Molecules in Hematology*, Recent Results
in Cancer Research 211, https://doi.org/10.1007/978-3-319-91439-8_8

in vitro antiproliferative and proapoptotic effects. In vivo studies have suggested limited cross-resistance between lenalidomide and pomalidomide. Moreover, pomalidomide achieved very convincing responses in relapsed and refractory multiple myeloma (RRMM) patients, including those, who are refractory to both lenalidomide and bortezomib. Since pomalidomide plus low-dose dexamethasone has shown better responses, progression-free survival (PFS) and overall survival (OS) than high-dose dexamethasone or pomalidomide alone, subsequent trials have pursued or are still investigating pomalidomide triplet combinations, using cyclophosphamide or other novel agents, such as proteasome inhibitors (PI: bortezomib, carfilzomib) or antibodies, like elotuzumab or daratumumab. Pomalidomide has also been assessed in AL amyloidosis, MPNs (myelofibrosis [MF]), Waldenstrom's macroglobulinemia, solid tumors (sarcoma, lung cancer), or HIV, and—for AL amyloidosis and MF—has already been proven to be remarkably active. Due to its potency, pomalidomide was approved for RRMM by the US Food and Drug Administration (FDA) and by the European Medicines Agency (EMA) in 2013 and for drug combination with low-dose dexamethasone in 2015. In June 2017, the FDA further expanded approval for pomalidomide in combination with daratumumab and low-dose dexamethasone for patients with RRMM.

Keywords

Pomalidomide · Multiple myeloma · Relapsed/refractory disease ·
Therapy options

1 Introduction

The accelerated approval in 2013 for the treatment of patients with RRMM, who had received at least two prior therapies, including lenalidomide and bortezomib, and had demonstrated disease progression on their last antimyeloma treatment, was based on the results of the CC-4047-MM-002 trial, a multicenter, randomized, open-label study in 221 patients with RRMM, who had previously received lenalidomide and bortezomib, but were refractory to their last myeloma treatment (Richardson et al. 2009). The treatment arms were pomalidomide alone or pomalidomide plus low-dose dexamethasone. The efficacy results demonstrated an overall response rate (ORR) of 7% in patients treated with pomalidomide alone as compared to 29% in those treated with pomalidomide plus low-dose dexamethasone. The median response duration was not evaluable (rather short) in the pomalidomide monotherapy arm versus 7.4 months in the pomalidomide plus low-dose dexamethasone arm. As MM is a so far incurable disease with an unfavorable clinical outcome under conventional chemotherapy (e.g., with melphalan or bendamustin alone), the introduction of novel agents, like PIs or IMiDs, demonstrated to substantially prolong survival in MM patients. Among these novel agents, especially pomalidomide constitutes a valuable option, including high-risk and/or refractory patients, since pomalidomide combinations have proven their potential and efficacy in PI- and IMiD-refractory patients.

2 Structure and Mechanism of Action

The structurally related parent compound of pomalidomide, namely thalidomide, was discovered to inhibit angiogenesis in 1994. Pomalidomide, the latest IMiD, suggests at least incomplete cross-resistance among thalidomide or lenalidomide, and—albeit all three IMiDs have similar structures—they differ markedly in their potency and side effects (Fig. 1). Further, structure–activity studies led to the first report in 2001 (D'Amato et al. 2001), demonstrating that pomalidomide was able to directly inhibit the tumor cell and vascular compartment of MM. Compared with thalidomide and lenalidomide, pomalidomide has stronger direct antiproliferative effects on myeloma tumor cells. Moreover, IMiDs have shown to have a pleiotropic mechanism of action: antiangiogenetic, anti-inflammatory and immunomodulatory activity on T cells, natural killer (NK) cells, monocytes (Mitsiades and Chen-Kiang 2013; Görgün et al. 2010; Gandhi et al. 2014), and effects induced on the bone marrow (BM) microenvironment (BMM) and cell proliferation (Fig. 2). In addition

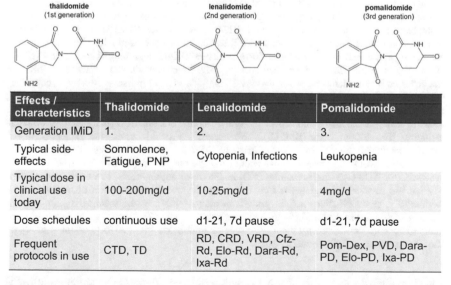

Effects / characteristics	Thalidomide	Lenalidomide	Pomalidomide
Generation IMiD	1.	2.	3.
Typical side-effects	Somnolence, Fatigue, PNP	Cytopenia, Infections	Leukopenia
Typical dose in clinical use today	100-200mg/d	10-25mg/d	4mg/d
Dose schedules	continuous use	d1-21, 7d pause	d1-21, 7d pause
Frequent protocols in use	CTD, TD	RD, CRD, VRD, Cfz-Rd, Elo-Rd, Dara-Rd, Ixa-Rd	Pom-Dex, PVD, Dara-PD, Elo-PD, Ixa-PD

Fig. 1 Thalidomide, lenalidomide, and pomalidomide structures. Albeit these three IMiDs are structurally similar, they are functionally different, resulting in different potencies. Pomalidomide is the most potent IMiD with approximately 100 times the strength of thalidomide and 10 times the potency of lenalidomide (Raza et al. 2017)

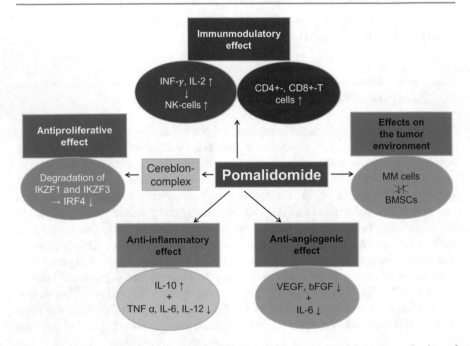

Fig. 2 Mechanism of action of pomalidomide. Pomalidomide has a pleiotropic mechanism of action. Binding to cereblon (CRBN) is an important component required for the antimyeloma activity of immunomodulatory drugs (IMiDs). CRBN forms an E3 ubiquitin ligase complex that ubiquitinates substrates targeting them for proteolysis. IMiDs potentiate the ubiquitination and proteolysis of two specific proteins, Ikaros (IKZF1) and Aiolos (IKZF3). They are important transcription factors for B cell differentiation. Knockdown of Ikaros and Aiolos in myeloma cells induces myeloma cell cytotoxicity and downregulation of interferon regulatory factor 4 (IRF4), which also is critical for myeloma cell survival. The immunomodulatory activity of IMiDs is characterized by an enhancement of CD4+ and CD8+ T cell co-stimulation. Moreover, enhancing interleukin 2 (IL-2) and interferon (IFN) production, the activity of natural killer cells (NK cells) is increased. Another important component of the mechanism of action of pomalidomide is the downregulation of the interaction between MM cells and the bone marrow (BM) microenvironment including BM stroma cells (BMSCs). This interaction could result, for example, in cell adhesion-mediated drug resistance. Furthermore, MM is characterized by an increased BM angiogenesis. IMiDs decrease vascular endothelial growth factor (VEGF) and basic fibroblast growth factor-2 (bFGF) levels resulting in an inhibition of angiogenesis. However, it is not clear whether this restraint of angiogenesis contributes to the overall tumor effect of IMiDs in MM. Additionally, pomalidomide inhibits proinflammatory cytokines, for example tumor necrosis factor α (TNF α), interleukin 6 (IL-6), and interleukin 12 (IL-12), increasing the levels of other interleukins with anti-inflammatory nature, such as interleukin 10 (IL-10) (Kortüm et al. 2015; Ríos-Tamayo et al. 2017; Zhu et al. 2013)

and like other drugs in this group, pomalidomide can decrease vascular endothelial growth factor (VEGF) and basic fibroblast growth factor-2 (bFGF) levels resulting in an inhibition of angiogenesis. MM is characterized by increased BM angiogenesis. However, it is not clear, whether this inhibition of angiogenesis contributes to the overall tumor effect of IMiDs in MM (Kortüm et al. 2015).

Additionally, pomalidomide inhibits proinflammatory cytokines (e.g., TNF α, IL-6, IL-12), increasing the levels of other interleukins with anti-inflammatory properties (such as IL-10) (Ríos-Tamayo et al. 2017).

The immunomodulatory activity of IMiDs is characterized by an enhancement of CD4+ and CD8+ T cell co-stimulation. Both lenalidomide and pomalidomide are more potent than thalidomide in inducing T cell proliferation and enhancing IL-2 and interferon γ (IFN γ) production (Zhu et al. 2013).

Indirect antimyeloma activity of IMiDs is postulated to be mediated by alteration of the interaction between MM cells and non-myeloma cells in the BMM, including BM stromal cells (BMSCs), osteoclasts, and immune cells. This interaction can result in cell adhesion-mediated drug resistance (CAM-DR). The crosstalk between MM cells and BMSCs can be altered by IMiDs, which may downregulate various cell surface adhesion molecules and decreases cell migration (Kortüm et al. 2015).

Another antiproliferative mode of action for thalidomide and its analogs is binding to cereblon (CRBN) (Lopez-Girona et al. 2012). CRBN forms an E3 ubiquitin ligase complex, that ubiquitinates substrates targeting them for proteolysis. IMiDs potentiate the ubiquitination and proteolysis of two specific proteins, Ikaros (IKZF1) and Aiolos (IKZF3), which are important transcription factors for B cell differentiation. Knockdown of Ikaros and Aiolos in myeloma cells induces myeloma cell cytotoxicity and leads to the downregulation of transcription factors like the interferon regulatory factor 4 (IRF4), which is also critical for myeloma cell survival (Kortüm et al. 2015). Albeit these findings, the precise molecular mechanism of action and all targets, through which IMiDs exert their antitumor effects, remain to be fully elucidated.

3 Preclinical Data

In vitro, IMiDs antagonize angiogenesis and expression of TNF-α and IL-6, while they facilitate production of IL-2 and IFN-γ and enhance T and NK cell proliferation and activity. Albeit all precise mechanisms of their action are not entirely revealed, IMiDs seem to induce downregulation of cytokine signaling (Görgün et al. 2010). Moreover, Görkün et al. demonstrated that the tumor suppressor molecule SOCS1 plays an important role in the tumor cell-immune cell-BMM interaction in MM. Importantly, lenalidomide and pomalidomide induced epigenetic modifications of SOCS1 gene in MM cells, as well as SOCS1-mediated modulation of the cytokine signaling in effector cells. Therefore, characterization of molecular mechanisms of IMiDs on immune cells in the BMM needs to be further defined to suggest that novel immune-based targeted therapies, such as the combination of IMiDs with epigenetic modulating drugs (e.g., histone deacetylase inhibitors [HDACi] and/or demethylating agents), may improve MM therapy. Given the promising clinical activity of pomalidomide even in lenalidomide-refractory MM, current efforts therefore attempt to delineate direct and epigenetic mechanisms to account for important differences (Görgün et al. 2010). Several preclinical and clinical studies have also demonstrated that threshold levels of CRBN expression are important to induce response to IMiDs (Schuster et al. 2012; Sehgal et al. 2015): CRBN depletion is initially cytotoxic to human myeloma cells, but surviving cells with stable CRBN depletion become highly resistant to both lenalidomide and pomalidomide, but not to the unrelated drugs bortezomib, dexamethasone, and/or melphalan. Acquired depletion of CRBN was described to be the primary genetic event of myeloma cell lines cultured to be sensitive or resistant to lenalidomide or pomalidomide. Gene expression changes induced by lenalidomide were substantially suppressed in the presence of CRBN depletion, demonstrating that CRBN is required for lenalidomide activity. Patients exposed and resistant to lenalidomide had lower CRBN levels in paired samples before and after therapy, suggesting that CRBN is an essential requirement for IMiD activity and possibly a useful biomarker for the clinical assessment of IMiDs' antimyeloma efficacy. Other recent studies have confirmed that threshold levels of CRBN expression are required for response to IMiD therapy (Schuster et al. 2012, Krönke). However, Seghal et al. suggested that baseline levels of Ikaros and Aiolos protein in tumor cells did not correlate with response or survival. They showed that pomalidomide led to rapid decline of Ikaros in T and NK cells in vivo, and, further, that therapy-induced activation of CD8+ T cells correlated with clinical response. These data suggest that pomalidomide leads to strong and rapid immunomodulatory effects involving both innate and adaptive immunities, even in heavily pretreated MM, which correlates with clinical antitumor effects. Another point of interest, which needs further investigation, is the possibility of resensitization of MM cells to pomalidomide and other antimyeloma agents, e.g., with use of the CXCR4 inhibitor plerixafor or others. CXCR4 is a metabotropic chemokine receptor with potent chemotactic activity. It may act as an inductor of the BM crosstalk, which leads to disease progression and CAM-DR. Prior data suggested that CXCR4, CXCR7, and their ligand CXCL12 may act as valid targets to antagonize CAM-DR in MM, and that antimyeloma combinations with the CXCL12 antagonist NOX-A12 or the CXCR4 inhibitor plerixafor may improve therapeutic responses due to adhesion interference of MM cells to BMSCs (Waldschmidt et al. 2017).

4 Biomarkers

Acquired depletion of CRBN has been demonstrated to be the primary genetic event of myeloma cell lines cultured to be sensitive or resistant to IMiDs. Gene expression changes induced by lenalidomide were substantially suppressed in the presence of CRBN depletion, demonstrating that CRBN is vital for IMiD activity. Zhu et al. also showed that patients exposed and resistant to lenalidomide had lower CRBN levels in paired samples before and after therapy, suggesting that CRBN is a useful biomarker for the clinical assessment of IMiDs' antimyeloma efficacy (Zhu et al. 2011). Other recent studies have confirmed that threshold levels of CRBN expression are required for response to IMiD therapy (Schuster et al. 2012).

Across six cohorts—of the phase II trials at Mayo in 345 MM patients receiving pomalidomide at doses of 2 or 4 mg/day (d)—confirmed responses of PR or better in 34%. Responses and duration of response (DOR) in those with high-risk molecular markers included (del)17p in 19 of 56 (34%): DOR 8.2 months; t(4;14): 6 of 24 (25%): DOR 4.8 months; t(14;16): 7 of 11 (64%): DOR 9.5 months and deletion 13 by cytogenetics: 13 of 37 (35%): DOR 8.2 months. In a multivariate analysis, LDH > ULN, number of prior regimens, and prior bortezomib therapy were predictive of a shorter time to progression and factors associated with a poor OS following initiation of pomalidomide therapy included ß2-microglobuline levels > 5.5 mg/l, LDH > ULN, number of prior regimens, and prior bortezomib therapy. In general and as true for almost all antimyeloma agents, number and types of prior regimens were the strongest predictors of pomalidomide response and survival, with best responses in patients who were the least heavily pretreated (Lacy 2013).

5 Clinical Data

The results of the CC-4047-MM-002 trial, a multicenter, randomized, open-label study with RRMM 221 patients, who had previously received lenalidomide and bortezomib and were refractory to their last line of treatment, led to pomalidomide's accelerated FDA approval in 2013 (Richardson et al. 2009). The treatment arms were pomalidomide alone or pomalidomide plus low-dose dexamethasone. The efficacy results showed superior ORR with pomalidomide/low-dose dexamethasone of 29% versus 7% with pomalidomide alone, with a substantial median response duration of 7.4 months.

A phase I dose-escalation study determined the maximum tolerated dose (MTD) of pomalidomide on days 1–21 of a 28-day cycle in 38 patients with RRMM (Richardson et al. 2013). Pretreatment had been substantial with a median of 6 prior therapies, including 63% who were refractory to both lenalidomide and bortezomib. There were four dose-limiting toxicities (grade 4 neutropenia) at 5 mg/d; therefore, the MTD was specified at 4 mg/d. Among the 38 patients enrolled (including 22 with added dexamethasone), 42% achieved minimal response (MR) or better, 21% PR or better, and 3% CR. Median duration of response, PFS, and OS were 4.6, 4.6, and 18.3 months, respectively.

The subsequent multicenter, phase II randomized study assessed two different pomalidomide dose schedules [4 mg for 21 vs. 28 days (21/28 vs. 28/28)] combined with dexamethasone in 84 advanced MM patients. The median number of prior therapy lines was again substantial with 5 and the ORR was 35% (arm 21/28) and 34% (arm 28/28), thus very similar, irrespective of the number of prior lines and level of refractoriness. Median duration of response, time to disease progression, and PFS were 7.3, 5.4, and 4.6 months, respectively. At 23 months of follow-up, median OS was 14.9 months (Leleu et al. 2013). This phase II trial suggested that 4 mg pomalidomide, given on days 1–21 of a 28-day cycle and combined with dexamethasone, was efficacious, well tolerated, allowed a "1-week-IMiD-rest" period and the blood count and patient to recuperate, which therefore determined the dose and schedule of choice.

5.1 High-Risk Patients

The International Myeloma Working Group (IMWG) published a consensus guideline on the treatment of MM patients with high-risk cytogenetics: Therein, cytogenetic abnormalities such as del(17p), t(4;14), t(14;16), t(14;20), gain(1q), and nonhyperdiploidy were specified as high risk, and patients with multiple abnormalities demonstrate more dismal therapy responses, earlier disease recurrence, and decreased PFS and OS (Sonneveld et al. 2016). Of note, pomalidomide in RRMM patients with high-risk cytogenetics was assessed in the phase III MM-003 study, an associated subanalysis and several phase II and phase I/II studies.

The MM-002-study was a multicenter, randomized, open-label dose-escalation study conducted to determine the MTD, safety, and efficacy of pomalidomide–dexamethasone in patients with RRMM, who had received both bortezomib and lenalidomide. The subanalysis reported on the use of pomalidomide versus pomalidomide–dexamethasone in patients with high-risk cytogenetics (Table 1), showing favorable responses, PFS, and OS also in high-risk patients (Richardson et al. 2012). Common grade 3/4 AEs (in >10% of patients) were neutropenia, thrombocytopenia, back pain, fatigue, renal failure, urinary tract infection, and leukopenia. Grade 3/4 adverse events (AEs) were similar in high- and standard-risk patients.

The MM-003 study was a phase III, multicenter, randomized, open-label study that compared the efficacy and safety of pomalidomide with low- versus high-dose dexamethasone in patients with MM, who were refractory after more than two previous treatments, including bortezomib and lenalidomide (San Miguel et al. 2013). Dimopoulos et al. updated these results with a median follow-up of

Table 1 Efficacy outcomes of the MM-002 study by cytogenetic profile (adapted from Richardson et al. 2012)

	High-risk cytogenetics[a] (n = 30)	Standard-risk cytogenetics (n = 57)
ORR n, (%)	7 (23)	23 (40)
Time to response[b], months (range)	1.2 (0.9–2.8)	1.9 (0.9–14.4)
Median DOR, months	4.9 (1.9–13.1)	10.1 (7.7-not reached)
Median PFS, months	3.1 (1.9–3.9)	5.5 (3.7–8.7)
Median OS, months	13.2 (4.7–19.8)	21.7 (12.4-not reached)

[a]High-risk cytogenetics defined as presence of del(17p13) and/or t(4p16/14q32)
[b]For patients that achieved ≥ PR
Abbreviations ORR = overall response rate, DOR = duration of response, PFS = progression-free response, OS = overall survival, PR = partial response

Table 2 Response rates among the MM-003 study patients based on cytogenetics (adapted from Dimopoulos et al. 2015)

	Modified high-risk cytogenetics[a]			Standard-risk cytogenetics		
	Pom–dex ($n = 77$)	High dex ($n = 35$)	p-value	Pom–dex ($n = 148$)	High dex ($n = 72$)	p value
ORR [%]	25	9	0.071	35	10	<0.001
≥ VGPR [%]	5	0	–	7	1	–
PR [%]	19	9	–	28	8	–

[a]del(17p)/t(4;14)

Abbreviations pom = pomalidomide, dex = low-dose dexamethasone, high dex = high-dose dexamethasone, ORR = overall response rate, VGPR = very good partial response, PR = partial response

15.4 months: Pomalidomide–dexamethasone significantly improved PFS as compared to high-dose dexamethasone alone, including high-risk patients with del(17p) or t(4;14). The median PFS in the pomalidomide–dexamethasone arm for patients with del(17p) was 4.6 months versus 1.1 months with high-dose dexamethasone and 2.8 months versus 1.9 months in patients with t(4;14). Among standard-risk patients, the median PFS with pomalidomide–dexamethasone was 4.2 months versus 2.3 months with high-dose dexamethasone. The median OS for patients with del(17p) was 12.6 months (pom–dex) versus 7.7 months (high dex) and 7.5 months versus 4.9 months in patients with t(4;14). For standard-risk patients, OS in the pom–dex arm was 14.0 months versus 9.0 months for patients with high-dose dexamethasone. However, it should be noted that 46% of high-risk patients and 64% of standard-risk patients enrolled in the high-dose dexamethasone arm subsequently received pomalidomide (Table 2); thus without this "crossover," the observed differences would have been even more striking (Dimopoulos et al. 2015).

5.2 Patients with Renal Failure

For patients with impaired renal function or renal failure, it is always a challenge to induce a suitable therapy, which is both efficient and well tolerated. Ramasamy et al. performed a phase II study (MM-013) of pomalidomide–dexamethasone in 81 patients with RRMM with moderate or severe renal impairment (RI), including patients on dialysis, who had received ≥ 1 prior treatment including lenalidomide. Patients were stratified in arm A with moderate RI (estimated glomerular filtration rate, eGFR ≥ 30 to < 45 ml/min), arm B with severe RI without dialysis (eGFR < 30), and arm C with severe RI requiring dialysis (eGFR < 30). The median number of cycles was 6 (range: 1–21), ORR was 32.1% (moderate RI: 39.4%, severe RI without dialysis: 32.4%, severe RI requiring dialysis: 14.3%), and median PFS was 6.5, 4.2, and 2.4 months, respectively. The median OS was 16.4 months in patients in arm A, 11.8 months in arm B, and 5.2 months in arm C.

The authors conclude that pomalidomide dosed at 4 mg on a 21/28-day schedule was a valuable therapy option and can be safely administered with low-dose dexamethasone in patients with moderate or severe RI, including those on hemodialysis (Ramasamy et al. 2015). Post hoc analysis and prospective evaluations of other clinical trials fortified this study (Siegel et al. 2012; Matous et al. 2014). Thus, pomalidomide is a suitable treatment option for patients with severe RI, even requiring dialysis. As pomalidomide can be eliminated from the blood circulation by hemodialysis, on dialysis days, patients should take their pomalidomide medication following hemodialysis (IMNOVID®: summary of product characteristics; Celgene, http://www.fachinfo.de; last revised: September 2016).

5.3 AL Amyloidosis and Other Disease Entities

Although previous studies could not show a survival advantage for patients with AL amyloidosis responding to salvage treatment with pomalidomide, Palladini et al. assessed the safety and efficacy in a phase II trial of pomalidomide–dexamethasone in 28 AL amyloidosis patients who were previously exposed to bortezomib, alkylators, and other immunomodulatory drugs. In a dose-escalation phase, three patients received 2 mg pomalidomide/d, with no dose-limiting toxicity and the remaining patients received 4 mg/d. Pomalidomide was administered continuously, and dexamethasone was given once per week at doses of 20 or 40 mg. Fifteen patients experienced grade 3/4 AEs; the most common were fluid retention and infections. Hematologic response was observed in 68% of patients (VGPR or CR in 29%), as well as a gratifying OS. Median time to response was short with 1 month. This trial confirmed that pomalidomide–dexamethasone was a rapidly active regime and may prolong survival in responding, heavily pretreated patients with AL amyloidosis (Palladini et al. 2017).

Pomalidomide is not only a relevant treatment option for MM or AL amyloidosis. There are also several clinical trials in other entities, like soft tissue sarcoma, medulloblastoma, sickle cell anemia, Waldenstrom's macroglobulinemia, myelofibrosis, Kaposi sarcoma. In the future, these trials will hopefully elucidate, whether and to what extent pomalidomide is a profitable treatment option in these challenging to treat diseases.

5.4 Pomalidomide in Combination Schedules

The introduction of novel agents and their combination have generated major advances in MM. Nevertheless, their immediate use in first-line and subsequent therapies makes the treatment of subsequent relapses a challenge, since MM may remain incurable and patients will ultimately acquire resistance to prior agents. Once patients are no longer responsive to IMiDs and bortezomib, the prognosis is grave and new agents, respectively the approval and use of well tolerable triplet or quadruple therapies, are needed. Furthermore, there is a lack of new therapies for patients with high-risk cytogenetics and RI, for which pomalidomide is a promising option. Currently, there are 139 trials that include pomalidomide and which are registered at ClinicalTrials.gov: 103 (103/139 = 74%) of these involve MM patients (out of currently 2228 clinical trials for the treatment of MM: 103/2220 = 4.6%).

5.4.1 Pomalidomide–Proteasome Inhibitor–Dexamethasone (P-VD) Combination

The combination of pomalidomide, bortezomib, and low-dose dexamethasone (P-VD) has been evaluated in several phase I/II clinical trials for the treatment of RRMM patients. Lacy et al. reported the results from a phase I/II study evaluating the safety and efficacy of P-VD in 50 patients with RRMM. In the phase I trial involving $n = 9$ patients, dose level I doses of pomalidomide 4 mg on days 1–21, bortezomib 1.0 mg/m^2 (1.3 mg/m^2 in dose level 2) i.v. on days 1, 8, 15, and 22, and dexamethasone 40 mg on days 1, 8, 15, and 22 in 28-day cycles were given. In the phase II part, 41 patients were treated. The median age was 66 years and 51% were female. The median number of prior treatment lines was 3, 100% had received prior lenalidomide, 68% had received prior SCT, 17% had received thalidomide, 56% alkylators, 57% bortezomib, and 25% were high risk by Mayo Stratification for Myeloma And Risk-Adapted Therapy (mSMART). Confirmed response occurred in 34/42 (81%) evaluable patients, including 3 stringent complete responses (sCR), 5 CRs, 8 VGPRs, and 18 PR. Among 11 evaluable high-risk patients, 9 (82%) achieved confirmed response. Median PFS was 17.7 months. At median follow-up of 9 months, 72% of patients were progression-free, 96% of patients were alive, and 66% had remained on study (Lacy et al. 2014). Richardson et al. presented another multicenter, open-label, randomized phase III study (MM-007; OPTIMISMM) comparing P-VD to bortezomib/low-dose dexamethasone (VD) alone in RRMM patients (EHA, June 2016), and this study has completed recruitment and is expected to confirm highly promising results with more extended treatment periods, PFS, and possibly also OS with P-VD versus VD alone (Richardson et al. 2015).

Furthermore, the combination of pomalidomide, carfilzomib, and low-dose dexamethasone (PCfzD) is evaluated in several phase I/II clinical trials for the treatment of RRMM (Bringhen et al., Jakubowiak et al., Rosenbaum et al., Shah et al.). Dosing varied for the combination in these trials, ORR for this combination ranged from 64 to 84%, and median PFS ranged from 9.2 to 16.8 months (Bringhen et al. 2016; Jakubowiak et al. 2017; Shah et al. 2015).

The results of these trials verify the benefit of new treatment combinations involving pomalidomide in triplets; therefore, the approval of P-VD and PCfzD in RRMM is being anticipated.

5.4.2 Pomalidomide–Cyclophosphamide–Dexamethasone (PCycloD) Combination

The combination of pomalidomide with cyclophosphamide and steroid (dexamethasone or prednisone) is a promising option to improve efficacy and treatment response in RRMM patients. The aim of a study performed by Baz et al. was to assess the safety and efficacy of adding oral weekly cyclophosphamide to the standard treatment pom–dex. A dose-escalation phase I study was performed to determine the recommended phase II dose of cyclophosphamide in combination with pom–dex (arm A). This was followed by a randomized, multicenter phase II study enrolling patients with lenalidomide-refractory MM. Patients were randomized (1:1) to receive pomalidomide 4 mg on days 1–21 of a 28-day cycle in combination with weekly dexamethasone 40 mg (20 mg, if patients were > 75 years or unable to tolerate 40 mg weekly) (arm B) or pomalidomide, cyclophosphamide, and dexamethasone (PCycloD), using cyclophosphamide with 400 mg orally on days 1, 8, and 15 (arm C). The primary endpoint was ORR. Eighty patients were enrolled (10 in the phase I part and 70 randomized in the phase II part: 36 in arm B and 34 in arm C). The ORR in arm B and C was 38.9% (95% CI: 23–54.8%) versus 64.7% (95% CI: 48.6–80.8%), and the median PFS was 4.4 (95% CI, 2.3–5.7) and 9.5 months (95% CI, 4.6–14), respectively. Toxicity was predominantly hematologic, but not statistically higher in arm C. The combination of PCycloD results in substantially improved ORR and PFS as compared to pom–dex alone in patients with lenalidomide-refractory MM and thus should be considered to enhance responses and prolong progression (Baz et al. 2016).

5.4.3 Pomalidomide–Antibody–Dexamethasone Combination

In June 2017, the FDA approved the anti-CD38 antibody (Ab) daratumumab in combination with pomalidomide and dexamethasone for the treatment of MM patients, who had received at least two prior therapies, including lenalidomide and a PI. Relevant for the approval was the trial of Chari et al. in which daratumumab–pom–dex (Dara-PD) was evaluated in RRMM patients with two or more prior lines of therapy, who were refractory to their last treatment. Patients received daratumumab 16 mg/kg at the recommended dosing schedule, pomalidomide 4 mg daily for 21 days of each 28-day cycles, and dexamethasone 40 mg weekly. Safety was the primary endpoint. ORR and minimal residual disease (MRD) by next-generation sequencing were secondary endpoints. Patients ($n = 103$) received a median of four (range: 1–13) prior therapies; 76% received three or more prior therapies. The safety profile of Dara-PD was similar to that of pom–dex alone, with the exception of daratumumab-specific infusion-related reactions (IRR: 50%) and a higher incidence of neutropenia, although without an increase in infections. The ORR was 60% and was generally consistent across subgroups (58% in double-refractory patients). Among patients with a CR or better, 29% were MRD negative at a threshold of 10^{-5}. At a median follow-up of 13.1 months, the median PFS was 8.8 (95% CI: 4.6–15.4) months and median OS was 17.5 (95% CI: 13.3-not reached) months. The estimated 12-month survival rate was 66% (95% CI: 55.6–74.8).

Aside from increased neutropenia, the safety profile of Dara-PD was consistent with that of the individual therapies. Deep, durable responses were observed in heavily pretreated patients (Chari et al. 2017).

Likewise, there are several trials ongoing proving the value of adding antibodies like elotuzumab and nivolumab to pom–dex in triplets or in quadruple combinations (pom–dex plus PI and Ab or pom–dex plus two abs). These combinations might further enhance responses, PFS, and OS, enrich the options in the treatment of RRMM patients, and enhance the possibilities of patient-individualized therapy approaches.

6 Toxicity

The most common side effects of pomalidomide reported in clinical trials have been fatigue and asthenia, neutropenia, anemia, constipation, nausea, diarrhea, dyspnea, upper respiratory tract infections, back pain, and pyrexia. In the comparative analysis of six sequential phase II trials at Mayo in 345 patients receiving pomalidomide at doses of 2 or 4 mg/d, most common toxicities (grade ≥ 3) were neutropenia (31%), anemia (16%), thrombocytopenia (12%), pneumonia (8%), and fatigue (8%). Venous thromboembolism (VTE) was seen in ten patients (3%; Lacy et al. 2012). Moreover, a brief review on two patients who developed pulmonary toxicity related to pomalidomide was consistent with previously published reports on pulmonary toxicity related to thalidomide and lenalidomide. It was suggested that this very rare toxicity should readily be recognized by clinicians in patients with pulmonary complaints and no identifiable infectious source and that timely withdrawal of the medication leads to rapid resolution of symptoms without long-term sequelae (Geyer et al. 2011). In general, pomalidomide induces less aesthesia and neuropathy than thalidomide and is more likely to induce neutropenia than thalidomide, but this side effect is usually well manageable with dose reduction. Subsets of MM patients, who are sensitive to the myelosuppressive effect of lenalidomide and have trouble tolerating even low doses, may do well with pomalidomide, suggesting that its myelosuppressive effect is less pronounced. Skin rash which might be observed with lenalidomide (Wäsch et al. 2012) is rarely seen with pomalidomide (Lacy 2013).

Pomalidomide is approved by the FDA and EMA with a boxed warning alerting patients and health care professionals that the drug can cause embryo-fetal toxicity and VTE. Because of this embryo-fetal risk, pomalidomide is available only through a restricted distribution program called the POMALYST Risk Evaluation and Mitigation Strategy (REMS) program. Prescribers must be certified with the POMALYSTREMS program by enrolling and complying with the REMS requirements. Patients must sign a patient–physician agreement form and comply with the REMS requirements. Female patients of reproductive potential who are not pregnant must comply with the pregnancy testing and contraception requirements. Males must comply with contraception requirements. Pharmacies must be certified with the POMALYSTREMS program, must only dispense to patients, who are authorized to receive pomalidomide, and comply with REMS (requirements on http://www.fda.gov).

7 Drug Interactions

CYP1A2 and CYP3A4 were identified as the most important enzymes metabolizing IMiDs. Further, pomalidomide is a substrate of p-glycoprotein (p-gp). It is not to be expected that pomalidomide causes drug interactions by inhibiting or inducing P450-isoenzymes, if it is administered simultaneously with other substrates of CYP1A2 or CYP3A4. Furthermore, the concomitant application of ketoconazole (strong CYP3A4 and p-gp inhibitor) and carbamazepine (strong CYP3A4/5 inductor) showed no significant impact on the exposition of pomalidomide. Indeed, co-administration of strong inhibitors of CYP1A2 (e.g., fluvoxamine, ciprofloxacin, or enoxacin) increases the plasma levels of pomalidomide. If concomitant treatment is unavoidable, the dose of pomalidomide should be decreased by 50%. Cigarette smoking may reduce pomalidomide exposure via CYP1A2 induction. Therefore, patients should be advised that smoking may reduce the efficacy of pomalidomide (IMNOVID®: summary of product characteristics; Celgene, http://www.fachinfo. de; last revised: September 2016).

8 Summary and Perspectives

Although new agents have significantly improved the prognosis in MM, novel therapies are constantly needed. Pomalidomide is effective and well tolerated in patients with advanced, refractory MM and potentially provides an unmet clinical need in patients with previously treated MM. The use of pomalidomide and low-dose dexamethasone, and their combination with other active agents, warrants further clinical testing. Moreover, the response in cytogenetically high-risk patients (Richardson et al. 2012) and with organ impairment, such as RI (Ramasamy et al. 2015), is currently confounded by low patient numbers and needs to be further investigated.

References

Baz RC, Martin TG 3rd, Lin HY, Zhao X, Shain KH, Cho HJ, Wolf JL, Mahindra A, Chari A, Sullivan DM, Nardelli LA, Lau K, Alsina M, Jagannath S (2016) Randomized multicenter phase 2 study of pomalidomide, cyclophosphamide, and dexamethasone in relapsed refractory myeloma. Blood 127(21):2561–2568

Bringhen S, Magarotto V, Liberati M et al (2016) A multicenter, open label phase I/II study of carfilzomib, pomalidomide and dexamethasone in relapsed and/or refractory multiple myeloma (MM) patients [Oral]. In: Oral presented at: 58th annual meeting and exposition of the American Society of Hematology (ASH); December 3–6, 2016; San Diego, CA, USA

Chari A, Suvannasankha A, Fay JW, Arnulf B, Kaufman JL, Ifthikharuddin JJ, Weiss BM, Krishnan A, Lentzsch S, Comenzo R, Wang J, Nottage K, Chiu C, Khokhar NZ, Ahmadi T, Lonial S (2017) Daratumumab plus pomalidomide and dexamethasone in relapsed and/or refractory multiple myeloma. Blood 130(8):974–981

D'Amato R, Lentzsch S, Anderson KC, Rogers MS (2001) Mechanism of action of thalidomide and 3-aminothalidomide in multiple myeloma. Semin Oncol 28:597–601

Dimopoulos MA, Weisel KC, Song KW, Delforge M, Karlin L, Goldschmidt H, Moreau P, Banos A, Oriol A, Garderet L, Cavo M, Ivanova V, Alegre A, Martinez-Lopez J, Chen C, Spencer A, Knop S, Bahlis NJ, Renner C, Yu X, Hong K, Sternas L, Jacques C, Zaki MH, San Miguel JF (2015) Cytogenetics and long-term survival of patients with refractory or relapsed and refractory multiple myeloma treated with pomalidomide and low-dose dexamethasone. Haematologica 100(10):1327–1333

Geyer HL, Viggiano RW, Lacy MQ, Witzig TE, Leslie KO, Mikhael JR, Stewart K (2011) Acute lung toxicity related to pomalidomide. Chest 140:529–533

Gandhi AK, Kang J, Havens CG et al (2014) Immunomodulatory agents lenalidomide and pomalidomide co-stimulate T cells by inducing degradation of T cell repressors Ikaros and Aiolos via modulation of the E3 ubiquitin ligase complex CRL4(CRBN.). Br J Haematol 164 (6):811–821

Görgün G, Calabrese E, Soydan E, Hideshima T, Perrone G, Bandi M, Cirstea D, Santo L, Hu Y, Tai YT, Nahar S, Mimura N, Fabre C, Raje N, Munshi N, Richardson P, Anderson KC (2010) Immunomodulatory effects of lenalidomide and pomalidomide on interaction of tumor and bone marrow accessory cells in multiple myeloma. Blood 116:3227–3237

IMNOVID®: summary of product characteristics; Celgene, http://www.fachinfo.de; last revised September 2016

Jakubowiak AJ, Rosenbaum CA, Stephens L et al (2017) Final results of phase (PH) 1/2 study of carfilzomib; pomalidomide; and dexamethasone (KPD) in patients (PTS) with relapsed/refractory multiple myeloma (RRMM): a multi-center MMRC study [Meeting Abstract]. In: Presented at: 22nd Congress of the European Hematology Association (EHA), June 22–25, 2017, Madrid, Spain. Poster#P680

Kortüm KM, Zhu YX, Shi CX, Jedlowski P, Stewart AK (2015) Cereblon binding molecules in multiple myeloma. Blood Rev 29:329–334

Lacy MQ, Kumar SK, LaPlant BR, Laumann K, Gertz MA, Hayman SR, Buadi FK, Dispenzieri A, Lust JA, Russell S, Dingli D, Zeldenrust SR, Fonseca R, Bergsagel PL, Stewart K, Roy V, Sher T, Chanan-Khan A, Reeder C, Rajkumar SV, Mikhael JR (2012) Pomalidomide plus low-dose dexamethasone (Pom/Dex) in relapsed myeloma: long term follow up and factors predicting outcome in 345 patients. Blood 120:201

Lacy MQ (2013) "IM iD" eally treating multiple myeloma. Blood 121:1926–1928

Lacy MQ, LaPlant BR, Laumann KM et al (2014) Pomalidomide, bortezomib, and dexamethasone for patients with relapsed lenalidomide refractory multiple myeloma. ASH Annual Meeting. Abstract 304. Presented December 8, 2014

Leleu X, Attal M, Arnulf B, Moreau P, Traulle C, Marit G, Mathiot C, Petillon MO, Macro M, Roussel M, Pegourie B, Kolb B, Stoppa AM, Hennache B, Bréchignac S, Meuleman N, Thielemans B, Garderet L, Royer B, Hulin C, Benboubker L, Decaux O, Escoffre-Barbe M, Michallet M, Caillot D, Fermand JP, Avet-Loiseau H, Facon T (2013) Pomalidomide plus low-dose dexamethasone is active and well tolerated in bortezomib and lenalidomide-refractory multiple myeloma: Intergroupe Francophone du Myélome 2009–02. Blood 121:1968–1975

Lopez-Girona A, Mendy D, Ito T et al (2012) Cereblon is a direct protein target for immunomodulatory and antiproliferative activities of lenalidomide and pomalidomide. Leukemia 26(11):2326–2335

Matous J, Siegel DS, Lonial S et al (2014) MM-008: a phase 1 trial evaluating pharmacokinetics and tolerability of pomalidomide + low-dose dexamethasone (LoDEX) in patients (Pts) with relapsed or refractory multiple myeloma and renal impairment [poster]. In: Poster presented at: 56th annual meeting and exposition of the American Society of hematology (ASH); December 6–9, 2014; San Francisco, CA, USA

Mitsiades CS, Chen-Kiang S (2013) Immunomodulation as a therapeutic strategy in the treatment of multiple myeloma. Crit Rev Oncol Hematol 88(Suppl 1):S5–S13

Palladini G, Milani P, Foli A, Basset M, Russo F, Perlini S, Merlini G (2017) A phase 2 trial of pomalidomide and dexamethasone rescue treatment in patients with AL amyloidosis. Blood 129(15):2120–2123

Ramasamy K, Dimopoulos MA, Van de Donk NWCJ, et al. (2015) Safety of treatment (Tx) with pomalidomide (POM) and low-dose dexamethasone (LoDEX) in patients (Pts) with relapsed or refractory multiple myeloma (RRMM) and renal impairment (RI), including those on dialysis [meeting abstract]. In: Presented at: 57th annual meeting and exposition of the American Society of Hematology (ASH); December 5–8, 2015, Orlando FL, USA. Abstract# 374

Raza S, Safyan RA, Lentzsch S (2017) Immunomodulatory drugs (IMiDs) in multiple myeloma. Curr Cancer Drug Targets 17(9):846–857

Ríos-Tamayo R, Martín-García A, Alarcón-Payer C, Sánchez-Rodríguez D, del Valle Díaz de la Guardia AM, García Collado CG, Jiménez Morales A, Jurado Chacón M, Cabeza Barrera J (2017) Pomalidomide in the treatment of multiple myeloma: design, development and place in therapy. Drug Des Devel Ther 11:2399–2408

Richardson P, Baz R et al (2009) A phase 1/2 multi-center, randomized, open label dose escalation study to determine the maximum tolerated dose, safety and efficacy of pomalidomide alone or in combination with low-dose dexamethasone in patients with relapsed and refractory multiple myeloma who have received prior treatment that includes lenalidomide and bortezomib. Blood 114:301

Richardson P, Jakubowiak A, Bahlis NJ, Siegel DS, Chen CI, Chen M, Zaki M, Larkins G, Anderson K (2012) Treatment outcomes with pomalidomide (POM) in combination with low-dose dexamethasone (LoDex) in patients with relapsed and refractory multiple myeloma (RRMM) and del(17p13) and/or t(4;14) (p16;q32) cytogenetic abnormalities who have received prior therapy with lenalidomide (LEN) and bortezomib (BORT). Blood 120:4053

Richardson PG, Siegel D, Baz R, Kelley SL, Munshi NC, Laubach J, Sullivan D, Alsina M, Schlossman R, Ghobrial IM, Doss D, Loughney N, McBride L, Bilotti E, Anand P, Nardelli L, Wear S, Larkins G, Chen M, Zaki MH, Jacques C, Anderson KC (2013) Phase 1 study of pomalidomide MTD, safety, and efficacy in patients with refractory multiple myeloma who have received lenalidomide and bortezomib. Blood 121:1961–1967

Richardson PG, Bensmaine A, Doerr T, Wang J, Zaki M (2015) MM-007: a phase 3 trial comparing the efficacy and safety of pomalidomide (POM) bortezomib (BORT) and low-dose-dexamethasone (LoDEX[PVD]) versus BORT and LoDEX (VD) in subjects with relapsed or refractory multiple myeloma (RRMM) [Poster]. In: Poster presented at: 2015 annual meeting of the American Society of Clinical Oncology (ASCO); May 29–June 2, 2015; Chicago, IL USA

San Miguel J, Weisel K, Moreau P et al (2013) Pomalidomide plus low-dose dexamethasone versus high-dose dexamethasone alone for patients with relapsed and refractory multiple myeloma (MM-003): a randomised, open-label, phase 3 trial. Lancet Oncol 14(11):1055–1066

Schuster SR, Kortuem KM, Zhu YX, Braggio E, Shi C-X, Bruins L, Schmidt J, Ahmann G, Kumar SK, Rajkumar SV, Mikhael JR, Roy V, LaPlant BR, Laumann K, Barlogie B, Shaughnessy JD Jr, Fonseca R, Bergsagel L, Lacy MQ, Stewart K (2012) Cereblon expression predicts response, progression free and overall survival after pomalidomide and dexamethasone therapy in multiple myeloma. Blood 120:194

Sehgal K, Das R, Zhang L, Verma R, Deng Y, Kocoglu M, Vasquez J, Koduru S, Ren Y, Wang M, Couto S, Breider M, Hansel D, Seropian S, Cooper D, Thakurta A, Yao X, Dhodapkar KM, Dhodapkar MV (2015) Clinical and pharmacodynamic analysis of pomalidomide dosing strategies in myeloma: impact of immune activation and cereblon targets. Blood 125(26):4042–4051

Shah JJ, Stadtmauer EA, Abonour R, Cohen AD, Bensinger WI, Gasparetto C, Kaufman JL, Lentzsch S, Vogl DT, Gomes CL, Pascucci N, Smith DD, Orlowski RZ, Durie BG (2015) Carfilzomib, pomalidomide, and dexamethasone for relapsed or refractory myeloma. Blood 126(20):2284–2290

Siegel DS, Richardson PG, Baz R, Chen M, Zaki M, Anderson KC (2012) Pomalidomide with low-dose dexamethasone in patients with relapsed and refractory multiple myeloma: impact of renal function on patient outcomes [Poster]. In: Poster presented at: 54th annual meeting of the American Society of Hematology (ASH); December 8–11, 2012, Atlanta, GA, USA

Sonneveld P, Avet-Loiseau H, Lonial S, Usmani S, Siegel D, Anderson KC, Chng WJ, Moreau P, Attal M, Kyle RA, Caers J, Hillengass J, San Miguel J, van de Donk NW, Einsele H, Bladé J, Durie BG, Goldschmidt H, Mateos MV, Palumbo A, Orlowski R (2016) Treatment of multiple myeloma with high-risk cytogenetics: a consensus of the International Myeloma Working Group. Blood 127(24):2955–2962

Waldschmidt JM, Simon A, Wider D, Müller SJ, Follo M, Ihorst G, Decker S, Lorenz J, Chatterjee M, Azab AK, Duyster J, Wäsch R, Engelhardt M (2017) CXCL12 and CXCR7 are relevant targets to reverse cell adhesion-mediated drug resistance in multiple myeloma. Br J Haematol 179(1):36–49

Wäsch R, Jakob T, Technau K, Finke J, Engelhardt M (2012) Stevens-Johnson/toxic epidermal necrolysis overlap syndrome following lenalidomide treatment for multiple myeloma relapse after allogeneic transplantation. Ann Hematol 91:287–289

Zhu YX, Braggio E, Shi CX, Bruins LA, Schmidt JE, Van Wier S, Chang XB, Bjorklund CC, Fonseca R, Bergsagel PL, Orlowski RZ, Stewart AK (2011) Cereblon expression is required for the antimyeloma activity of lenalidomide and pomalidomide. Blood 118:4771–4779

Zhu YX, Kortuem KM, Stewart AK (2013) Molecular mechanism of action of immune-modulatory drugs thalidomide, lenalidomide and pomalidomide in multiple myeloma. Leuk Lymphoma 54(4):683–687

Enasidenib

Alwin Krämer and Tilmann Bochtler

Contents

A. Krämer (✉) · T. Bochtler
Clinical Cooperation Unit Molecular Hematology/Oncology, German Cancer Research Center
(DKFZ), University of Heidelberg, Heidelberg, Germany
e-mail: a.kraemer@dkfz.de

A. Krämer · T. Bochtler
Department of Internal Medicine V, University of Heidelberg, Heidelberg, Germany

© Springer International Publishing AG, part of Springer Nature 2018
U. M. Martens (ed.), *Small Molecules in Hematology*, Recent Results
in Cancer Research 211, https://doi.org/10.1007/978-3-319-91439-8_9

Abstract

Enasidenib is an orally available, selective, potent, small molecule inhibitor of mutant isocitrate dehydrogenase 2 (IDH2). Neomorphic mutations in IDH2 are frequently found in both hematologic malignancies and solid tumors and lead to the production of the oncometabolite (R)-2-hydroxyglutarate. Increased levels of (R)-2-hydroxyglutarate cause histone and DNA hypermethylation associated with blocked differentiation and tumorigenesis. In PDX mice transplanted with human IDH2-mutant acute myeloid leukemia cells, enasidenib treatment led to normalization of (R)-2-hydroxyglutarate serum levels, differentiation of leukemic blasts and increased survival. Early clinical data in patients with relapsed/refractory IDH2-mutant acute myeloid leukemia show that enasidenib is well tolerated and induces durable complete remissions as a single agent in about 20% of cases. One notable drug-related adverse effect is differentiation syndrome. On the basis of these results the compound has recently been approved for the treatment of relapsed/refractory IDH2-mutant acute myeloid leukemia in the USA. Although no data are available yet, clinical trials on the treatment of patients with several types of IDH2-mutant solid tumors including gliomas, chondrosarcomas and cholangiocarcinomas are currently being performed.

Keywords

Isocitrate dehydrogenase · IDH · Acute myeloid leukemia · AML
Glioblastoma · Ketoglutarate · 2-hydroxyglutarate · Hypermethylation
AG-221

1   Introduction

Neomorphic somatic mutations in both isocitrate dehydrogenase 1 (IDH1) and IDH2 are frequently found in several types of human malignancies including glioma (Parsons et al. 2008; Yan et al. 2009), acute myeloid leukemia (AML) (Mardis et al. 2009), myeloproliferative neoplasms (Green and Beer 2010), myelodysplastic syndromes (Thol et al. 2010a, b), chondrosarcomas (Amary et al. 2011), cholangiocarcinomas (Borger et al. 2012), lymphomas (Cairns et al. 2012; Odejide et al. 2014), melanomas (Shibata et al. 2011), and thyroid cancer (Murugan et al. 2010). Whereas IDH1 mutations are more frequent in solid tumors, mutations in IDH2 prevail in hematological malignancies, with about 12% of patients with AML carrying an IDH2 mutation (Krämer and Heuser 2017). Mutations in IDH2 almost exclusively occur at arginine 172 or arginine 140 (Paschka et al. 2010; Thol et al. 2010a, b) and affect the enzymes active site, where IDH2 substrates isocitrate and $NADP^+$ bind (Gross et al. 2010; Sellner et al. 2010; Ward et al. 2010).

IDH1 and IDH2 catalyze the oxidative decarboxylation of isocitrate to α-ketoglutarate. Mutant IDH loses this normal activity with concomitant gain of a neomorphic function leading to the conversion of α-ketoglutarate to the oncometabolite (R)-2-hydroxyglutarate. Increased levels of (R)-2-hydroxyglutarate competitively inhibit α-ketoglutarate-dependent enzymes, thereby inducing histone and DNA hypermethylation and a consecutive block in cellular differentiation promoting tumorigenesis (Figueroa et al. 2010; Losman et al. 2013; Lu et al. 2012). Consequently, levels of (R)-2-hydroxyglutarate are substantially increased in sera of patients with IDH-mutant AML (Balss et al. 2012, 2016; Chaturvedi et al. 2017; DiNardo et al. 2013; Fathi et al. 2012; Janin et al. 2014; Sellner et al. 2010).

2 Structure and Mechanism of Action (Ideally with IC50 Values of Targeted Kinases)

Enasidenib (former AG-221) or 2-methyl-1-((4-(6-(trifluoromethyl)-pyridin-2-yl)-6-((2-(trifluoromethyl)-pyridin-4-yl)amino)-1,3,5-triazin-2-yl)amino)propan-2-ol is an orally available, selective, potent, small molecule inhibitor of mutant IDH2 (Fig. 1). Somatic IDH2 mutations in human tumors are heterozygous. Because IDH2 forms homodimers, the mutant enzyme exists as a mixture of mutant homodimers and mutant–wildtype heterodimers, with the heterodimer producing (R)-2-hydroxyglutarate more efficiently than mutant homodimers (Pietrak et al. 2011). Co-crystallization of enasidenib with mutant IDH2 revealed that the inhibitor binds in an allosteric manner at the dimer interface (Wang et al. 2013). IC_{50} values for inhibition of IDH2-R140Q and IDH2-R172 K heterodimers were in the range of 0.11–0.31 μM in in vitro kinase assays and 0.01–0.53 μM in intact cells, depending on the cell lines used (Yen et al. 2017). For comparison, IC_{50} values for inhibition of the IDH2 wildtype homodimer, the IDH1 wildtype homodimer, and the IDH1-R132H heterodimer were 39.8, 1.1 and 77.6 μM in in vitro kinase assays. IC_{50} values for a panel of 25 unrelated kinases were all >10 μM.

Fig. 1 Chemical structure of enasidenib

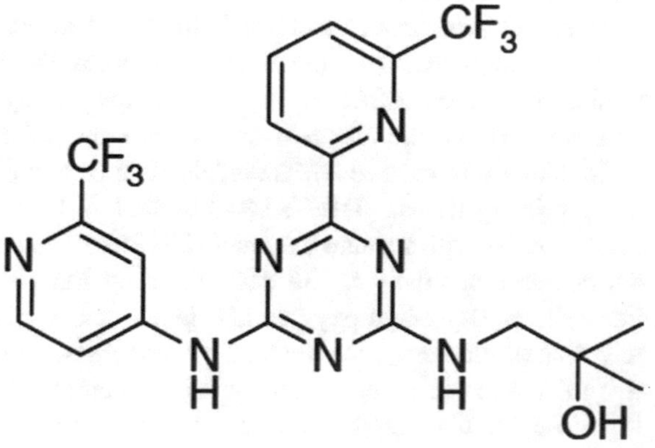

In cell lines and primary human AML cells, inhibition of mutant IDH2 by enasidenib reduced (R)-2-hydroxyglutarate levels and restored hematopoietic differentiation in vitro (Wang et al. 2013; Yen et al. 2017). Enasidenib also inhibited growth factor-independent proliferation and reversed histone H3 hypermethylation induced by expression of mutant IDH2-R140Q in TF-1 erythroleukemia cells (Yen et al. 2017). In contrast, the compound did not induce apoptosis in cell lines or primary AML cells. Accordingly, IDH2-mutant AML cells exposed to enasidenib ex vivo produce mature, functioning neutrophils with conserved mutant IDH2 allele frequency, indicating that they are derived from maturation of leukemic blasts (Yen et al. 2017).

3 Preclinical Data

Preclinical data in mice are available for IDH2-mutant AML and glioblastoma cells. In a subcutaneous mouse xenograft model using glioblastoma U87MG cells engineered to express mutant IDH2-R140Q, enasidenib led to maximum (R)-2-hydroxyglutarate reduction 12 h after dosing of 96.2% in plasma and 97.1% in tumors at 50 mg/kg (Yen et al. 2017).

In mice competitively transplanted with normal bone marrow and bone marrow cells from transgenic animals carrying mutant IDH2-R140Q and FLT3-ITD alleles, 100 mg/kg enasidenib twice daily markedly reduced (R)-2-hydroxyglutarate serum levels as well, attenuated aberrant DNA methylation, and induced differentiation of leukemic cells in vivo, again—similar to the ex vivo situation—without a major reduction in mutant allele burden (Shih et al. 2014, 2017). Importantly and in contrast to these results, combined inhibition of IDH2-R140Q and FLT3-ITD with enasidenib and quizartinib (AC220) led to more profound demethylation, a reduction in mutant allele burden and consequent recovery of non-malignant hematopoiesis (Shih et al. 2017).

In mice transplanted with murine hematopoietic cells co-transduced with IDH2-R140Q, NRAS-G12D, and DNMT3A-R882H, 40 mg/kg enasidenib twice daily reduced (R)-2-hydroxyglutarate serum levels by >95%, decreased disease burden, and significantly increased survival (Kats et al. 2017). With the exception of an initial increase in the number of leukemic cells in the peripheral blood reminiscent of differentiation syndrome, the dosing schedule was well tolerated with no obvious side effects over a 4-week treatment period.

In addition to genetic AML models, data from patient-derived xenograft models using primary human IDH2-R140Q-mutant AML cells have been reported. When these animals with sustained human CD45+ cell counts were treated with 30 mg/kg enasidenib twice daily for 38 days, the drug caused near normal serum as well as intracellular (R)-2-hydroxyglutarate levels and surface expression of several differentiation markers, accompanied by a decrease in human CD45+ blast counts in several tissues (Yen et al. 2017). When compared to vehicle or treatment with low-dose Ara-C (2 mg/kg given for 5 days), 45 mg/kg once daily enasidenib led to a statistically significant survival advantage, again accompanied by reductions in (R)-2-hydroxyglutarate levels and cell differentiation but constant mutant IDH2-R140Q allele frequencies (Yen et al. 2017). As lower drug doses not associated with a survival benefit did not cause increased expression of differentiation markers, onset of differentiation seems to be key to survival of mice treated with enasidenib.

4 Clinical Data

Clinical data for inhibition of mutant IDH2 with enasidenib are currently only available for patients with hematological malignancies. In a single first-in-human phase I/II trial, maximum tolerated dose (MTD), pharmacokinetics, pharmacodynamics, safety, and clinical activity of enasidenib have recently been reported in 239 patients with advanced IDH2-mutant myeloid malignancies (NCT01915498; Stein et al. 2017a). One hundred and thirteen patients received increasing doses of enasidenib in the dose-escalation phase, and 126 patients were treated with a fixed dose of 100 mg enasidenib once daily in the expansion part of the trial. Enasidenib (100 mg) once daily dosing was chosen because of robust steady-state drug concentrations, median plasma (R)-2-hydroxyglutarate level suppression of 93, 28, and 90.4% for IDH2-R140Q, IDH2-R172K, and all mutations, respectively, and clinical activity. After multiple doses, enasidenib demonstrated an extended half-life of approximately 137 h.

Of the total cohort of 239 patients, the largest subgroup of 176 individuals suffered from relapsed or refractory AML. The remaining 63 patients suffered from refractory anemia with excess blasts. The median age of the AML cohort and the total study population was 67 (range 19–100) and 70 (range 19–100) years, respectively. Seventy-five percent of all patients had IDH2-R140 and 24% had IDH2-R172 mutations. Of the 176 relapsed/refractory AML patients, 94 patients (53%) had received two or more prior chemotherapy regimens. Overall response rate (ORR) and complete remission rate for patients with relapsed/refractory AML in this study were 40.3 and 19.3%. ORR for IDH2-R140- and IDH2-R172-mutant patients was 35.4 and 53.3%, while rates of complete remission were 17.7 and 24.4%, respectively, suggesting equivalent clinical responses of the two mutation types to enasidenib treatment despite a more variable extent of (R)-2-hydroxyglutarate suppression in IDH2-R170-mutant AML. Accordingly, the extent of (R)-2-hydroxyglutarate serum level suppression did not correlate with clinical response. Ten percent of the patients proceeded to allogeneic stem cell transplantation. In 48.3% of patients, the best outcome after a median of four enasidenib treatment cycles was stable disease. Some of these stable disease patients in addition to a subset of patients with partial remission experienced restoration of normal hematopoiesis with normalization of platelet and neutrophil counts (Stein 2016; Stein et al. 2017a). In accordance with preclinical data, remissions were a consequence of differentiation rather than induction of cell death and may thereby explain the lower frequency of infections in patients responding to enasidenib treatment (Amatangelo et al. 2017) as well as hematopoietic recovery occurring typically without intervening bone marrow aplasia or hypoplasia (Stein et al. 2017a).

In contrast to standard chemotherapy but similar to hypomethylating agents, delayed responses did occur several months after enasidenib initiation in several patients. Median time to first response was 1.9 months. In the absence of disease progression, patients should therefore receive multiple enasidenib treatment cycles before concluding refractoriness to the compound. Also, transiently increased blast counts after enasidenib initiation have been noted that did not per se signal disease progression (Döhner et al. 2017).

At AML diagnosis, the variant allele frequency (VAF) of IDH2 mutations was highly variable, ranging from low-level subclonality to full heterozygous clonality. Notably, no correlation between mutant IDH2 VAF at diagnosis and response to enasidenib was found (Amatangelo et al. 2017). With regard to changes in mutant IDH2 VAF from diagnosis to best response, the majority of patients did not show a significant decrease in VAF irrespective of clinical response, fitting to induction of differentiation as major mechanism of enasidenib action as described above (Amatangelo et al. 2017; Stein et al. 2017a). Nevertheless, in a subset of patients molecular remissions were achieved with mutant IDH2 allele burden becoming undetectable with response. However, no significant difference in event-free survival was observed between patients achieving molecular remissions and patients in complete hematologic remission without molecular remission (Amatangelo et al. 2017). Co-occurring mutations in NRAS and other MAPK pathway components were associated with primary resistance to mIDH2 inhibition by enasidenib.

Median overall survival among patients with IDH2-mutated relapsed/refractory AML in this trial was 9.3 months, while patients attaining partial or complete remission achieved a median survival of 19.7 months. Median event-free survival duration was 6.4 months (Stein et al. 2017a).

In a recent subgroup analysis of the trial, both response rates and survival times for 37 patients older than 60 years with previously untreated mIDH2 AML were similar as compared with the total study population (Pollyea et al. 2017). ORR was 37.8% with a CR rate of 19%. Median overall survival among all 37 patients and for responding patients was 10.4 and 19.8 months, respectively.

In addition to enasidenib monotherapy, initial phase I results on the combination of enasidenib with either azacitidine or standard induction chemotherapy have been recently released. As a clinical rationale for combining enasidenib with azacitidine, both compounds reduce DNA methylation, azacitidine via inhibition of DNA methyltransferases, and enasidenib by suppressing (R)-2-hydroxyglutarate levels and thereby restoring the function of α-ketoglutarate-dependent TET family enzymes. Of six patients with newly diagnosed mIDH2 AML that have received azacitidine plus enasidenib 100 mg ($n = 3$) or 200 mg ($n = 3$), the ORR was 3/6 (50%) with 2 (33%) patients achieving CR (DiNardo et al. 2017). Thirty-eight patients with newly diagnosed mIDH2 AML (median age 63, range 32–76) received 100 mg enasidenib once daily combined with standard induction chemotherapy (daunorubicin 60 mg/m^2/day or idarubicin 12 mg/m^2/day × 3 days with cytarabine 200 mg/m^2/day × 7 days) (Stein et al. 2017b). After induction, patients received ≤ 4 cycles of consolidation chemotherapy while continuing the mIDH2 inhibitor. Patients were allowed to continue on maintenance enasidenib for ≤ 2 years from the start of induction. Among 37 efficacy-evaluable enasidenib-treated patients, a response of CR, CRi, or CRp was achieved in 12/18 (67%) patients with de novo AML and 11/19 (58%) patients with sAML. Fourteen patients received ≥ 1 cycle of consolidation therapy, and eight patients proceeded to HSCT.

Despite a median survival of about 20 months in patients who respond to enasidenib, most patients eventually relapse (Stein et al. 2017a). In contrast to targeted therapies with tyrosine kinase inhibitors, a recent study showed that of all 12 relapse samples studied, none harbored second site resistance mutations in IDH2 (Quek et al. 2017). Importantly, 2-hydroxyglutarate (2HG) levels remained suppressed in most patients after developing resistance, suggesting that enasidenib indeed remains effective in inhibiting mIDH2. Instead, persisting mIDH2 clones acquired additional mutations or aneuploidy as possible bypass pathways. Specifically, (i) acquisition of IDH1 codon R132 mutations which resulted in a rise in 2HG ($n = 2$), (ii) deletion of chromosome 7q ($n = 4$), (iii) gain of function mutations in genes implicated in cell proliferation (FLT3, CSF3R) ($n = 3$), and (iv) mutations in hematopoietic transcription factors (GATA2, RUNX1) ($n = 2$) were found to have evolved in mIDH2 subclones at relapse as potential resistance conferring mechanisms.

5 Toxicity

In the above phase I/II in mIDH2 relapsed/refractory AML patients, enasidenib was well tolerated, and the MTD was not reached at a dose of 650 mg once per day (Stein et al. 2017a). Eighty-two percent of patients experienced treatment-related adverse events, the most common ones being indirect hyperbilirubinemia and nausea. Enasidenib-related grade 3–4 adverse events occurred in 41% of the patients, most frequently indirect hyperbilirubinemia and differentiation syndrome. The most common treatment-related serious adverse events (TEAEs) were differentiation syndrome (8%), leukocytosis (4%), tumor lysis syndrome (3%), nausea (2%), and hyperbilirubinemia (2%). A total of 18 patients developed serious differentiation syndrome with a median time to onset of 48 days and two deaths. In the majority of patients, differentiation syndrome was manageable with systemic corticosteroids but required enasidenib dosing interruption in 10/23 patients. Leukocytosis can be treated by concomitant application of hydroxyurea. As described above already, enasidenib seems not to cause bone marrow aplasia and associated severe infections as the drug leads to myeloid differentiation rather than cell death. Accordingly, enasidenib-related grade 3–4 hematologic adverse events (10%) and infections (1%) were infrequent.

In combination with azacitidine, the most frequent TEAEs were hyperbilirubinemia, nausea, cytopenia, and febrile neutropenia (DiNardo et al. 2017). Enasidenib combined with induction chemotherapy was generally well tolerated (Stein et al. 2017b). One dose-limiting toxicity was observed (persistent grade 4 thrombocytopenia). The most frequent grade ≥ 3 non-hematologic treatment-emergent adverse events during induction therapy were febrile neutropenia (63%), hypertension (11%), colitis (8%), and maculopapular rash (8%). Thirty- and 60-day mortality rates were 5% and 8%, respectively. Median times for ANC recovery to $\geq 500/\mu L$ were 34 days and 33 days for platelet recovery to >50,000/μL. In patients with sAML, there was an increased time to platelet count recovery (median 50 days).

6 Summary and Perspective

Enasidenib (former AG-221) is an orally available mutant IDH2 inhibitor that has been—on the basis of a single phase I/II clinical trial without a comparison group—approved in the USA for the treatment of adults with relapsed or refractory AML and an IDH2 mutation as detected by an FDA-approved test. Single-agent enasidenib treatment induces complete remissions in about 20% of patients with mIDH2 relapsed/refractory AML and is well tolerated. Mode of action is induction of differentiation, thereby avoiding bone marrow aplasia but also failing to induce molecular remissions in the majority of cases. Why about 60% of patients do not achieve remission despite the presence of an IDH2 mutation remains currently unclear. In contrast to tyrosine kinase inhibitor treatment, no secondary site IDH2 mutations were found to explain resistance development. Enasidenib is at various stages of clinical testing in other countries for AML, myelodysplastic syndromes, and solid tumors. A multicenter, randomized phase III trial of enasidenib versus conventional care regimens in older subjects with late stage AML harboring an IDH2 mutation (NCT02577406, IDHENTIFY) has been started and is ongoing. In light of the encouraging results in elderly, previously untreated patients, the Beat AML Master Trial (NCT03013998) examines the role of enasidenib monotherapy in this population. Combining enasidenib with chemotherapy and azacitidine in AML is currently analyzed in two additional clinical trials (NCT02677922; NCT02632708). Also, combining enasidenib with FLT3 inhibition might be rewarding, as suggested by preclinical data (Shih et al. 2017). Furthermore, a potential role for the compound in IDH2-mutated angioimmunoblastic T-cell lymphomas (AITL) and solid tumors is being evaluated (NCT02273739).

References

Amantangelo MD, Quek L, Shih A, Stein EM, Roshal M, David MD et al (2017) Enasidenib induces acute myeloid leukemia cell differentiation to promote clinical response. Blood 130:732–741

Amary MF, Bacsi K, Maggiani F, Damato S, Halai D, Berisha F et al (2011) IDH1 and IDH2 mutations are frequent events in central chondrosarcoma and central and periosteal chondromas but not in other mesenchymal tumours. J Pathol 224:334–343

Balss J, Pusch S, Beck AC, Herold-Mende C, Krämer A, Thiede C et al (2012) Enzymatic assay for quantitative analysis of (D)-2-hydroxyglutarate. Acta Neuropathol 124:883–891

Balss J, Thiede C, Bochtler T, Okun JG, Saadati M, Benner A et al (2016) Pretreatment D-2-hydroxyglutarate serum levels negatively impact on outcome in IDH1-mutated acute myeloid leukemia. Leukemia 30:782–788

Borger DR, Tanabe KK, Fan KC, Lopez HU, Fantin VR, Straley KS et al (2012) Frequent mutation of isocitrate dehydrogenase (IDH) 1 and IDH2 in cholangiocarcinoma identified through broad-based tumor genotyping. Oncologist 17:72–79

Cairns RA, Iqbal J, Lemonnier F, Kucuk C, de Leval L, Jais JP et al (2012) IDH2 mutations are frequent in angioimmunoblastic T-cell lymphoma. Blood 119:1901–1903

Chaturvedi A, Herbst L, Pusch S, Klett L, Goparaju R, Stichel D et al (2017) Pan-mutant-IDH1 inhibitor BAY1436032 is highly effective against human IDH1 mutant acute myeloid leukemia in vivo. Leukemia (Epub ahead of print). https://doi.org/10.1038/leu.2017.46

DiNardo CD, Propert KJ, Loren AW, Paietta E, Sun Z, Levine RL et al (2013) Serum 2-hydroxyglutarate levels predict isocitrate dehydrogenase mutations and clinical outcome in acute myeloid leukemia. Blood 121:4917–4924

DiNardo CD, Stein AS, Fathi AT, Montesinos P, Odenike O, Kantarjian HM et al (2017) Mutant isocitrate dehydrogenase (mIDH) inhibitors, enasidenib or ivosidenib, in combination with azacitidine (AZA): preliminary results of a phase 1b/2 study in patients with newly diagnosed acute myeloid leukemia (AML). ASH, Abstract, p 639

Döhner H, Estey E, Grimwade D et al (2017) Diagnosis and management of AML in adults: 2017 ELN recommendations from an international expert panel. Blood 129:424–447

Fathi AT, Sadrzadeh H, Borger DR, Ballen KK, Amrein PC, Attar EC et al (2012) Prospective serial evaluation of 2-hydroxyglutarate, during treatment of newly diagnosed acute myeloid leukemia, to assess disease activity and therapeutic response. Blood 120:4649–4652

Figueroa ME, Abdel-Wahab O, Lu C, Ward PS, Patel J, Shih A et al (2010) Leukemic IDH1 and IDH2 mutations result in a hypermethylation phenotype, disrupt TET2 function, and impair hematopoietic differentiation. Cancer Cell 18:553–567

Green A, Beer P (2010) Somatic mutations of IDH1 and IDH2 in the leukemic transformation of myeloproliferative neoplasms. N Engl J Med 362:369–370

Gross S, Cairns RA, Minden MD, Driggers EM, Bittinger MA, Jang HG et al (2010) Cancer-associated metabolite 2-hydroxyglutarate accumulates in acute myelogenous leukemia with isocitrate dehydrogenase 1 and 2 mutations. J Exp Med 207:339–344

Janin M, Mylonas E, Saada V, Micol JB, Renneville A, Quivoron C, Koscielny S et al (2014) Serum 2-hydroxyglutarate production in IDH1- and IDH2-mutated de novo acute myeloid leukemia: a study by the Acute Leukemia French Association group. J Clin Oncol 32:297–305

Kats LM, Vervoort SJ, Cole R, Rogers AJ, Gregory GP, Vidacs E et al (2017) A pharmacogenomic approach validates AG-221 as an effective and on-target therapy in IDH2 mutant AML. Leukemia 31:1466–1470

Krämer A, Heuser M (2017) IDH-Inhibitoren. Onkologe 23:632–638

Losman JA, Looper RE, Koivunen P, Lee S, Schneider RK, McMahon C et al (2013) (R)-2-hydroxyglutarate is sufficient to promote leukemogenesis and its effects are reversible. Science 339:1621–1625

Lu C, Ward PS, Kapoor GS, Rohle D, Turcan S, Abdel-Wahab O et al (2012) IDH mutation impairs histone demethylation and results in a block to cell differentiation. Nature 483:474–478

Mardis ER, Ding L, Dooling DJ, Larson DE, McLellan MD, Chen K et al (2009) Recurring mutations found by sequencing an acute myeloid leukemia genome. N Engl J Med 361: 1058–1066

Murugan AK, Bojdani E, Xing M (2010) Identification and functional characterization of isocitrate dehydrogenase 1 (IDH1) mutations in thyroid cancer. Biochem Biophys Res Commun 393:555–559

Odejide O, Weigert O, Lane AA, Toscano D, Lunning MA, Kopp N et al (2014) A targeted mutational landscape of angioimmunoblastic T-cell lymphoma. Blood 123:1293–1296

Parsons DW, Jones S, Zhang X, Lin JC, Leary RJ, Angenendt P et al (2008) An integrated genomic analysis of human glioblastoma multiforme. Science 321:1807–1812

Paschka P, Schlenk RF, Gaidzik VI, Habdank M, Kronke J, Bullinger L et al (2010) IDH1 and IDH2 mutations are frequent genetic alterations in acute myeloid leukemia and confer adverse prognosis in cytogenetically normal acute myeloid leukemia with NPM1 mutation without FLT3 internal tandem duplication. J Clin Oncol 28:3636–3643

Pietrak B, Zhao H, Qi H, Quinn C, Gao E, Boyer JG et al (2011) A tale of two subunits: how the neomorphic R132H IDH1 mutation enhances production of αHG. Biochemistry 50:4804–4812

Pollyea DA, Tallman MS, De Botton S, DiNardo CD, Kantarjian HM, Collins RH et al (2017) Enasidenib monotherapy is effective and well-tolerated in patients with previously untreated mutant IDH2 (mIDH2) acute myeloid leukemia (AML). ASH, Abstract, p 638

Quek L, David M, Kennedy A, Metzner M, Amatangelo M, Shih AH et al (2017) Clonal heterogeneity in differentiation response and resistance to the IDH2 inhibitor enasidenib in acute myeloid leukemia. ASH, Abstract, p 724

Sellner L, Capper D, Meyer J, Langhans CD, Hartog CM, Pfeifer H et al (2010) Increased levels of 2-hydroxyglutarate in AML patients with IDH1-R132H and IDH2-R140Q mutations. Eur J Haematol 85:457–459

Shibata T, Kokubu A, Miyamoto M, Sasajima Y, Yamazaki N (2011) Mutant IDH1 confersan in vivo growth in a melanoma cell line with BRAF mutation. Am J Pathol 178:1395–1402

Shih AH, Shank KR, Meydan C, Intlekofer AM, Ward P, Thompson CB et al (2014) AG-221, a small molecule mutant IDH2 inhibitor, remodels the epigenetic state of IDH2-mutant cells and induces alterations in self-renewal/differentiation in IDH2-mutant AML model in vivo. Blood 124 (abstract 437)

Shih AH, Meydan C, Shank K, Garrett-Bakelman FE, Ward P, Intlekofer AM et al (2017) Combination targeted therapy to disrupt aberrant oncogenic signaling and reverse epigenetic dysfunction in IDH2- and TET2-mutant acute myeloid leukemia. Cancer Discov 7:494–505

Stein EM (2016) Molecular pathways: IDH2 mutations—co-opting cellular metabolism for malignant transformation. Clin Cancer Res 22:16–19

Stein EM, DiNardo CD, Pollyea DA, Fathi AT, Roboz GJ, Altman JK et al (2017a) Enasidenib in mutant IDH2 relapsed or refractory acute myeloid leukemia. Blood 130:722–731

Stein EM, DiNardo CD, Mims AS, Savona MR, Pratz K, Stein AS et al (2017b) Ivosidenib or enasidenib combined with standard induction chemotherapy is well tolerated and active in patients with newly diagnosed AML with IDH1 or IDH2 mutation: initial results from a phase 1 trial. ASH, Abstract, p 726

Thol F, Damm F, Wagner K, Göhring G, Schlegelberger B, Hölzer D et al (2010a) Prognostic impact of IDH2 mutations in cytogenetically normal acute myeloid leukemia. Blood 116: 614–616

Thol F, Weissinger EM, Krauter J, Wagner K, Damm F, Wichmann M et al (2010b) IDH1mutations in patients with myelodysplastic syndromes are associated with an unfavorable prognosis. Haematologica 95:1668–1674

Wang F, Travins J, DeLaBarre B, Penard-Lacronique V, Schalm S, Hansen E et al (2013) Targeted inhibition of mutant IDH2 in leukemia cells induces cellular differentiation. Science 340: 622–626

Ward PS, Patel J, Wise DR, Abdel-Wahab O, Bennett BD, Coller HA et al (2010) The common feature of leukemia-associated IDH1 and IDH2 mutations is a neomorphic enzyme activity converting alpha-ketoglutarate to 2-hydroxyglutarate. Cancer Cell 17:225–234

Yan H, Parsons DW, Jin G, McLendon R, Rasheed BA, Yuan W et al (2009) IDH1 and IDH2 mutations in gliomas. N Engl J Med 360:765–773

Yen K, Travins J, Wang F, David MD, Artin E, Straley K et al (2017) AG-221, a first-in-class therapy targeting acute myeloid leukemia harboring oncogenic IDH2 mutations. Cancer Discov 7:478–493

Midostaurin: A Multiple Tyrosine Kinases Inhibitor in Acute Myeloid Leukemia and Systemic Mastocytosis

Richard F. Schlenk and Sabine Kayser

Contents

R. F. Schlenk (✉)
NCT-Trial Center, German Cancer Research Center, Heidelberg, Germany
e-mail: richard.schlenk@nct-heidelberg.de

S. Kayser
Department of Internal Medicine V, University Hospital of Heidelberg, Heidelberg, Germany

S. Kayser
Clinical Cooperation Unit Molecular Hematology/Oncology, German Cancer Research
Center (DKFZ), University of Heidelberg, Heidelberg, Germany

© Springer International Publishing AG, part of Springer Nature 2018
U. M. Martens (ed.), *Small Molecules in Hematology*, Recent Results
in Cancer Research 211, https://doi.org/10.1007/978-3-319-91439-8_10

Abstract

Midostaurin (PKC412, Rydapt®) is an oral multiple tyrosine kinase inhibitor. Main targets are the kinase domain receptor, vascular endothelial-, platelet derived-, and fibroblast growth factor receptor, stem cell factor receptor c-KIT, as well as mutated and wild-type FLT3 kinases. Midostaurin was approved by the Food and Drug Administration (FDA) and the European Medical Agency (EMA) for acute myeloid leukemia with activating *FLT3* mutations in combination with intensive induction and consolidation therapy as well as aggressive systemic mastocytosis (ASM), systemic mastocytosis with associated hematological neoplasm (SM-AHN) or mast cell leukemia (MCL). Several clinical trials are active or are planned to further investigate the role of midostaurin in myeloid malignancies and mastocytosis.

Keywords

Multikinase inhibitor · AML with activating FLT3 mutations · Systemic mastocytosis

1 Introduction

Midostaurin (N-benzoyl-staurosporine, also known as PKC412 and CGP41251, Fig. 1) is an indolocarbazole and was initially developed as a protein kinase C (PKC) inhibitor (Fabbro et al. 2000; Propper et al. 2001; Andrejauskas-Buchdunger and Regenass 1992). During the drug development process, it has been identified as a multi-targeted tyrosine kinase inhibitor (TKI), with activity against a variety of kinases, including the kinase domain receptor (KDR, a type III receptor tyrosine kinase), vascular endothelial growth factor receptor 2 (VEGFR-2), platelet derived- (PDGFR), and fibroblast growth factor receptor (FGFR), stem cell factor receptor (c-KIT), as well as mutated and wild-type fms-related tyrosine (FLT3) kinases (Propper et al. 2001; Andrejauskas-Buchdunger and Regenass 1992; Weisberg et al. 2002). Midostaurin reversibly binds to the catalytic domain of these kinases and inhibits downstream signaling pathways resulting in growth arrest and enhanced apoptosis (Propper et al. 2001; Weisberg et al. 2002; Karaman et al. 2008). It has a broad anti-proliferative activity against various cell lines in vitro (Weisberg et al. 2002; Ikegami et al. 1995) and was able to reverse the P-glycoprotein-mediated multidrug resistance of tumor cells in vitro (Budworth et al. 1996; Utz et al. 1994). Exposure of cells to midostaurin in vitro resulted in a dose-dependent increase in the G2/M phase of the cell cycle arrest and increased polyploidy, apoptosis and enhanced sensitivity to ionizing radiation (Zaugg et al. 2001).

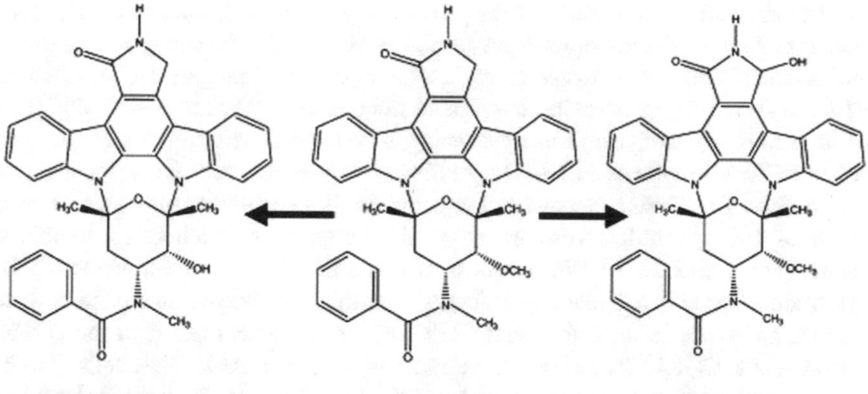

CGP62221   **PKC412**   **CGP52421**

Fig. 1 Chemical structure of midostaurin (PKC412) and its metabolites according to Propper et al. (2001). CGP6221 and CGP52421 are generated from PKC412 via P450 liver enzyme metabolism

2 FLT3 Mutations in AML

In AML, activating *FLT3* mutations are present in about 20–30% of newly diagnosed patients and are among the most frequent molecular abnormalities (Papaemmanuil et al. 2016; Nagel et al. 2017). FLT3 is a member of the class III receptor tyrosine kinase family and has an established role in normal growth and differentiation of hematopoietic precursor cells (Hannum et al. 1994). Physiologically, the FLT3 receptor dimerizes at the plasma membrane upon ligand binding, leading to a conformational change in its activation loop that allows adenosine triphosphate access to the FLT3 active site. This is followed by autophosphorylation and activation of numerous downstream signaling pathways (Griffith et al. 2004; Gu et al. 2011; Hayakawa et al. 2000). Mutations of the *FLT3* gene lead to ligand-independent activation and dysregulation of downstream pathways such as PI3 K/AKT, MAPK/ERK, and STAT5 (Gilliland and Griffin 2002; Rosnet et al. 1991; Meshinchi and Appelbaum 2009). These pathways inhibit apoptosis and differentiation and promote proliferation. Their high frequency in AML, location on the cell surface, and association with an adverse prognosis make *FLT3* mutations an attractive target (Kayser and Schlenk 2017; Kayser and Levis 2017).

3 Activity of Midostaurin in Cell Cultures and Murine Models

The antitumor activity of midostaurin was evaluated on murine and human tumor models (Ikegami et al. 1995). In a preclinical human tumor xenograft models, midostaurin 200 mg/kg once daily for 4 weeks showed a broad antitumor activity.

In addition, midostaurin inhibited the growth of gastric, colorectal, breast and lung cancer cell lines with inhibition rates of 58–80%. In 2002, Weisberg et al. showed that administration of midostaurin successfully prevented progressive leukemia in *FLT3*-ITD-expressing retroviral transfected mice models (Weisberg et al. 2002). In an in vitro pharmacodynamic analysis using 10 primary AML samples, which were either *FLT3* wild-type or *FLT3*-ITD positive ($n = 5$, each), one of the major active metabolites, CGP52421, was even more cytotoxic than midostaurin over a dose range of 100–500 nM, corresponding to the range over which FLT3 inhibition occurs (Levis et al. 2006). When midostaurin and CGP52421 were combined in the cytotoxic assay at levels that approximate what might be present in a patient, there was no difference in the effect with CGP52421 alone as compared to the combination. Thus, CGP52421 seemed to be more cytotoxic to AML blast cells than its parent compound, midostaurin, which might be related to its lower selectivity. Enhanced activity of midostaurin was reported with a histone deacetylase inhibitor (Bali et al. 2004) or with a heat-shock-protein 90 inhibitor (George et al. 2004) for AML cell lines. The combination of midostaurin with eight conventional antileukemic agents (cytarabine, doxorubicin, idarubicin, mitoxantrone, etoposide, 4-hydroperoxycyclophosphamide, methotrexate and vincristine) using three cell lines with *FLT3* mutations and five with *FLT3* wild-type revealed synergistic anti-proliferative activity of midostaurin with all agents studied except methotrexate for *FLT3*-mutated cell lines (Furukawa et al. 2007).

4 Pharmacokinetics and Drug Metabolism in Humans

Single-dose pharmacokinetic studies in six healthy volunteers (five men, one woman; age range, 22–51 years) demonstrated rapid oral absorption of midostaurin with time to maximum concentration at 1–3 h (He et al. 2017). The maximum plasma drug concentration and area under the concentration-time curve increased with dose, but under-proportionally, especially after long-term treatment. In humans, midostaurin is predominantly metabolized by CYP3A4 into two major active circulating metabolites: CGP62221 (due to O-demethylation) and CGP52421 (due to hydroxylation) (Propper et al. 2001). In plasma, midostaurin and its metabolites are highly protein-bound, ranging from 98 to 99%. Due to the high plasma protein binding, elimination of midostaurin from plasma is slow with a terminal half-life of about 20 h, and half-lifes of CGP62221 and CGP52421 with 33 and 495 h, respectively (He et al. 2017). The pharmacokinetic analysis from a phase-II PKC412 trial reported by Stone et al. suggested that, in most patients, PKC412 (and its active metabolite, CGP62221) reached micromolar concentrations during the first week of treatment with subsequent rapid decline (Stone et al. 2005). In contrast, the concentration of the other major metabolite, CGP52421, rose continuously through day 28 and remained relatively stable thereafter. Interestingly, the plasma concentration of CGP52421 at steady state was roughly sevenfold higher compared to that of either midostaurin or CGP62221. In addition, the metabolite CGP52421 accumulates in plasma during repetitive treatment cycles and its half-life is with >1 month longer as compared to midostaurin and CGP62221 (Levis et al. 2006). Major excretion of midostaurin and its metabolites is by feces, whereas urinary excretion plays only a minor role based on data of healthy adults (He et al. 2017).

5 Clinical Data

5.1 Midostaurin in Solid Tumors

A phase-I dose-escalation study in 33 patients with advanced solid malignancies was conducted with midostaurin given at doses ranging from 25 to 225 mg/day in combination with 5-fluorouracil 200 $mg/m^2/day$, given daily with a 21-day protracted continuous intravenously (i.v.) infusion repeated every 4 weeks (Eder et al. 2004). No significant toxicities were observed with doses up to 150 mg/day. Among nine patients treated with 225 mg/day of midostaurin, one experienced grade 3 fatigue and nausea, another developed grade 3 hyperglycemia, and three had grade 2 emesis and stomatitis, leading to early treatment discontinuation. However, response was rather disappointing with only two minor responses consisting of a 40–45% tumor reduction (gallbladder carcinoma and breast cancer, respectively). There was no evidence of a pharmacokinetic interaction between 5-fluorouracil and midostaurin.

In addition, midostaurin was evaluated in combination with gemcitabine and cisplatin in $n = 23$ patients with non-small-cell lung cancer (Monnerat et al. 2004). The schedule included escalating doses ranging from 25 to 150 mg/day of midostaurin, given every day of a 4-week cycle with cisplatin 100 mg/m^2 on day 2 and gemcitabine 1000 mg/m^2 on days 1, 8, and 15. Dose-limiting toxicities were observed at a dose of 150 mg/day, and the next lower dose tested of 50 mg/day was therefore considered as the recommended phase-II dose. Among 33 cycles in eight patients, toxicity consisted of grade 1–2 diarrhea (12.5%) and asthenia (50%) with only one patient experiencing grade 3 headache at this dose level. Again, response was only marginal (3 partial responses). In 2011, a single-arm, phase-I trial was initiated to evaluate the safety and efficacy of midostaurin 50 mg twice daily (bid) in combination with 5-fluorouracil and radiotherapy for 8 cycles in $n = 19$ patients with locally advanced rectal cancer in the USA, but so far, results are pending (ClinicalTrails.gov identifier: NCT01282502). Taken together, only little activity was identified for midostaurin in solid tumors.

5.2 Midostaurin in AML (Phase-I/II)

Data from a phase-I trial of midostaurin in a variety of solid tumors revealed that myelosuppression was not a dose-limiting toxicity at the recommended phase-II dose of 75 mg orally three times a day (Propper et al. 2001). Results from a phase-I trial with single-agent midostaurin in relapsed or refractory AML or older de novo AML patients with *FLT3* mutations, who were otherwise ineligible for chemotherapy, revealed a peripheral blast count decrease of at least 50% in the majority (70%) of the patients (Stone et al. 2005). Autophosphorylation of FLT3 in blast cells of responding patients was inhibited by >90% by day 3. Midostaurin was generally well tolerated; the most common toxicities were grade 1 and 2 nausea (48%), vomiting (41%), diarrhea (26%), and fatigue (7%). Although elimination of peripheral blast counts was extremely rapid in these patients, the median response duration was short (median, 13 weeks; range, 9-47 weeks). This early progression was associated with a 50–75% decrease of midostaurin plasma levels by day 28 due to autoinduction of its own metabolism via CYP3A4. In addition, in an index AML patient, a new drug-resistant *FLT3* mutation in the tyrosine kinase domain (TKD) has been described (Heidel et al. 2006). Therefore, both, pharmacokinetic mechanisms and appearance of resistance mutations may contribute to a short duration of the response with midostaurin as single agent. Thus, combination of midostaurin with standard chemotherapy in AML patients was a logic consequence (Stone et al. 2012). In this trial, midostaurin has been evaluated in a phase-I/II study in combination with standard induction chemotherapy with daunorubicin and cytarabine as well as consolidation with high-dose cytarabine in first line, *FLT3*-mutated but also in *FLT3* wild-type patients younger than 61 years (Stone et al. 2012). Midostaurin in combination with intensive induction chemotherapy was evaluated in different schedules, concomitantly versus sequential as well as continuously versus on/off. Initially, Midostaurin 100 mg twice daily in combination with chemotherapy was administered on either a concomitant dose schedule starting on day 1 of a 28-day cycle or sequentially starting on day 8. After the first 14 patients, prolonged exposure was deemed too toxic and the study was amended to limit treatment to 14 days per chemotherapy course (days 1–7 and 15–21 of the concomitant schedule; days 8–21 of the sequential schedule). Given intolerance of the 14-day-per-cycle exposure to midostaurin 100 mg twice daily, the study was again amended to reduce the dose of midostaurin to 50 mg twice daily in both the 14-day concomitantly and sequentially schedules. Tolerability improved for patients who received midostaurin 50 mg twice daily for 14 days per cycle in both the concomitant and sequential arms. The sequential schedule was finally chosen for further evaluation based (i) on the slightly higher degree of tolerability in the sequential arm, (ii) the fact that a pharmacokinetic interaction between midostaurin and daunorubicin could not be excluded, and (iii) results from other studies showing a possible antagonism if a FLT3 inhibitor was given before chemotherapy (Levis et al. 2004). With this dose schedule, an overall complete remission (CR) rate of 80% (CR rate in 74% of the *FLT3*-wild-type patients and in 92% of the *FLT3*-mutated patients) was achieved. Together with the promising overall survival (OS) data in patients with *FLT3*-mutated AML of 85 and 62% at one and two years, respectively, these encouraging results provided rational for the subsequent randomized phase-III trial in *FLT3*-mutated AML (CALGB 10603/RATIFY) (Stone et al. 2017).

So far not addressed was the optimal duration of TKI therapy. Intermittent dosing (e.g., from day 8 to 21) does not lead to continuous target inhibition. In parallel, FLT3 ligand (FL) levels were shown to increase dramatically following intensive chemotherapy and gradually with each course of chemotherapy (Sato et al. 2011). High FL levels upward shifted the cytotoxicity IC50 of FLT3 inhibitors by twofold–fourfold. Thus, FL upregulation may be an important driver of resistance, in particular when the inhibitor is given intermittently.

A still ongoing phase-II trial in adult AML patients (≥ 18 and ≤ 70 years) with *FLT3*-ITD evaluating midostaurin in combination with intensive induction-, consolidation-including allogeneic hematopoietic cell transplantation (HCT) and maintenance therapy with single-agent midostaurin was initiated in June 2012. All patients were intended to receive consolidation therapy in a prioritized manner consisting of either allogeneic HCT from matched related or unrelated donor as first priority or high-dose cytarabine (HiDAC, age-adapted dosing) as second priority. Both regimens include a one-year maintenance of midostaurin, starting at the earliest at day 30 and at the latest day 100 after allogeneic HCT, or in case of HiDAC consolidation throughout consolidation followed directly by maintenance therapy. After recruitment of $n = 147$ patients, the study was amended including a sample size increase to 284 patients and a dose reduction of sevenfold based on the lower bound of the confidence interval of the ratio (area under the curve) midostaurin with ketoconazole/AUC midostaurin without ketoconazole) was implemented (Dutreix et al. 2013) in case of co-medication with strong CYP3A4 inhibitors (e.g., posaconazole). Median age was 54 years (range, 18–70 years). CR rate after double induction therapy was 76%, regardless of age. Within this trial, 146 patients received an allogeneic HCT. The cumulative incidence of relapse (CIR) and death after transplant were 13% and 16% without differences between younger and older patients ($p = 0.97$, $p = 0.41$, respectively). CIR in patients starting maintenance therapy was 20% one year after start of maintenance without difference between allogeneic HCT and HiDAC ($p = 0.99$). In addition, no difference in CIR was identified in patients after consolidation with allogeneic HCT or HiDAC according to dose reduction of midostaurin during first induction therapy ($p = 0.43$, $p = 0.98$, respectively). Median OS was 25 months without any difference according to age group (younger patients, 18–60 years, 26 months; older patients, 61–70 years, 23 months; $p = 0.15$). The final results of this trial are currently pending (ClinicalTrials.gov identifier: NCT01477606) (Schlenk et al. 2016).

5.3 Midostaurin in AML (Phase-III)

Recently, the pivotal large international multicenter randomized double-blinded phase-III trial (CALGB 10603, RATIFY, clinicaltrials.gov: NCT00651261) investigating the efficacy of midostaurin versus placebo as adjunct to conventional chemotherapy in young adult (18–59 years) patients with *FLT3*-mutated AML was published (Stone et al. 2017). Within the screening period, *FLT3* mutations (including *FLT3*-ITD and *FLT3*-TKD mutation) were determined centrally prior to enrollment into the clinical part of the study in one of nine academic laboratories around the world with results being available within the timeframe of 48 h after sample receipt in the laboratory. The trial was activated in May 2008, and after screening of 3270 patients, a total of 717 younger adult *FLT3*-mutated AML patients (18–60 years) were randomized until October 2011. The study scheme was based on the phase-II results (Stone et al. 2012) and included the combination of midostaurin or placebo 50 mg bid on days 8–21 to standard intensive 7 + 3 induction chemotherapy (cytarabine 200 mg/m^2/day on days 1–7 by i.v. continuously and daunorubicin 60 mg/m^2/day on days 1–3) as well as 4 cycles of HiDAC (3 g i.v. twice daily over 3 h on days 1, 3, 5) as consolidation therapy. A one-year maintenance therapy with midostaurin or placebo was intended after completion of consolidation therapy.

Although not specifically mandated, allogeneic HCT was performed in 25% ($n = 167$) in first CR and overall including allogeneic HCT after induction failure and after relapse in 57% ($n = 429$) of the patients. OS, the primary endpoint of the study, was significantly improved by midostaurin with a hazard ratio of 0.78 (95%-CI: 0.63–0.96, p value: 0.009), translating in a median survival of 74.7 months in the midostaurin arm (range, 31.5 months not reached) as compared to 25.6 months in the placebo arm (range, 18.6–42.9 months), respectively. Interestingly, this improvement was regardless of the type of *FLT3* mutation (ITD or TKD) or the *FLT3*-ITD allelic ratio (cutoff 0.7). Based on these results, the US Food and Drug Administration (FDA) has approved midostaurin (Rydapt®; Novartis Pharmaceuticals, Inc.) on April 28th, 2017 for the treatment of adult newly diagnosed *FLT3*-mutated AML. A companion diagnostic test for the detection of *FLT3* mutations ("LeukoStrat CDx FLT3 Mutation Assay"), developed by Invivoscribe Technologies Inc., was also approved. According to the FDA label, the recommended dose of midostaurin (available in 25 mg capsules) is 50 mg twice daily on days 8–21 of each cycle of induction with cytarabine and daunorubicin and days 8–21 of each cycle of consolidation with HiDAC. The label notes that the drug is not indicated for single-agent treatment of AML. The currently used dosage form is 25 mg soft gelatine capsules, which should be stored at room temperature (25 °C; 77 °F). A 25 mg/ml oral solution is available for pediatric investigation, but is currently not approved. In Europe, the marketing authorization was granted by the European Medicines Agency (EMA) on July 20th, 2017 including also single-agent maintenance therapy for patients in CR. Though approved, the debate is still ongoing how midostaurin impacts OS and about the role of maintenance therapy. In an explorative analysis including CRs according to the protocol and CRs occurring beyond day 60, Midostaurin improved the CR rate significantly after induction therapy ($p = 0.04$). In terms of prevention of relapse, midostaurin was most effective in patients who received an allogeneic HCT in first CR. These patients had an in trend better survival ($p = 0.07$) and a significant lower CIR ($p = 0.02$), if again all patients achieving a CR after induction therapy were analyzed (Stone et al. 2017b). In contrast, patients who received chemotherapy as consolidation therapy had a comparable CIR rate whether they received midostaurin or not. In addition, those patients who proceeded to maintenance therapy (midostaurin, $n = 105$;

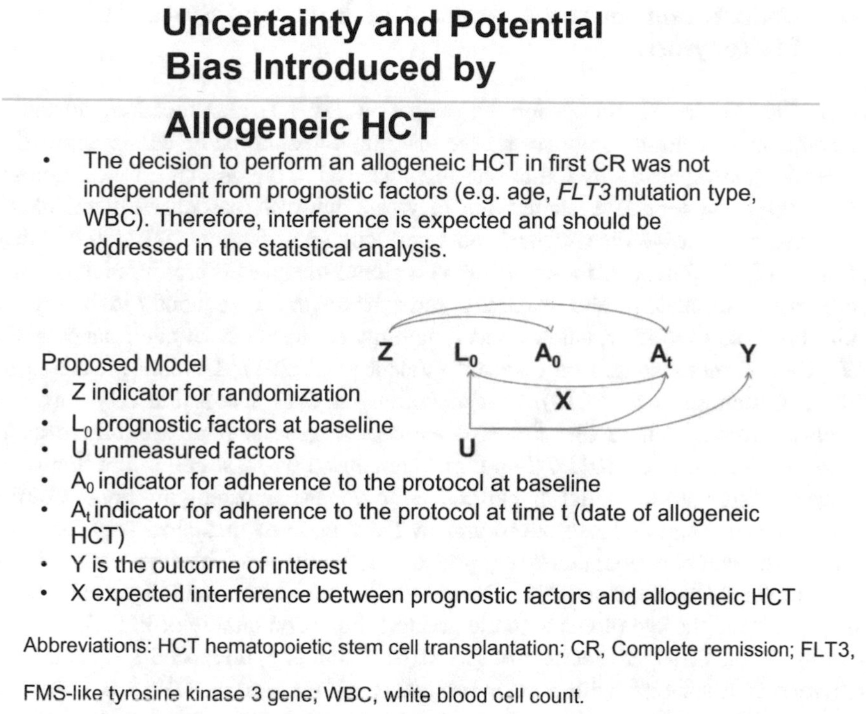

Uncertainty and Potential Bias Introduced by

Allogeneic HCT

- The decision to perform an allogeneic HCT in first CR was not independent from prognostic factors (e.g. age, *FLT3* mutation type, WBC). Therefore, interference is expected and should be addressed in the statistical analysis.

Proposed Model
- Z indicator for randomization
- L_0 prognostic factors at baseline
- U unmeasured factors
- A_0 indicator for adherence to the protocol at baseline
- A_t indicator for adherence to the protocol at time t (date of allogeneic HCT)
- Y is the outcome of interest
- X expected interference between prognostic factors and allogeneic HCT

Abbreviations: HCT hematopoietic stem cell transplantation; CR, Complete remission; FLT3, FMS-like tyrosine kinase 3 gene; WBC, white blood cell count.

Fig. 2 Adapted model from Hernán and Robins (2017). HCT hematopoietic stem cell transplantation; CR Complete remission; FLT3 FMS-like tyrosine kinase 3 gene; WBC white blood cell count

placebo, $n = 69$) had no significant benefit of midostaurin in terms of disease-free survival ($p = 0.49$) and OS ($p = 0.38$) (Larson et al. 2017). Taken together, these data indicate that the addition of midostaurin to first induction therapy is most important to induce the observed beneficial effect including the reduced relapse rate in patients after allogeneic HCT in first CR. In contrast, subgroup analyses currently do not indicate a clear benefit for midostaurin in combination with consolidation chemotherapy and/or as maintenance. An issue so far not addressed in the analysis of the RATIFY trial is the causal inference induced by allogeneic HCT (Hernán and Robins 2017). Based on the subgroup analysis, focusing on maintenance therapy (Larson et al. 2017) patients with lower risk (e.g., *FLT3*-TKD mutations) received more frequently maintenance therapy suggesting that patients with high-risk parameters (e.g., high allelic *FLT3*-ITD ratio) may have more frequently received an allogeneic HCT in first CR. To address this issue, a re-analysis on a per protocol basis of the data using appropriated statistical methods for causal inference (Hernán and Robins 2017) may lead to further exciting insides (Fig. 2). Furthermore, the different effects on event-free survival and OS according to gender also warrant further analysis (Stone et al. 2017) and need to be addressed in additional prospective studies.

5.4   Midostaurin for the Treatment of Advanced Systemic Mastocytosis

According to the World Health Organization (WHO) classification, advanced systemic mastocytosis comprises rare hematologic neoplasms including aggressive systemic mastocytosis, systemic mastocytosis with an associated hematologic neoplasm (also termed systemic mastocytosis with an associated hematologic non-mast cell lineage disease) and mast cell leukemia (Horny et al. 2008; Valent et al. 2017). Hallmark of mastocytosis is a clonal, neoplastic proliferation of mast cells that accumulate in one or more organ systems, most frequently involving the skin, bone marrow, liver, spleen, and lymph nodes. In >80% of adult patients, the *KIT* D816V mutation can be detected (Valent et al. 2017; Garcia-Montero et al. 2006; Kristensen et al. 2011). This mutation encodes a constitutively activated receptor tyrosine kinase that drives disease pathogenesis (Garcia-Montero et al. 2006; Kristensen et al. 2011). Symptoms are caused by mast cell infiltration (e.g., urticaria pigmentosa, portal hypertension, cytopenias, osteolytic bone lesions, hypersplenism, and malabsorption) and by the release of mediators (e.g., anaphylaxis, flushing, abdominal cramping, pruritus, and fatigue) with a high variability of the symptoms (Valent et al. 2017). Recent studies have identified fatigue and fear of anaphylaxis as the symptoms with the greatest impact on quality of life (QoL) (Van Anrooij et al. 2016; Siebenhaar et al. 2016). Clinically, advanced systemic mastocytosis is associated with a poor prognosis with a median OS of 3.5 years in patients with aggressive systemic mastocytosis, 2 years in those with systemic mastocytosis with an associated hematologic neoplasm, and less than 6 months in those with mast cell leukemia (Cohen et al. 2014; Lim et al. 2009a, b; Georgin-Lavialle et al. 2013). Cladribine and interferon alfa have been associated with limited response and duration of response in small, retrospective studies (Delaporte et al. 1995; Tefferi et al. 2001; Kluin-Nelemans et al. 2003; Hauswirth et al. 2004; Pardanani et al. 2004; Lim et al. 2009; Barete et al. 2015). Since 2006, imatinib at a dose of 400 mg/daily is approved by the FDA for the treatment of aggressive systemic mastocytosis in patients without *KIT* D816V or with unknown *KIT* mutation status (Quintas-Cardama et al. 2006), this indication is applicable to only ∼10% of patients (Garcia-Montero et al. 2006; Kristensen et al. 2011).

The multikinase inhibitor midostaurin inhibits both non-mutant and mutant *KIT* D816V and is currently the first and only FDA approved TKI as monotherapy for advanced systemic mastocytosis with *KIT* mutations (Gotlib et al. 2016). Based on promising activity of midostaurin in case reports (Gotlib et al. 2005), it was evaluated in a single-arm, phase-II trial in $n = 116$ patients with advanced systemic mastocytosis at a dose of 100 mg twice daily (Gotlib et al. 2016). Eighty-nine patients were eligible for primary efficacy; of those, $n = 16$ had aggressive systemic mastocytosis, $n = 57$ systemic mastocytosis with an associated hematologic neoplasm, and $n = 16$ mast cell leukemia. Overall, $n = 77$ of the 89 (87%) patients harbored a *KIT* D816V mutation. The overall response rate was 60%; 45% of the patients had a major response, which was defined as complete resolution of at least one type of mastocytosis-related organ damage. Additionally, midostaurin was associated with clinically significant benefits with respect to patient-reported symptoms and quality of life which probably had been related to combined inhibitory effects on the proliferation of neoplastic mast cells and mediator release (Gotlib NEJM 2016). Response rates were similar regardless of the subtype of advanced systemic mastocytosis or exposure to previous therapy. The median OS was 28.7 months (95%-CI, 18.1 to not reached), and the median progression-free survival was 14.1 months. Among the 16 patients with mast cell leukemia, the median OS was 9.4 months (95%-CI, 7.5 to not reached). Dose reduction owing to toxic effects occurred in 56% of the patients; re-escalation to the starting dose was feasible in 32% of those patients. The most frequent adverse events were low-grade nausea, vomiting, and diarrhea. New or worsening grade 3 or 4 neutropenia, anemia, and thrombocytopenia occurred in 24, 41, and 29% of the patients, respectively. Based on these results, midostaurin was approved by the FDA and EMA for the treatment of this detrimental disease with otherwise limited treatment options.

6 Common and Serious Side Effects

The most common side effects of midostaurin are nausea, vomiting, fatigue, headache, diarrhea, and anorexia (Stone et al. 2017a). In most cases, vomiting occurred within 1 h of midostaurin intake and subsided when treatment was withdrawn. Treatment with antiemetics was tried with variable success. Other adverse events include abdominal cramps, constipation, anorexia, anemia, leukopenia, neutropenia, thrombocytopenia, impaired liver function, dyslipidemia, hyperglycemia, impaired glucose tolerance, hyperthyroidism, pain, hypertension, rash, sweating, urinary tract infection, cough, viral infection, taste alteration, pruritus, dizziness, arthralgia, mucositis, edema, insomnia, dysuria, pneumonia, fever, infection.

Specific grade 3 or higher adverse events that had been reported during treatment in AML patients within the phase-III trial (CALGB 10603/RATIFY) were a higher rate of grade 3/4 rash/desquamation (Stone et al. 2017). Otherwise, no difference between midostaurin as compared to placebo was identified indicating that midostaurin was well tolerated.

7 Interactions with Strong Inhibitors of Cytochrome P450

Since midostaurin is metabolized by CYP3A4 to active compounds (He et al. 2017), dose interactions were evaluated in three phase-I healthy volunteer drug–drug interaction studies. A single dose of 50 mg midostaurin was coadministered with the potent CYP3A4 inhibitor ketoconazole (400 mg daily for 10 days) or CYP3A4 inducer rifampicin (600 mg daily for 14 days). Additionally, the effects of midostaurin as a single dose (100 mg) and multiple doses (50 mg twice daily) on midazolam (a sensitive CYP3A4 probe) concentration were evaluated. The plasma concentrations of midostaurin and its two active metabolites, CGP62221 and CGP52421, were determined using a sensitive liquid chromatography/tandem mass spectrometry method (Dutreix et al. 2013). Within this study, the exposure of midostaurin increased by more than tenfold (90%-CI, 7.4–14.5) due to CYP3A4 inhibition by ketoconazole, and induction of CYP3A4 by rifampicin decreased midostaurin exposure by more than tenfold. Midostaurin did not appreciably affect the concentrations of midazolam at single or multiple doses. Therefore, CYP3A4 inhibitors are thought to represent the most significant potential for drug interaction with midostaurin. In addition, the coadministration of paracetamol (per oral and i.v. administration) together with midostaurin should be avoided due to rare cases of TKI-induced inhibition of paracetamol glucuronidation, which may lead to severe and fatal liver toxicity (Liu et al. 2011; Claridge et al. 2010; Craig et al. 2011).

8 Effect of Midostaurin on Cardiac Intervals

Some TKIs have been shown to affect cardiac repolarization, as detected by heart rate-corrected QT (QTc) prolongation (Chu et al. 2007; Levis et al. 2012; DeAngelo et al. 2006; Tolcher et al. 2011). Therefore, the effect of midostaurin on cardiac repolarization has been evaluated in a randomized phase-I study in a parallel design with active (moxifloxacin) and placebo control arms in 192 healthy volunteers (Del Corral et al. 2012). Midostaurin or placebo were administered at a dose of 75 mg twice daily for 2 days and 75 mg once daily for 1 day. In the 4-day evaluation period, only about one-third of the participants (35%) experienced a mostly mild adverse event (97% were grade 1). No grade 3 or 4 adverse events were reported. Thus, midostaurin demonstrated a good safety profile in healthy volunteers, with no prolonged cardiac repolarization or other changes on the electrocardiogram. In addition, none of the clinical studies have suggested a substantive risk for cardiac abnormalities with midostaurin (Stone et al. 2017a; Schlenk et al. 2016).

9 Summary and Perspectives

Midostaurin (Rydapt®) was approved by the FDA and EMA for AML with activating *FLT3* mutations as detected by an FDA-approved test in the USA in combination with intensive induction and postremission therapy at a dosage of 50 mg twice daily. In addition, it was approved as monotherapy for aggressive systemic mastocytosis (ASM), systemic mastocytosis with associated hematological neoplasm (SM-AHN), or mast cell leukemia (MCL) at a dosage of 100 mg/twice daily.

In *FLT3*-mutated AML, the role of midostaurin as adjunct to intensive induction therapy is based on the data from the double-blinded, randomized CALGB 10603/RATIFY trial well established and this is particularly true for patients proceeding to allogeneic HCT in first CR. In contrast, the impact of midostaurin during HiDAC consolidation and single-agent midostaurin maintenance therapy is based on additional subset analyses presented at ASH 2017 less clear and needs additional investigations. Furthermore, causal inference induced by allogeneic HCT may have a significant impact on outcome and should spur further post hoc analysis. Since its clinical benefit was independent from the type of *FLT3* mutation (TKD, ITD low allelic ration, ITD high allelic ratio), an evaluation of midostaurin in *FLT3*-wild-type AML is already underway.

In advanced systemic mastocytosis, midostaurin significantly moved the field forward. Currently, midostaurin is the only approved multikinase inhibitor in patients with ASM, but new treatment strategies for alternative targets are needed.

References

Andrejauskas-Buchdunger E, Regenass U (1992) Differential inhibition of the epidermal growth factor-, platelet-derived growth factor-, and protein kinase C-mediated signal transduction pathways by the staurosporine derivative CGP 41251. Cancer Res 52(19):5353–5358

Bali P, George P, Cohen P et al (2004) Superior activity of the combination of histone deacetylase inhibitor LAQ824 and the FLT-3 kinase inhibitor PKC412 against human acute myelogenous leukemia cells with mutant FLT-3. Clin Cancer Res 10(15):4991–4997

Barete S, Lortholary O, Damaj G et al (2015) Long-term efficacy and safety of cladribine (2-CdA) in adult patients with mastocytosis. Blood 126(8):1009–1016

Budworth J, Davies R, Malkhandi J, Gant TW, Ferry DR, Gescher A (1996) Comparison of staurosporine and four analogues: their effects on growth, rhodamine 123 retention and binding to P-glycoprotein in multidrug-resistant MCF-7/Adr cells. Br J Cancer 73(9):1063–1068

Chu TF, Rupnick MA, Kerkela R et al (2007) Cardiotoxicity associated with tyrosine kinase inhibitor sunitinib. Lancet (9604);370:2011–2019

Claridge LC, Eksteen B, Smith A et al (2010) Acute liver failure after administration of paracetamol at the maximum recommended daily dose in adults. BMJ 341:c6764

Cohen SS, Skovbo S, Vestergaard H et al (2014) Epidemiology of systemic mastocytosis in Denmark. Br J Haematol 166(4):521–528

Craig DG, Bates CM, Davidson JS et al (2011) Overdose pattern and outcome in paracetamol-induced acute severe hepatotoxicity. Br J Clin Pharmacol 71(2):273–282

DeAngelo DJ, Stone RM, Heaney ML et al (2006) Phase 1 clinical results with tandutinib (MLN518), a novel FLT3 antagonist, in patients with acute myelogenous leukemia or high-risk myelodysplastic syndrome: safety, pharmacokinetics, and pharmacodynamics. Blood 108 (12):3674–3681

Delaporte E, Piérard E, Wolthers BG et al (1995) Interferon-alpha in combination with corticosteroids improves systemic mast cell disease. Br J Dermatol 132(3):479–482

Del Corral A, Dutreix C, Huntsman-Labed A et al (2012) Midostaurin does not prolong cardiac repolarization defined in a thorough electrocardiogram trial in healthy volunteers. Cancer Chemother Pharmacol 69(5):1255–1263

Dutreix C, Munarini F, Lorenzo S, Roesel J, Wang Y (2013) Investigation into CYP3A4-mediated drug-drug interactions on midostaurin in healthy volunteers. Cancer Chemother Pharmacol 72 (6):1223–1234

Eder JP Jr, Garcia-Carbonero R, Clark JW et al (2004) A phase I trial of daily oral 4'- N -benzoyl-staurosporine in combination with protracted continuous infusion 5-fluorouracil in patients with advanced solid malignancies. Invest New Drugs 22(2):139–150

Fabbro D, Ruetz S, Bodis S et al (2000) PKC412-a protein kinase inhibitor with a broad therapeutic potential. Anticancer Drug Des 15(1):17–28

Furukawa Y, Vu HA, Akutsu M et al (2007) Divergent cytotoxic effects of PKC412 in combination with conventional antileukemic agents in FLT3 mutation-positive versus - negative leukemia cell lines. Leukemia 21(5):1005–1014

Garcia-Montero AC, Jara-Acevedo M, Teodosio C et al (2006) KIT mutation in mast cells and other bone marrow hematopoietic cell lineages in systemic mast cell disorders: a prospective study of the Spanish Network on Mastocytosis (REMA) in a series of 113 patients. Blood 108 (7):2366–2372

George P, Bali P, Cohen P et al (2004) Cotreatment with 17-allylaminodemethoxygeldanamycin and FLT-3 kinase inhibitor PKC412 is highly effective against human acute myelogenous leukemia cells with mutant FLT-3. Cancer Res 64(10):3645–3652

Gilliland DG, Griffin JD (2002) The roles of FLT3 in hematopoiesis and leukemia. Blood 100 (5):1532–1542

Georgin-Lavialle S, Lhermitte L, Dubreuil P, Chandesris MO, Hermine O, Damaj G (2013) Mast cell leukemia. Blood 121(8):1285–1295

Gotlib J, Berubé C, Growney JD et al (2005) Activity of the tyrosine kinase inhibitor PKC412 in a patient with mast cell leukemia with the D816V KIT mutation. Blood 106(8):2865–2870

Gotlib J, Kluin-Nelemans HC, George TI et al (2016) Efficacy and safety of midostaurin in advanced systemic mastocytosis. N Engl J Med 374(26):2530–2541

Griffith J, Black J, Faerman C et al (2004) The structural basis for autoinhibition of FLT3 by the juxtamembrane domain. Mol Cell 13(2):169–178

Gu TL, Nardone J, Wang Y, et al (2011) Survey of activated FLT3 signaling in leukemia. PLoS One6:e19169

Hannum C, Culpepper J, Campbell D et al (1994) Ligand for FLT3/FLK2 receptor tyrosine kinase regulates growth of haematopoietic stem cells and is encoded by variant RNAs. Nature 368 (6472):643–648

Hauswirth AW, Simonitsch-Klupp I, Uffmann M et al (2004) Response to therapy with interferon alpha-2b and prednisolone in aggressive systemic mastocytosis: report of five cases and review of the literature. Leuk Res 28(3):249–257

Hayakawa F, Towatari M, Kiyoi H et al (2000) Tandem-duplicated Flt3 constitutively activates STAT5 and MAP kinase and introduces autonomous cell growth in IL-3-dependent cell lines. Oncogene 19(5):624–631

He H, Tran P, Tedesco V et al (2017) Midostaurin, a novel protein kinase inhibitor for the treatment of acute myelogenous leukemia: insights from human absorption, metabolism, and excretion studies of a BDDCS II drug. Drug Metab Dispos 45(5):540–555

Horny MP, Metcalfe DD, Bennett JM (2008) Mastocytosis. In: Swerdlow SH, Campo E (eds) WHO classification of tumors of hematopoietic and lymphoid tissues. International Agency for Research and Cancer, Lyon, France, pp 54–63

Hernán MA, Robins JM (2017) Per-protocol analyses of pragmatic trials. N Engl J Med 377 (14):1391–1398

Ikegami Y, Yano S, Nakao K et al (1995) Antitumor activity of the new selective protein kinase C inhibitor 4'-N-benzoyl staurosporine on murine and human tumor models. Arzneimit-telforschung 45(11):1225–1230

Karaman MW, Herrgard S, Treiber DK et al (2008) A quantitative analysis of kinase inhibitor selectivity. Nat Biotechnol 26(1):127–132

Kayser S, Schlenk RF (2017) Targeting the FLT3 mutation in acute myeloid leukemia. Eur Oncol Haematol 13(2). Epub ahead of print

Kayser S, Levis MJ (2017) Advances in targeted therapy for acute myeloid leukaemia. Br J Haematol. 2017 Nov 28. https://doi.org/10.1111/bjh.15032. [Epub ahead of print] Review

Kluin-Nelemans HC, Oldhoff JM, Van Doormaal JJ et al (2003) Cladribine therapy for systemic mastocytosis. Blood 102(13):4270–4276

Kristensen T, Vestergaard H, Møller MB (2011) Improved detection of the KIT D816V mutation in patients with systemic mastocytosis using a quantitative and highly sensitive real-time qPCR assay. J Mol Diagn 13(2):180–188

Larson RA et al (2017) An analysis of maintenance therapy and post-midostaurin outcomes in the international prospective randomized, placebo-controlled, double-blind trial (CALGB 10603/RATIFY [Alliance]) for newly diagnosed acute myeloid leukemia (AML) patients with FLT3 mutations blood 2017:ASH 2017

Levis M, Pham R, Smith BD et al (2004) In vitro studies of a FLT3 inhibitor combined with chemotherapy: sequence of administration is important to achieve synergistic cytotoxic effects. Blood 104(4):1145–1150

Levis M, Brown P, Smith BD, Stine A, Pham R, Stone R et al (2006) Plasma inhibitory activity (PIA): a pharmacodynamic assay reveals insights into the basis for cytotoxic response to FLT3 inhibitors. Blood 108(10):3477–3483

Levis MJ, Perl AE, Dombret H et al (2012) Final results of a phase 2 open-label, monotherapy efficacy and safety study of quizartinib (AC220) in patients with FLT3-ITD positive or negative relapsed/refractory acute myeloid leukemia after second-line chemotherapy or hematopoietic stem cell transplantation. Blood 120(12):673

Lim KH, Tefferi A, Lasho TL et al (2009a) Systemic mastocytosis in 342 consecutive adults: survival studies and prognostic factors. Blood 113(23):5727–5736

Lim KH, Pardanani A, Butterfield JH, Li CY, Tefferi A (2009b) Cytoreductive therapy in 108 adults with systemic mastocytosis: outcome analysis and response prediction during treatment with interferon-alpha, hydroxyurea, imatinib mesylate or 2-chlorodeoxyadenosine. Am J Hematol 84(12):790–794

Liu Y, Ramirez J, Ratain MJ (2011) Inhibition of paracetamol glucuronidation by tyrosine kinase inhibitors. Br J Clin Pharmacol 71(6):917–920

Meshinchi S, Appelbaum FR (2009) Structural and functional alterations of FLT3 in acute myeloid leukemia. Clin Cancer Res 15(13):4263–4269

Monnerat C, Henriksson R, Le Chevalier T et al (2004) Phase I study of PKC412 (N-benzoyl-staurosporine), a novel oral protein kinase C inhibitor, combined with gemcitabine and cisplatin in patients with non-small-cell lung cancer. Ann Oncol 15(2):316–323

Nagel G, Weber D, Fromm E et al (2017) German-Austrian AML Study Group (AMLSG). Epidemiological, genetic, and clinical characterization by age of newly diagnosed acute myeloid leukemia based on an academic population-based registry study (AMLSG BiO). Ann Hematol 96(12):1993–2003

Papaemmanuil E, Gerstung M, Bullinger L et al (2016) Genomic classification and prognosis in acute myeloid leukemia. N Engl J Med 374(23):2209–2221 2016 Jun 9

Pardanani A, Hoffbrand AV, Butterfield JH, Tefferi A (2004) Treatment of systemic mast cell disease with 2-chlorodeoxyadenosine. Leuk Res 28(2):127–131

Propper DJ, McDonald AC, Man A, Thavasu P, Balkwill F, Braybrooke JP et al (2001) Phase I and pharmacokinetic study of PKC412, an inhibitor of protein kinase C. J Clin Oncol 19 (5):1485–1492

Quintas-Cardama A, Aribi A, Cortes J et al (2006) Novel approaches in the treatment of systemic mastocytosis. Cancer 107(7):1429–1439

Rosnet O, Marchetto S, deLapeyriere O et al (1991) Murine Flt3, a gene encoding a novel tyrosine kinase receptor of the PDGFR/CSF1R family. Oncogene 6(9):1641–1650

Sato T, Yang X, Knapper S et al (2011) FLT3 ligand impedes the efficacy of FLT3 inhibitors in vitro and in vivo. Blood 117(12):3286–3293

Schlenk RF, Fiedler W, Salih H et al (2016) Impact of age and midostaurin-dose on response and outcome in acute myeloid leukemia with FLT3-ITD: interim-analyses of the AMLSG 16-10 Trial (NCT01477606). Blood 128(22):449 (abstract)

Siebenhaar F, Von Tschirnhaus E, Hartmann K et al (2016) Development and validation of the mastocytosis quality of life questionnaire: MCQoL. Allergy 71(6):869–877

Stone RM, DeAngelo DJ, Klimek V et al (2005) Patients with acute myeloid leukemia and an activating mutation in FLT3 respond to a small-molecule FLT3 tyrosine kinase inhibitor, PKC412. Blood 105(1):54–60

Stone RM, Fischer T, Paquette R et al (2012) Phase IB study of the FLT3 kinase inhibitor midostaurin with chemotherapy in younger newly diagnosed adult patients with acute myeloid leukemia. Leukemia 26(9):2061–2068

Stone RM, Mandrekar SJ, Sanford BL et al (2017a) Midostaurin plus chemotherapy for acute myeloid leukemia with FLT3 mutation. N Engl J Med 377(5):454–464

Stone RM et al (2017b) The addition of midostaurin to standard chemotherapy decreases cumulative incidence of relapse (CIR) in the international prospective randomized, placebo-controlled, double-blind trial (CALGB 10603/RATIFY [Alliance]) for newly diagnosed acute myeloid leukemia (AML) patients with FLT3 mutations. Blood 2017:ASH 2017

Tefferi A, Li C-Y, Butterfield JH, Hoagland HC (2001) Treatment of systemic mastcell disease with cladribine. N Engl J Med 344(4):307–309

Tolcher AW, Appleman LJ, Shapiro GI et al (2011) A phase I open-label study evaluating the cardiovascular safety of sorafenib in patients with advanced cancer. Cancer Chemother Pharmacol 67(4):751–764

Utz I, Hofer S, Regenass U et al (1994) The protein kinase C inhibitor CGP 41251, a staurosporine derivative with antitumor activity, reverses multidrug resistance. Int J Cancer 57(1):104–110

Valent P, Akin C, Hartmann K, Nilsson G, Reiter A, Hermine O et al (2017) Advances in the classification and treatment of mastocytosis: current status and outlook toward the future. Cancer Res 77(6):1261–1270

Van Anrooij B, Kluin-Nelemans JC, Safy M et al (2016) Patient-reported disease-specific quality-of-life and symptom severity in systemic mastocytosis. Allergy 71(11):1585–1593

Weisberg E, Boulton C, Kelly LM et al (2002) Inhibition of mutant FLT3 receptors in leukemia cells by the small molecule tyrosine kinase inhibitor PKC412. Cancer Cell 1(15):433–443

Zaugg K, Rocha S, Resch H et al (2001) Differential p53-dependent mechanism of radiosensitization in vitro and in vivo by the protein kinase C-specific inhibitor PKC412. Cancer Res 61 (2):732–738

Venetoclax: Targeting BCL2 in Hematological Cancers

Annika Scheffold, Billy Michael Chelliah Jebaraj
and Stephan Stilgenbauer

Contents

A. Scheffold · B. M. C. Jebaraj · S. Stilgenbauer (✉)
Department of Internal Medicine III, Ulm University,
Albert Einstein Allee 23, 89081 Ulm, Germany
e-mail: Stephan.Stilgenbauer@uniklinik-ulm.de

A. Scheffold
e-mail: annika.scheffold@uni-ulm.de

© Springer International Publishing AG, part of Springer Nature 2018
U. M. Martens (ed.), *Small Molecules in Hematology*, Recent Results
in Cancer Research 211, https://doi.org/10.1007/978-3-319-91439-8_11

Abstract

Over the last years, targeted anti-cancer therapy with small-molecule inhibitors and antibodies moved to the forefront as a strategy to treat hematological cancers. These novel agents showed outstanding effects in treatment of patients, often irrespective of their underlying genetic features. However, evolution and selection of subclones with continuous treatment leads to disease relapse and resistance toward these novel drugs. Venetoclax (ABT-199) is a novel, orally bioavailable small-molecule inhibitor for selective targeting of *B-cell lymphoma 2* (BCL2). Venetoclax is in clinical development and shows high efficacy and safety in particular in the treatment of chronic lymphocytic leukemia (CLL), but preliminarily also in acute myeloid leukemia (AML) and acute lymphoblastic leukemia (ALL). The most important and impressive outcomes of venetoclax treatment include a rapid induction of apoptosis and drastic reduction of the tumor bulk within a few hours after administration. Venetoclax was approved by the FDA and EMA in 2016 for patients with previously treated CLL with del (17p13) and patients failing B cell receptor signaling inhibitors (EMA only), on the basis of a single-arm phase II trial demonstrating a tremendous response rate of 79% with complete remission in 20% of cases and an estimated 1-year progression-free survival of 72%. This review focuses on the mode of action, the preclinical models, and outcomes from various clinical trials with venetoclax in different hematologic cancers as well as future development.

Keywords

Venetoclax · BCL2 inhibitors · Hematologic cancer

1   Background: The Balance between Anti-apoptotic and Pro-apoptotic Proteins

BCL2 family proteins play a major role in the regulation of cell death, and BCL2 has been the first anti-apoptotic gene discovered in 1985 (Tsujimoto et al. 1985). The BCL2 family is highly conserved and contains more than a dozen proteins that are key regulators of the mechanism of intrinsic programmed cell death. The BCL2 family is clustered into three main functional groups, the pro-survival and anti-apoptotic proteins BCL2, MCL1, BCL-XL and BCL-W (O'Connor et al. 1998; Gibson et al. 1996; Boise et al. 1993; Opferman et al. 2005; Opferman et al. 2003), the multi-BH domain pro-apoptotic proteins BAX and BAK and the pro-apoptotic

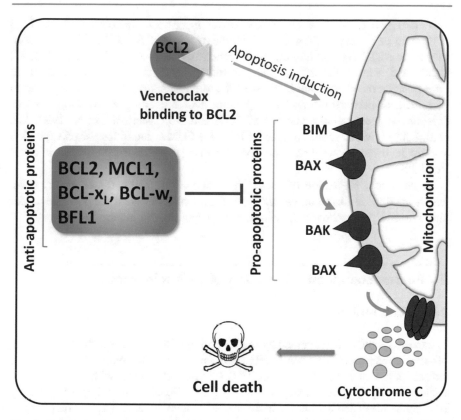

Fig. 1 Overview of pro- and anti-apoptotic molecules. **a** Cell death signals trigger BID and BIM to activate BAX and BAK, which in turn initiate MOMP and lead to apoptosis. **b** Anti-apoptotic molecules, including BCL2, antagonize both activator and effector molecules and block the apoptotic cascade. **c** Cell death signals also activate sensitizer molecules, which antagonize anti-apoptotic molecules and release the block on apoptosis. This physiologic role is pharmacologically recapitulated by BH3-mimetic drugs such as venetoclax

BH3-only proteins BIM, tBID; BAD, PUMA; NOXA and HRK (Inohara et al. 1997; Datta et al. 2002; Oda et al. 2000; O'Connor et al. 1998; Wei et al. 2000; Korsmeyer et al. 2000) that trigger and execute the 'suicidal' cell death. In healthy cells, the balance between cell survival and cell death requires the dynamic binding interactions between the pro-apoptotic and anti-apoptotic proteins (Fig. 1). However, in various malignancies, the anti-apoptotic proteins are frequently overexpressed, leading to defective apoptosis (Robertson et al. 1996).

In cancers, anti-apoptotic BCL2 is upregulated by various mechanisms. The t(14;18) chromosomal translocation which is a genetic hallmark of follicular lymphoma (a subtype of indolent non-Hodgkin lymphoma) includes juxtapositioning of *BCL2* in the IGHV locus, activating *BCL2* at the transcriptional level (Tsujimoto et al. 1985). Amplification of chromosome 18q21 resulting in high BCL2 levels is observed in small-cell lung cancers (SCLC) (Monni et al. 1997) and mantle cell lymphoma (MCL) (Bentz et al. 2000). In chronic lymphocytic leukemia (CLL), the most common cytogenetic abnormality is the del(13q14), the minimally deleted region of which includes the *BCL2* repressors, microRNAs 15 and 16 (Cimmino et al. 2005). Moreover, hypomethylation of *BCL2* in CLL also contributes to *BCL2* upregulation due to epigenetic dysregulation (Hanada et al. 1993; Cahill and Rosenquist 2013). On the other hand, defects in expression of pro-apoptotic members result in a loss of the tumor suppressive function and lead to an imbalance between pro-and anti-apoptotic BCL2 family proteins. Homozygous deletions or inactivating mutations of BAX and BID (Meijerink et al. 1998; Lee et al. 2004) or defective expression of BID and PUMA due to loss of p53 function also tip the balance toward anti-apoptotic proteins (Sturm et al. 2000; Miyashita and Reed 1995).

In summary, prevention of apoptosis is one of the hallmarks of cancer cells, which in addition to sustaining survival of the malignant clone, impacts treatment outcome and progression of the disease (Hanahan and Weinberg 2011).

2 Pharmacology and Evolution of BH3 Mimetics

2.1 BCL2 Inhibitors

In cancer, apoptosis is prevented by the formation of a heterodimer through binding of the pro-apoptotic protein's BH3 domain into the hydrophobic cleft of anti-apoptotic proteins. The era of BCL2 inhibitors started with the design of anti-sense oligonucleotides to knockdown BCL2 (Reed et al. 1990), followed by BH3 mimetics which bind to the hydrophobic groove of the anti-apoptotic proteins, stabilizing the pro-apoptotic proteins to carry out their function (Fig. 2a).

Oblimersen, the antisense oligonucleotide that was designed to specifically target BCL2 showed only limited efficacy either in monotherapy (O'Brien et al. 2005) or in combination with chemotherapy (O'Brien et al. 2009). Inhibitors of BCL2 derived from natural substances such as AT-101 (Balakrishnan et al. 2009) and synthetic inhibitors such as obatoclax showed modest responses in CLL patients (Brown et al. 2015).

ABT-737 was a highly specific small-molecule inhibitor of BCL-x_L, BCL2, and BCL-W with EC50 of 78.7, 30.3, and 197.8 nM in cell-free assays. The drug was designed by a strategy of combining screening using nuclear magnetic resonance, structure-based design, and combinatory chemical synthesis (Oltersdorf et al. 2005). Preclinical data showed ABT-737 to trigger BAX- and BAK-mediated apoptosis in various cancer cell lines and xenograft models (van Delft et al. 2006). Refractoriness to ABT-737 treatment was associated with the upregulation of MCL1 (van Delft et al. 2006). However, the therapeutic use of ABT-737 was limited due to its lack of oral bioavailability and the induction of thrombocytopenia, and higher incidences of transaminitis were observed in the treatment owing to a lower binding affinity of the drugs to BCL2 (Wilson et al. 2010).

A precursor of ABT-199 is navitoclax (ABT-263), a first-in-class dual inhibitor of BCL2 and BCL-x_L. Navitoclax is structurally related to ABT-737 and inhibits

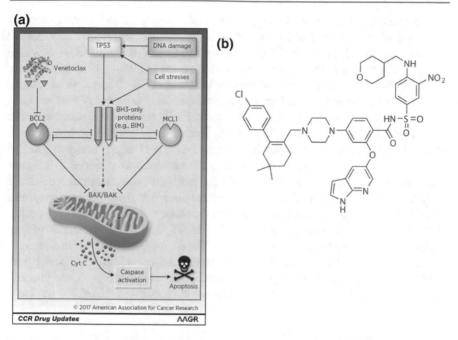

Fig. 2 **a** Summary of molecules which interplay in mitochondrial apoptosis. Venetoclax acts as a BH3 mimetic and inhibits BCL2. The activation of BAX and BAK and their delocalization to the outer mitochondrial membrane induces cytochrome c release by depolarization and caspase activation. In healthy cells, BCL2 represses the activation of BAX and BAK. Figure is adopted from Roberts et al. (2017). **b** Chemical structure of venetoclax ($C_{45}H_{50}ClN_7O_7S$(4-(4-{[2-(2-(4-chlorophenyl)-4,4-dimethylcyclohex-2*H*-pyrrolo[2,3-*b*]pyridine-5-yloxy)benzamide))

BCL2 and BCL-x_L with EC50 values of 60 and 20 nM, respectively (Tse et al. 2008). Navitoclax has been evaluated in clinical phase I and II trials in B-cell lymphomas as well as in solid tumors (Gandhi et al. 2011; Tolcher et al. 2015); however, the strong inhibition of BCL-x_L induced a rapid decrease in circulating platelets due to a direct toxic effect. This concentration-dependent grade 3 and 4 thrombocytopenia affected treatment with high drug doses (Gandhi et al. 2011; Kaefer et al. 2014). Navitoclax was explored in a phase I study in relapsed/refractory CLL. In this trial, nine of 29 patients achieved a response with a median PFS of 25 months (Roberts et al. 2012). A phase 2 study of rituximab with or without navitoclax in untreated CLL reported ORR of 55% (Kipps et al. 2015). However, due to the thrombocytopenia, navitoclax never entered clinical phase III trials in spite of being proven efficient in BCL2 dependent malignancies (Roberts et al. 2012).

Venetoclax (ABT-199, GDC-0199) is a selective, potent, orally bioavailable BCL2 inhibitor. The structural formula is $C_{45}H_{50}ClN_7O_7S$ (4-(4-{[2-(2-(4-chlorophenyl)-4,4-dimethylcyclohex-2*H*-pyrrolo[2,3-*b*]pyridine-5-yloxy)benzamide)), with a molecular mass of M_r = 868.4 g/mol (Fig. 2b). In comparison to navitoclax, venetoclax lacks a thiophenyl unit located at the P4 hotspot which re-engineers the BH3-binding domain. The pharmacokinetics of venetoclax is described by a $K_i < 0.01$ nM in cell-free assays, and it has 4800 times higher potency for BCL2 than for BCL-x_L($K_i = 48$ nM) and BCL-W ($K_i = 245$ nM) (Fig. 2). There is no activity described targeting MCL-1 ($K_i > 444$ nM) (Souers et al. 2013). The half-life time of venetoclax is 16–19 h (Roberts et al. 2016). ABT-199 was studied in various cellular models and primary patient samples ex vivo, where it induced apoptosis and its sensitivity strongly correlated with the expression of BCL2 (Anderson et al. 2016; Fischer et al. 2015; Varadarajan et al. 2013). The dosing in clinical trials is performed daily and ranges between 300 and 900 mg/day. The peak plasma concentration of venetoclax is achieved 5–8 h after drug uptake. If venetoclax is taken with a fat meal, the mean maximum observed plasma concentration (Cmax) and area under the plasma concentration—time curve (AUC) are fourfold increased as its intestinal uptake and absorbance are accelerated. Venetoclax is metabolized by CYP3A4/5 and is a substrate of the P-glycoprotein pump (Agarwal et al. 2016). The use of CYP3A inhibitors leads to an accumulation and dose increase and therefore should be avoided (Agarwal et al. 2016, 2017). Due to the high degree of specificity and comparatively lower toxicity, only venetoclax among all the BCL2 inhibitors successfully reached the market.

2.2 MCL1 Inhibitors

MCL1 is an anti-apoptotic member of the BCL2 family of proteins. MCL1 is frequently upregulated in various cancers and hence considered as a promising therapeutic target. Moreover, transcriptional upregulation or amplification of MCL1 is described to be an important mechanism, driving resistance to BCL2 inhibitors (Beroukhim et al. 2010). As MCL1 has a binding pocket for BAK, several compound screens have been performed to develop competitive inhibitors to disrupt this interaction (Varadarajan et al. 2013). However, MCL1 inhibition is known to be embryonically lethal (Rinkenberger et al. 2000), and MCL1 is also important for survival of hematopoietic stem cells (Opferman et al. 2005), which might limit the therapeutic window due to toxicity. After TW-37 which showed potential efficacy in in vitro models by disruption of MCL1 binding to BAK (Varadarajan et al. 2013), development of an amenable inhibitor had been challenging. Recent findings presented S63845 with potent anti-tumor activity in vitro and in vivo (Kotschy et al. 2016). The inhibitor binds to the BH3 binding groove of MCL1 and was efficacious in the pre-clinical setting in different hematopoietic cancers such as multiple myeloma, acute myeloid leukemia, and lymphomas as well as in solid cancers. Interestingly, S63845 showed no adverse effect on hematopoietic progenitor cells which points to MCL1 as a treatment option for MCL1 dependent tumors and in drug combination with BCL2 inhibitors (Kotschy et al. 2016) (Table 1).

Table 1 Properties of BCL2 and MCL1 inhibitors and their assessment in clinical trials

BH3 mimetic	Proposed targets	Affects platelets ex vivo	Clinical trial	Approval	Reference
ABT-737	BCL2, BCL-x$_L$	Yes	NCT01440504	No	Oltersdorf et al. (2005)
ABT-263	BCL2, BCL-x$_L$	Yes	NCT00406809	No	Tse et al. (2008)
ABT-199	BCL2	No	NCT01794520 NCT02677324 NCT03128879 NCT02471391	Yes	Souers et al. (2013)
WEHI-539	BCL-x$_L$	No	No	No	Lessene et al. (2013)
BM-1197	BCL-x$_L$	No	No	No	Bai et al. (2014)
AT-101	pan-BCL2	No	NCT01977209	No	Albershardt et al. (2011)
Obatoclax (GX15-070)	pan-BCL2	No	NCT00719901 NCT00521144	No	Albershardt et al. (2011), Nguyen et al. (2007)
BXI-62/72	BCL-x$_L$	No	NCT02494583 NCT02335411 NCT02149225	No	Park et al. (2013)
MIM1, UMI-77	MCL1	No	No	No	Cohen et al. (2012), Abulwerdi et al. (2014)
S63845	MCL1		NCT02979366	Pending	Kotschy et al. (2016)

3 Preclinical Studies Using Venetoclax

A number of preclinical studies reported the tremendous effects of venetoclax in vitro. The major mode of action of venetoclax is the activation of BAK and BAX and subsequent mitochondrial cytochrome C release leading to apoptosis. Treatment with venetoclax was reported in various cellular models to functionally validate its mode of action. Jurkat T-cells lacking BAX showed no response to treatment with different concentrations of venetoclax (Vogler et al. 2013). Apoptosis induction by venetoclax in peripheral blood samples from CLL cases was confirmed by externalization of phosphatidylserine. Comparison of venetoclax with ABT-737 and ABT-263 to analyze their susceptibility to affect platelets showed markedly reduced toxicity of venetoclax in comparison to ABT-737 or ABT-263 (Vogler et al. 2013).

Furthermore, during preclinical development, high single-agent cell-killing was demonstrated in non-Hodgkin's lymphoma (NHL) cell lines including those from diffused large B-cell lymphoma (DLBCL), mantle cell lymphoma (MCL), and follicular lymphoma (FL). Notably, NHL cell lines carrying the t(14;18) BCL2 gain showed higher sensitivity toward ABT-199 treatment than cell lines without the alteration (Souers et al. 2013). Multiple myeloma cell lines showed sensitivity to venetoclax correlating with the expression profile of BCL2, BCL-x_L, and MCL1 which were predictive for treatment response. Interestingly, the co-expression of BCL2 and BCL-x_L resulted in resistance to venetoclax monotherapy but still showed response to BCL-x_L inhibitors.

Remarkable effects were also demonstrated for ABT-199 treatment of AML and pediatric ALL cell lines (Fischer et al. 2015). Also, studies using xenografts of AML (Pan et al. 2014), ALL (Frismantas et al. 2017), and B-cell lymphomas with venetoclax as monotherapy or in combination with rituximab and bendamustine (Souers et al. 2013) highlighted the efficacy of venetoclax as well as its safety in combination treatments. In line with these findings, studies using MLL-rearranged ALL primary samples in vitro (Alford et al. 2015) and in vivo (Khaw et al. 2016) demonstrated the potent single-agent activity of venetoclax in these tumor entities.

In CLL, treatment with ibrutinib, a novel small-molecule inhibitor of BTK showed impressive clinical activity with durable responses (Byrd et al. 2014; Byrd et al. 2015); however, subsets of patients did not achieve deep remission or cure. To address a possible synergism between venetoclax and ibrutinib, ex vivo serial samples of CLL patients under ibrutinib treatment were treated with venetoclax. The combination resulted in high cytotoxicity in vitro and confirmed a possible synergy between venetoclax and ibrutinib. Of functional relevance, the decrease of MCL1 and BCL-x_L mediated by ibrutinib augmented the response to inhibition of BCL2 through venetoclax, strongly endorsing for a clinical trial with this combination therapy (Cervantes-Gomez et al. 2015).

Importantly, on the other hand, various studies were performed to assess the safety profile of venetoclax and their impact on non-tumor hematopoietic lineages using genetically modified murine models. Pre-B-cells and immature B-cells were found to highly depend on BCL-x_L (Motoyama et al. 1995) with a low expression of BCL2 in these subsets; however, a gradual switch in BCL2 expression in pro-B-cell precursors directed their maturation (Merino et al. 1994). In order to validate the mode of action of ABT-199 on normal lymphocyte subsets, knockout mice models carrying knockouts of apoptotic players (Bim, Bax, Bak, Puma, Noxa) were analyzed (Khaw et al. 2014).

Analysis of the in vitro sensitivity of lymphocyte subsets identified human peripheral B-cells of healthy donors to be more sensitive to venetoclax treatment than CD4+ or CD8+ T-cells and granulocytes. These data were also confirmed by analyzing murine lymphocyte subsets (Khaw et al. 2014). In contrast to cells of the B-cell lineage, the T-cell lineage and granulocytes were resistant to venetoclax treatment. In-depth analysis of T-cell subsets revealed a higher susceptibility of double-negative (CD4- CD8-) thymocytes and mature peripheral T-cells than CD4 and CD8 subsets to venetoclax treatment, correlating with their reliance on BCL2 (Gratiot-Deans et al. 1994; Veis et al. 1993).

4 Clinical Efficacy of Venetoclax in Hematological Malignancies

4.1 Venetoclax for Treatment of Poor-Risk CLL

CLL is a B-cell malignancy, where clonal CD5+ CD19+ CD23+ B-cells are present in the peripheral blood and infiltrate lymphoid organs such as lymph nodes, spleen, and bone marrow. The mechanisms underlying CLL pathogenesis are not fully resolved, and the clinical course of CLL is highly diverse. Recently, there was a paradigm change in treatment of CLL from chemoimmunotherapy-based treatments to the use of small-molecule inhibitors targeting key survival mechanisms especially in cases with high-risk genetic aberrations. The three main FDA/EMA approved small-molecule inhibitors with proven efficacy are ibrutinib, targeting BTK; idelalisib, targeting PI3K-δ; and venetoclax targeting BCL2.

4.2 Phase I and Phase II Trials with Venetoclax as a Single-Agent in CLL

In spite of variations in BCL2 expression levels between patient samples, almost all CLL tumors express high levels of BCL2 primarily due to the prevalence of del (13q14), harboring the BCL2 repressors, miR-15 and miR-16 (Cimmino et al. 2005).

A phase I first-in-human dose escalation clinical trial was initiated to determine the dosings of venetoclax in patients with relapsed/refractory CLL, SLL, or B-NHL (Roberts et al. 2016). To address the safety and pharmacokinetic profile, the first group was treated with an escalating dose, in which 56 patients received treatment with eight different doses ranging from initial doses between 20 and 50 mg venetoclax and received a weekly increase up to 1200 mg per day. In the second group, 60 patients were treated in a stepwise weekly ramp-up of up to 400 mg per day. Treatment with venetoclax resulted in an overall response rate (ORR) of 79% in the relapsed/refractory CLL with poor prognostic clinical factors (ORR of 77% in the dose escalation cohort, ORR of 82% in the expansion cohort) (Roberts et al. 2016). Strikingly, with venetoclax treatment, a rapid reduction of absolute lymphocyte counts occurred within 6–24 h after a single 20 mg dosing, where apoptotic CLL cells were detected in peripheral blood. Reduction in tumor burden was detected in blood, lymph nodes, and bone marrow; however, tumor lysis syndrome (TLS) occurred only in two patients with lymphadenopathy. Twenty percentage of patients achieved complete remission, and among them, 5% were negative for MRD by flow cytometry, which has never been observed with BTK or PI3 K inhibitors treatments (Woyach and Johnson 2015). Notably, tumor lysis syndrome emerged as dose-limiting toxicity in these early data and dedicated risk mitigation strategies have been implemented including a slow ramp-up dosing and prophylactic measures to allow for save treatment initiation (for details please see below).

In the dose escalation protocol, 60 patients were treated with a weekly dose ramp-up of 20–400 mg daily and no tumor lysis syndrome was observed. Progression-free survival of 69% was reported after 15 months. The grade 3/4 adverse effects included neutropenia in 40% of the patients and grade 1/2 adverse effects were associated with the gastrointestinal system. Nevertheless, infections due to neutropenia remained lower compared to treatment with chemoimmunotherapy. The efficacy of venetoclax was irrespective of the cytogenetics and TP53 mutation status. After a median observation time of 17 months, 41 patients (35%) showed progressive disease and among these 18 patients (16%) developed Richter's transformation.

Due to the promising results in poor-risk CLL, a pivotal phase II clinical trial was initiated, accruing relapsed/refractory CLL patients with del(17p). In this multicenter open-label study, 107 patients were enrolled between 2013 and 2014 and treated with venetoclax with a weekly dose escalation from 20 to 400 mg over 4 weeks (20, 50, 100, 200, 400 mg) and continued until disease progression. Overall response after an observation time of 12 months was 79.4% (85 of 107 patients), and in 8% of patients, complete remission was achieved. Estimated PFS and OS after 12 months were 72 and 86.7%, respectively (Fig. 3) (Stilgenbauer et al. 2016).

Responses were durable, and majority of the patients showed reduction in absolute lymphocyte count, target lymph node lesion diameter, and bone marrow infiltrate at a median of 0.3 months of treatment (Fig. 4). Management of tumor lysis syndrome was by prophylaxis. Laboratory TLS was observed in five patients during dose escalation and in one patient in the third week; however, no clinical

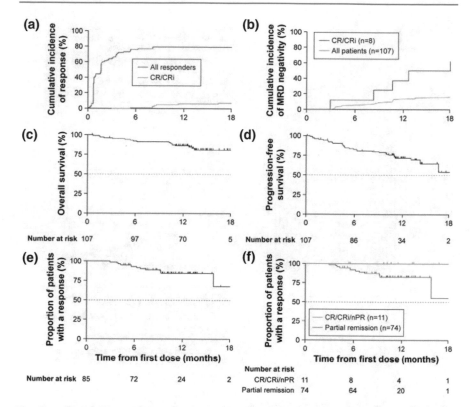

Fig. 3 a Cumulative incidence of overall response and CR by independent review-committee assessment. **b** Cumulative incidence of minimal residual disease-negative status in peripheral blood for all patients and for patients achieving CR or CRi by independent review-committee assessment. Kaplan–Meier curves for **c** overall survival, **d** progression-free survival (*n* = 107), **e** duration of overall response for all responders by independent review-committee assessment (*n* = 85), and **f** duration of overall response for all responders separated by response subgroups (independently assessed). CR: complete remission; Cri: CR with incomplete recovery of blood counts; nPR: nodular partial response (Stilgenbauer et al 2016; Huber et al. 2017)

TLS appeared in these cases. The most common adverse effect of higher grade was neutropenia in 40% of patients, which was handled with dose reductions, G-CSF administration, or prophylactic antibiotic regimens. The results of this pivotal trial led to FDA approval of venetoclax in April 2016 for the treatment of previously treated CLL patients with the 17p deletion (Deeks 2016).

To date, limited clinical data is available regarding the sequential use of the novel drugs or synergism of inhibitors in combinations. Various drug combinations are currently being tested to improve response rates and with an aim for deep remission or even cure.

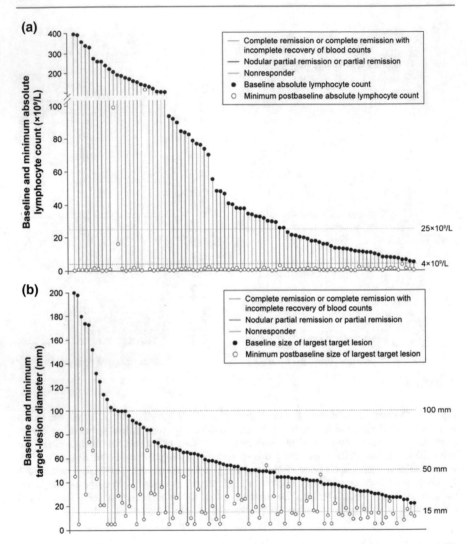

Fig. 4 Absolute change from baseline in peripheral absolute lymphocyte count in patients with a baseline absolute lymphocyte count $> 5 \times 10^9$ cells/L ($n = 87$) (**a**) and unidimensional nodal diameter ($n = 96$) (**b**). Thresholds of 4×10^9 cells/L (**a**) and 15 mm (**b**) corresponded to requirements for complete remission. Line length indicates absolute best change from baseline; each line represents one patient, with patients arranged in descending order of baseline measurement. Nodal measurements were computed tomography scan-derived, consisting unidimensional diameters of largest target lesions for patients who had at least one follow-up computed tomography scan on study. Response categories were assessed by an independent review committee (Stilgenbauer et al 2016; Huber et al. 2017)

4.3 Venetoclax in Combination Therapy for the Treatment of CLL

Since the combination of venetoclax with rituximab enhanced the efficacy of venetoclax in preclinical models, a phase Ib study was initiated where relapsed/refractory CLL patients were continuously treated with venetoclax and received a single dose of rituximab every six weeks. Primary aim of the combination study was to address the maximum tolerable dose and safety of the combination, and further objectives were to assess the pharmacokinetic profile, efficacy, overall response, and PFS (Seymour et al. 2017). Twenty-five (51%) of 49 patients had a complete remission and 28 (57%) patients achieved undetectable bone marrow MRD. The most common adverse effects included grade 1/2 gastrointestinal events and grade 3/4 neutropenia in 26 (53%) patients, similar to that of venetoclax monotherapy. Remarkably, 42 (86%) patients responded (ORR) to the combination, and a 2-year progression-free survival was achieved in 82% (Seymour et al. 2017).

Most recently, the first randomized phase III data on venetoclax became available from the MURANO trial. This showed profound improvement in PFS (primary endpoint), clinical response rate, MRD response, and OS in relapsed/refractory CLL patients treated with venetoclax plus rituximab (VR) compared to bendamustine and rituximab (BR). Of the 389 patients enrolled, 27% had a del(17p13), 60% received one prior therapy, and 15% were refractory to fludarabinc. At intcrim analysis (median follow-up of 23.8 months), PFS was significantly prolonged for VR compared to BR arm (median PFS not reached vs. 17 months, Fig. 5). The ORR for VR was 93.3% compared to 68% for BR, and CR/CRi was achieved in 26.8% versus 8.2%, respectively. MRD negativity was attained in 83.5% of cases treated with VR compared to 23.1% treated with BR. Comparable number of fatal AEs (5%) and Richter's transformation (3%) was observed in both treatment arms. The dramatic efficacy of VR treatment combined with favorable tolerability will lead to approval of this combination therapy for relapsed/refractory CLL (Seymour et al. 2017) (Fig. 5).

Furthermore, a prospective, open-label multicenter randomized phase 3 trial was initiated to compare the efficacy of obinutuzumab combined with venetoclax versus obinutuzumab with chlorambucil (Clb) in the front line treatment of CLL patients with comorbidity (CLL14 trial of the GCLLSG). The safety run-in phase of the trial included 12 patients who received the experimental arm (obinutuzumab with venetoclax). The safety and efficacy of 6 weekly cycles of obinutuzumab and daily treatment with venetoclax appeared well tolerated and showed excellent efficacy; therefore, the randomized phase III trial is currently fully accrued, and follow-up is ongoing (Fischer et al. 2015).

Several lines of evidence support the combination of venetoclax with other small-molecule inhibitors in CLL. Ongoing clinical phase II trials are recruiting participants for combination treatment of ibrutinib, venetoclax, and obinutuzumab for first-line treatment of CLL (CLL13, GAIA trial; NCT02950051). The study protocol compares several combinations such as standard chemotherapy (FCR/BR)

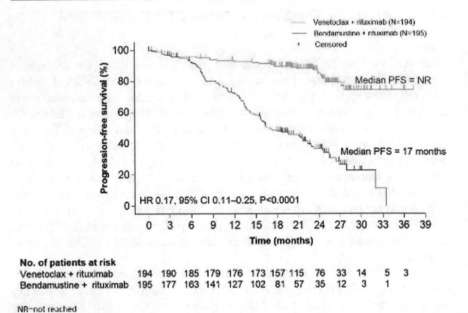

Fig. 5 Progression-free survival of the interim analysis of the pivotal phase III MURANO trial. The combination of venetoclax with rituximab showed a dramatic prolongation of PFS in comparison to bendamustine and rituximab (Seymour et al. 2017)

versus rituximab with venetoclax (RVe) versus obinutuzumab with venetoclax versus obinutuzumab with ibrutinib and venetoclax (GIVe) in previously untreated fit patients without del(17p13) or *TP53* mutation (NCT02758665). Furthermore, the combination of venetoclax with ibrutinib (NCT02756897) is being studied for the treatment of relapsed/refractory CLL. In the CLL-BAG trial, the sequential regimen of bendamustine for debulking of tumor cells is followed by ABT-199 and GA101-induction and -maintenance therapy. Interim results after the induction phase report tremendous success with an overall response rate in 97% of treated patients and 89% of patients were MRD-negative (NCT02401503) (Cramer et al. 2017). Even more impressive results are expected from these trials on treatment-naïve patients as well as relapsed/refractory diseases (Table 2).

4.4 Venetoclax for the Treatment of Acute Lymphoblastic Leukemia (ALL)

Treatment of pediatric B-cell precursor ALL (BCP-ALL) has evolved to be more and more successful over the past decades as survival rates of patients have improved to more than 80% (Pui et al. 2015). However, decreased tolerance to therapy (toxicity) and minimal residual disease positivity with subsequent relapse remain issues associated with poor outcome. As BCP-ALL is a very heterogeneous

Table 2 Selection of the important clinical trials in chronic lymphatic leukemia and their adverse effects (grade 3/4)

Trial name/population	Treatment	Phase	Identifier	N	ORR [%]	Reference	Adverse effects grade 3/4
Relapsed/refractory CLL	Venetoclax monotherapy	I	NCT01328626	116	79%	Roberts et al. (2016) NEJM	Neutropenia 41% (48) Thrombocytopenia 12% (14) TLS (dose expansion cohort 10/56)
Relapsed/refractory CLL with del (17p)	Venetoclax monotherapy	II	NCT01889186	107	79.4% (85)	Stilgenbauer et al. (2016) Lancet Oncology	Neutropenia 40% (43) Anemia 18% (19) Thrombocytopenia 15% (16) Infection 20% (21)
Relapsed/refractory CLL	Venetoclax + rituximab	Ib	NCT01682616	49	51% (25)	Seymour et al. (2017) Lancet Oncology	Neutropenia 53% (26) Thrombocytopenia 16% (8) Anemia 14% (7) TLS 4% (2)
Untreated CLL, run-in phase CLL14	Obinutuzumab combined with venetoclax versus obinutuzumab with chlorambucil	III	NCT02242942	13	58% (7)	Fischer et al. (2015) Blood	Neutropenia 58% (7) Infections 16.7% (2) Diarrhea 8.3% (1) Leukopenia 8.3% (1) Thrombocytopenia 16.7% (2) Laboratory TLS 16.7% (2)
CLL2-BAG (untreated CLL or relapsed/refractory CLL)	Bendamustine, then venetoclax + GA101	II	NCT02401503	66	97% (interim result)	Cramer et al. (2017) Hematol. Oncol.	

(continued)

Table 2 (continued)

Trial name/population	Treatment	Phase	Identifier	N	ORR [%]	Reference	Adverse effects grade 3/4		
								V + R	B + R
MURANO (relapsed/refractory CLL with/without del (17p))	Venetoclax + rituximab versus bendamustine + rituximab	III	NCT02005471	389	97.3% (interim result)	Seymour et al. (2017) Blood	Neutropenia	112 (57.7%)	73 (38.8%)
							Anemia	21 (10.8%)	26 (13.8%)
							Thrombocytopenia	11 (5.7%)	19 (10.1%)
							Febrile neutropenia	7 (3.6%)	18 (9.6%)
							Pneumonia	10 (5.2%)	15 (8.0%)
CLL2-GIVe (untreated CLL with TP53 deletion (17p-) and/or mutation	Venetoclax + ibrutinib + obinutuzumab	II	NCT02758665		recruiting	German CLL Study Group			

disease, ideal biomarkers for early stratification of patients into groups which would potentially benefit from treatment with venetoclax are required. In particular, the prognosis of Philadelphia chromosome-positive acute lymphoblastic leukemia (Ph (+) ALL) remains unfavorable. Ph(+) ALL occurs in 25% of adults and in only 3% of pediatric ALL patients (Liu-Dumlao et al. 2012). The current treatment regimen includes multi-chemotherapy which is complemented with the kinase inhibitors imatinib or dasatinib. A pre-clinical trial in xenograft mice demonstrated that the combination of dasatinib and venetoclax is synergistic and tolerable in vivo and that the anti-leukemic effects were vastly improved (Leonard et al. 2016).

Two clinical trials are planned to study the efficacy of venetoclax monotherapy in ALL. A phase I study to address the safety and pharmacokinetics of venetoclax monotherapy in pediatric and young adult patients will recruit patients with relapsed/refractory ALL (NCT03236857). Another open-label phase I dose-escalating study will recruit participants and analyze safety and pharmacokinetics of venetoclax, navitoclax, and chemotherapy in relapsed acute lymphoblastic leukemia (NCT03181126).

4.5 Treatment of Non-Hodgkin's Lymphomas (NHL) and Multiple Myeloma (MM) with Venetoclax

Non-Hodgkin's lymphoma describes a group of B- and T-cell lymphomas, which range from indolent to aggressive types. The low-grade or indolent subtypes include follicular lymphoma (FL) and CLL, while the high-grade or aggressive NHLs include diseases such as diffuse large B-cell lymphoma (DLBCL) and mantle cell lymphoma (MCL). While the standard chemo-immuno therapy has improved the outcome of patients diagnosed with aggressive non-Hodgkin's lymphomas, treatment after disease relapse remains challenging.

Venetoclax monotherapy is being assessed in a clinical trial for pediatric and young patients with NHL (NCT03236857), and even further clinical trials are planned to study venetoclax in combination (NCT03181126). A clinical phase III trial is currently investigating in the combination of venetoclax and ibrutinib in MCL patients (NCT03112174). An ongoing phase I single-arm study investigates the combination of venetoclax with bendamustine and rituximab. After completion of the treatment cycles with bendamustine, rituximab, and venetoclax, venetoclax is continued as monotherapy for two more years. In a phase I first in human trial of 106 recruited patients with relapsed/refractory FL (29), DLBCL (34), MCL (28), Waldenstroem macroglobulinea (4), marginal zone lymphoma (3) and DLBCL derived from Richter's syndrome (3), an ORR of 44% and median PFS of 6 months was achieved. 14 patients had a complete response, 33 patients showed a partial response, and 32 patients had a stable disease. In this dose escalation study, the MCL cases achieved durable response with 800mg while 1200mg was the effective single agent dose of venetoclax for FL and DLBCL patients (Davids et al. 2017).

A follow-up phase II single-arm study is currently recruiting participants for the combination of venetoclax with obinutuzumab in relapsed/refractory DLBCL. Here, the combination treatment is repeated for three cycles, and if complete or partial responses are obtained, the patients will receive stem cell transplantation (NCT02987400). Several trials aiming for the combination treatment of venetoclax with rituximab or obinutuzumab, cyclophosphamide, etoposide, prednisone, and others are under investigation.

Venetoclax demonstrated cell killing in multiple myeloma cell lines and primary tumor cells (Kumar et al. 2015), and several clinical studies with venetoclax are currently ongoing for the treatment of multiple myeloma. Relapsed/refractory patients receive combinations of venetoclax and current standard therapy with dexamethasone and bortezomib (NCT02755597; NCT01794507). Other trials combine venetoclax with daratumumab, a CD38 antibody (NCT03314181). In the monotherapy approach, 21% of patients responded to venetoclax treatment. Notably, 40% of these patients carried the t(11;14) translocation, were refractory to bortezomib and lenalidomide, and were treated with at least four prior regimens (Kumar et al. 2015). Due to good safety and efficacy, a phase Ib trial was initiated to study the combination treatment of venetoclax with bortezomib and dexamethasone. Sixty-six heavily pretreated patients were enrolled. The overall response rate was 66%, and the median time to progression was 9.7 months. The results were irrespective of the t(11;14) status, with manageable adverse effects and an acceptable safety profile (Moreau et al. 2017).

4.6 Venetoclax for Treatment of Myeloid Malignancies

Acute myeloid leukemia is an aggressive malignancy of the myeloid progenitor cells. AML cases have variable outcome after chemotherapy due to the enormous clinical and molecular heterogeneity. Over decades, the induction therapy of combined anthracycline plus cytarabine cytotoxic agents has remained the standard of treatment with little improvement in survival with the additions of novel agents. Though the manipulation of intensity and duration of treatment modestly improved survival incertain patient subsets, a consolidation chemotherapy often including stem cell transplant remains necessary (Fernandez et al. 2009). Venetoclax demonstrated high efficiency in preclinical AML models as well as synergy with anthracyclines (Teh et al. 2017).

Venetoclax achieved remarkable results in early clinical trials in AML. The M13-387 phase Ib trial evaluated the safety and the maximum tolerable dose of venetoclax in treatment naïve elderly AML patients not eligible for standard induction chemotherapy. Patients were treated in two arms, a ramp-up of venetoclax with decitabine or 5-azacitidine. Nineteen of 22 patients completed the first 28-day cycle with venetoclax. The response to treatment was 75% in the decitabine and 70% in the 5-azacitidine arms (DiNardo et al. 2015). Also, venetoclax as a single agent in heavily pretreated AML patients resulted in an overall response rate of 19% (Konopleva et al. 2016). Based on these results, further clinical trials were initiated for the treatment of AML. A phase III study was initiated to assess treatment with Venetoclax in combination with azacitidine, where patients not eligible for intensive therapy were randomized to venetoclax with azacitidine or placebo with azacitidine arms. Interim results present an impressive overall response rate of 69% with a complete response (CR) of 60% in high-risk AML patients (NCT03236857; DiNardo et al. 2015).

5 Venetoclax in Solid Tumors

As various cancers show dependency on anti-apoptotic BCL2 family members for their survival, the use of venetoclax extends beyond that of hematologic malignancies.

BCL2 is overexpressed in 85% of estrogen receptor-positive (ER) breast cancers. ER was found to bind two estrogen response elements (EREs) in the coding regions of BCL2, thereby enhancing BCL2 expression in these tumors (Perillo et al. 2000). Preclinical data generated in ER-positive breast cancer xenografts showed venetoclax to be highly efficacious. Also, venetoclax was found to synergize with PI3K and mTOR inhibitors enhancing its apoptotic effect (Vaillant et al. 2013). To explore more effective therapeutic strategies, safety and efficiency of venetoclax were tested in a phase Ib study in ER^+ $BCL2^+$ breast cancer patients. The results were heterogeneous, as four patients had a partial response and five has a stable disease with a clinical benefit rate of 69%. Venetoclax treatment of ER+ breast cancers is further being validated in phase II clinical trials which are ongoing (NCT02391480).

Small-cell lung cancer (SCLC) is a high proliferating cancer with a low doubling time, rapid metastasis, and quick relapse after treatment. First-line chemotherapy with platinum-based agents and etoposide remains without long-term success, and multiple-targeted approaches using receptor tyrosine kinase (RTK) inhibitors are being investigated. Though the RTK inhibitors were of therapeutic relevance, the curative potential was minimal (Niederst et al. 2013). Assessment of the efficacy of venetoclax in SCLC treatment is still in the pre-clinical phase. The expression of BCL2 was comprehensively assessed in different lung cancer cell lines, and BCL2 inhibitors were found to synergize with anthracyclines providing a promising strategy for treatment (Inoue-Yamauchi et al. 2017). Venetoclax was also addressed in combination with BET inhibitor ABBV-075, since BET is known to regulate key oncogenes as MYC, CCND2, and BCL2L1 and enhance complex formation of pro-apoptotic BIM and BCL2 (Lam et al. 2017). The combination treatment proved to be highly synergistic and therefore might be a possible rationale for treatment of SCLC patients with high BCL2 expression.

6 Toxicity and Adverse Effects Associated with BCL2 Inhibitor Treatments

6.1 Thrombocytopenia

BH3 mimetics such as ABT-767 and ABT-263 inhibit BCL2, as well as BCL-x_L and BCL-W. Since thrombocytes depend on BCL-x_L for survival, treatment with these inhibitors leads to reduction in platelets and dose-dependent thrombocytopenia due to direct toxic anti-platelet effects. Assessment of safety and tolerability of navitoclax documented the prevalence of thrombocytopenia in different tumor entities. In a clinical trial on 39 SCLC patients, 41% developed grade III–VI thrombocytopenia upon treatment with navitoclax (Rudin et al. 2012). In a phase II study of CLL patients, 36% of patients suffered from grad III–IV thrombocytopenia (Kipps et al. 2015). This mode of action of these drugs on platelets was clarified to be mediated by apoptosis cell death, as well as decreased calcium flux, reducing the activation of platelets (Vogler et al. 2013). To circumvent severe thrombocytopenia, the initial dose of navitoclax was kept low within the first seven days of treatment. However, these side effects limited the clinical development of navitoclax. Venetoclax being a highly specific for BCL2 with lower affinity toward BCL-x_L did not induce dose-dependent thrombocytopenia.

6.2 Tumor Lysis Syndrome (TLS)

The tumor lysis syndrome is one of the major risk issues in venetoclax treatment, owing to the very high potency of the drug. Due to the rapid response, with abrupt onset at 6–8 h following dosing, venetoclax is prone to induce tumor lysis syndrome, depending on tumor mass, comorbidities (in particular renal function), and treatment dose (Cheson et al. 2017). TLS results from rapid cell death, wherein tumor cells release their metabolites, nucleic acids, and intracellular ions into the blood stream, thereby potentially inducing metabolic dysfunction. The efflux of cellular metabolites leads to a disbalance of the blood homeostasis with an increase in uric acid, potassium, and phosphoric acid and decrease in calcium levels. If the renal excretion is affected or delayed, an accumulation of these metabolites occurs in blood. The incidence of TLS is increased in tumors with a high tumor burden or high cell turnover (Cheson et al. 2017; Crombie and Davids 2017). The most common criteria for subdivision into clinical and laboratory TLS were defined in 2004 by Cairo et al. (2004). Laboratory TLS includes at least two or more biochemical variables being increased or reduced by a factor of more than 25%; furthermore, TLS appears within three days prior or seven days after initiation of therapy. TLS causes hyperuricemia, hyperkalemia, hyperphosphatemia, and hypocalcemia and can lead to acute renal failure and cardiac events of life-threatening potential. If laboratory TLS is accompanied by clinically relevant events such as creatinine increase, seizures, or cardiac dysfunction, a clinical TLS is diagnosed. Prophylaxis and treatment of TLS includes hydration, diuresis, monitoring of electrolytes, and prevention of hypouricemia with allopurinol or rasburicase (Howard et al. 2011).

For treatment with venetoclax, a treatment risk stratification is implemented where patients are grouped according to their TLS risk. Low risk for TLS is defined by small nodal disease, a low ALS $< 25 \times 10^9$/L. Medium risk includes an ALS $> 25 \times 10^9$/L or a lymph node with more than 5 cm diameter. The high-risk group for TLS is a radiological tumor > 10 cm in diameter and a ALS $> 25 \times 10^9$/L (Roberts et al. 2016). Therapy with venetoclax is initiated with a low starting dose, and patients pass through a weekly dose ramp-up from 20 to 50, 100, 200, and 400 mg to ensure safety and tolerability. Laboratory monitoring of blood counts and clinical chemistry is mandatory during treatment initiation, and immediate action is required in case of relevant abnormalities. Detailed information and guidance on TLS management are beyond the scope of this article and are available in the prescription information of venetoclax. Meticulous adherence to the guidelines is required to deliver venetoclax therapy safely.

7 Venetoclax Drug Interactions

7.1 Interaction with CYP3A4 Inhibitors

The routes of elimination of venetoclax were tested by administration of a 200 mg single dose of ^{14}C (100 µCi) venetoclax to four healthy volunteers. The recovery of total radioactive dose (100% ± 5%) was through feces as the major route of drug elimination. The major metabolite M27 was formed by oxidation cytochrome P450 isoform 3A4 (CYP3A4) (Choo et al. 2014; Li et al. 2016). Since various drugs such as protease inhibitors, anti-fungal agents, macrolide antibiotics, and anti-depressants are described to be inhibitors of CYP3A4, possibility of drug interactions was tested using ketoconazole as a representative agent. Twelve NHL patients were enrolled for a phase I, open-label study, where patients received venetoclax and ketoconazole, the strong CYP3A4 inhibitor. Inhibition of CYP3A4 led to a significant increase in the mean maximum observed plasma concentration Cmax and area under the plasma concentration-time curve (AUC∞) by 2.3-fold and 6.4-fold, respectively.

Similarly, also, simultaneous treatment with venetoclax and CYP3A4 inducers such as Rifampin led to an increase in the AUC and Cmax of venetoclax (Agarwal et al. 2016). These studies suggest the need to avoid concomitant use of strong and moderate inhibitors or inducers of CYP3A4 during the venetoclax ramp-up phase in patients (Agarwal et al. 2017). Also, venetoclax dosage should be reduced by 25–50% when co-administering the CYP3A4 modulators after dose escalation.

7.2 Interaction with P-Glycoprotein Inhibitors

Venetoclax has been described to be a substrate of P-glycoproteins (P-gp) based on in vitro studies. Also, venetoclax was shown to inhibit P-glycoprotein at the transcriptional and protein levels (Weiss et al. 2016). In a clinical trial in healthy volunteers, the effect of venetoclax on the pharmacokinetics of digoxin, a P-gp inhibitor was evaluated. Co-administration of digoxin and venetoclax increased digoxin maximum observed plasma concentration (Cmax) by 35% and area under the plasma concentration-time curve (AUC0–∞) by 9%. The study indicated that venetoclax can increase the concentrations of P-gp substrates. The study suggested administration of narrow therapeutic index P-gp substrates, six hours prior to venetoclax to minimize the potential interaction.

8 Biomarkers of Resistance to Venetoclax Treatment

Biomarkers are important to predict the response and efficacy to venetoclax therapy and for early assignment of combination or alternative treatments for effective therapy.

Due to the high specificity of venetoclax, upregulation of alternative anti-apoptotic is described to confer resistance to therapy. Several preclinical and ex vivo studies analyzed the ratio between BCL2 and MCL1 which was of clinical importance to predict venetoclax treatment response. Studies of multiple myeloma xenografts showed that the overexpression of BCL2 and MCL1 led to resistance toward BCL2 inhibitors treatment (Punnoose et al. 2016). Upregulation of BCL-x_L or MCL1 or both is also contributing to venetoclax resistance in lymphoma cell lines (Tahir et al. 2017).

Functional analysis of the cell's response to venetoclax using BH3 profiling of primary CLL cells showed a significant association between apoptotic priming by venetoclax ex vivo to clinical response to venetoclax. Precisely, the extent of mitochondrial depolarization by a BIM BH3 peptide in vitro correlated with percentage reduction of CLL in the blood following venetoclax treatment suggesting its use as a potential biomarker for early risk stratification (Anderson et al. 2016).

Furthermore, acquired missense mutations in the BH3 binding groove of resistant cell lines were detected to interfere with drug binding capacity. Also, acquired mutations in the pro-apoptotic BAX gene limiting its anchoring to the mitochondria were also described to interfere with apoptosis induction by venetoclax (Fresquet et al. 2014).

9 Summary and Future Perspectives

The EMA and FDA approval of venetoclax, a novel, and highly specific BCL2 inhibitor already indicates its high therapeutic potential in CLL and potentially also in various other malignancies. Venetoclax demonstrated tremendous success in treatment of poor risk, relapsed/refractory CLL, and in the future may be revolutionizing treatment of various other hematological malignancies. With precision medicine evolving to a real-world paradigm, there is an absolute need for novel and specific targeted therapies. The use of targeted combination therapies will further improve the landscape of treatment options for patients who are refractory to conventional therapies and may eventually lead to novel approaches en route toward the cure of cancer.

References

Abulwerdi F et al (2014) A novel small-molecule inhibitor of mcl-1 blocks pancreatic cancer growth in vitro and in vivo. Mol Cancer Ther 13:565–75

Agarwal SK, Hu B, Chien D, Wong S, Salem A (2016) Evaluation of Rifampin's transporter inhibitory and CYP3A inductive effects on the pharmacokinetics of venetoclax, a BCL-2 inhibitor: results of a single- and multiple-dose study. J Clin Pharmacol 56:1335–1343

Agarwal SK et al (2017) Effect of ketoconazole, a strong CYP3A inhibitor, on the pharmacokinetics of venetoclax, a BCL-2 inhibitor, in patients with non-Hodgkin lymphoma. Br J Clin Pharmacol 83:846–854

Albershardt TC et al (2011) Multiple BH3 mimetics antagonize antiapoptotic MCL1 protein by inducing the endoplasmic reticulum stress response and up-regulating BH3-only protein NOXA. J Biol Chem 286:24882–24895

Alford SE et al (2015) BH3 inhibitor sensitivity and Bcl-2 dependence in primary acute lymphoblastic leukemia cells. Cancer Res 75:1366–1375

Anderson MA et al (2016) The BCL2 selective inhibitor venetoclax induces rapid onset apoptosis of CLL cells in patients via a TP53-independent mechanism. Blood 127:3215–3224

Bai L et al (2014) BM-1197: a novel and specific Bcl-2/Bcl-xL inhibitor inducing complete and long-lasting tumor regression in vivo. PLoS ONE 9:e99404

Balakrishnan K, Burger JA, Wierda WG, Gandhi V (2009) AT-101 induces apoptosis in CLL B cells and overcomes stromal cell-mediated Mcl-1 induction and drug resistance. Blood 113:149–153

Bentz M et al (2000) t(11;14)-positive mantle cell lymphomas exhibit complex karyotypes and share similarities with B-cell chronic lymphocytic leukemia. Genes, Chromosom Cancer 27:285–294

Beroukhim R et al (2010) The landscape of somatic copy-number alteration across human cancers. Nature 463:899–905

Boise LH et al (1993) bcl-x, a bcl-2-related gene that functions as a dominant regulator of apoptotic cell death. Cell 74:597–608

Brown JR et al (2015) Obatoclax in combination with fludarabine and rituximab is well-tolerated and shows promising clinical activity in relapsed chronic lymphocytic leukemia. Leuk Lymphoma 56:3336–3342

Byrd JC et al (2015) Three-year follow-up of treatment-naïve and previously treated patients with CLL and SLL receiving single-agent ibrutinib. Blood 125

Byrd JC et al (2014) Ibrutinib versus ofatumumab in previously treated chronic lymphoid leukemia. N Engl J Med 371:213–223

Cahill N, Rosenquist R (2013) Uncovering the DNA methylome in chronic lymphocytic leukemia. Epigenetics 8:138–148

Cairo MS, Bishop M (2004) Tumour lysis syndrome: new therapeutic strategies and classification. Br J Haematol 127:3–11

Cervantes-Gomez F et al (2015) Pharmacological and protein profiling suggests venetoclax (ABT-199) as optimal partner with ibrutinib in chronic lymphocytic leukemia. Clin Cancer Res 21:3705–3715

Cheson BD et al (2017) Tumor lysis syndrome in chronic lymphocytic leukemia with novel targeted agents. Oncologist 22:1283–1291

Choo EF et al (2014) The role of lymphatic transport on the systemic bioavailability of the BCL-2 protein family inhibitors navitoclax (ABT-263) and ABT-199. Drug Metab Dispos 42:207–212

Cimmino A et al (2005) miR-15 and miR-16 induce apoptosis by targeting BCL2. Proc Natl Acad Sci 102:13944–13949

Cohen NA et al (2012) A competitive stapled peptide screen identifies a selective small molecule that overcomes MCL-1-dependent leukemia cell survival. Chem Biol 19:1175–1186

Cramer P et al (2017) Bendamustine (B), followed by obinutuzumab (G) and venetoclax (A) in patients with chronic lymphocytic leukemia (Cll): Cll2-bag trial of the german CLL study group (GCLLSG). Hematol Oncol 35:25–27

Crombie J, Davids MS (2017) Venetoclax for the treatment of patients with chronic lymphocytic leukemia. Futur Oncol 13:1223–1232

Datta SR et al (2002) Survival factor-mediated BAD phosphorylation raises the mitochondrial threshold for apoptosis. Dev Cell 3:631–643

Davids MS, Roberts AW, Seymour JF, Pagel JM, Kahl BS, Wierda WG, Puvvada S, Kipps TJ, Anderson MA, Salem AH, Dunbar M, Zhu M, Peale F, Ross JA, Gressick L, Desai M, Kim SY, Verdugo M, Humerickhouse RA, Gordon GB, Gerecitano JF (2017) Phase I first-in-human study of venetoclax in patients with relapsed or refractory non-hodgkin lymphoma. J Clin Oncol 35(8):826–833

Deeks ED (2016) Venetoclax: first global approval. Drugs 76:979–987

DiNardo C et al (2015) A phase 1b study of venetoclax (ABT-199/GDC-0199) in combination with decitabine or azacitidine in treatment-naive patients with acute myelogenous leukemia who are ≥ to 65 years and not eligible for standard induction therapy. Blood 126

Fernandez HF et al (2009) Anthracycline dose intensification in acute myeloid leukemia. N Engl J Med 361:1249–1259

Fischer K et al (2015) Results of the safety run-in phase of CLL14 (BO25323): a prospective, open-label, multicenter randomized phase III trial to compare the efficacy and safety of obinutuzumab and venetoclax (GDC-0199/ABT-199) with obinutuzumab and chlorambucil in patients w…. Blood 126

Fischer U et al (2015) Genomics and drug profiling of fatal TCF3-HLF − positive acute lymphoblastic leukemia identifies recurrent mutation patterns and therapeutic options. Nat Genet 47:1020–1029

Fresquet V, Rieger M, Carolis C, Garcia-Barchino MJ, Martinez-Climent JA (2014) Acquired mutations in BCL2 family proteins conferring resistance to the BH3 mimetic ABT-199 in lymphoma. Blood 123:4111–4119

Frismantas V et al (2017) Ex vivo drug response profiling detects recurrent sensitivity patterns in drug-resistant acute lymphoblastic leukemia. Blood 129:e26–e37

Gandhi L et al (2011) Phase I study of navitoclax (ABT-263), a novel Bcl-2 family inhibitor, in patients with small-cell lung cancer and other solid tumors. J Clin Oncol 29:909–916

Gibson CJ, Davids MS (2015) BCL-2 antagonism to target the intrinsic mitochondrial pathway of apoptosis. Clin Cancer Res 21:5021–5029

Gibson L et al (1996) bcl-w, a novel member of the bcl-2 family, promotes cell survival. Oncogene 13:665–675

Gratiot-Deans J, Merinot R, Nurezt G, Turkau LA (1994) Bcl-2 expression during T-cell development: early loss and late return occur at specific stages of commitment to differentiation and survival. 91, 10685–10689

Hanada M, Delia D, Aiello A, Stadtmauer E, Reed JC (1993) bcl-2 gene hypomethylation and high-level expression in B-cell chronic lymphocytic leukemia. Blood 82:1820–1828

Hanahan D, Weinberg RA (2011) Hallmarks of cancer: the next generation. Cell 144:646–674

Howard SC, Jones DP, Pui C-H (2011) The tumor lysis syndrome. N Engl J Med 364:1844–1854

Huber H, Edenhofer S, Estenfelder S, Stilgenbauer S (2017) Profile of venetoclax and its potential in the context of treatment of relapsed or refractory chronic lymphocytic leukemia. Onco Targets Ther 10:645–656

Inohara N, Ding L, Chen S, Núñez G (1997) Harakiri, a novel regulator of cell death, encodes a protein that activates apoptosis and interacts selectively with survival-promoting proteins Bcl-2 and Bcl-X(L). EMBO J 16:1686–1694

Inoue-Yamauchi A et al (2017) Targeting the differential addiction to anti-apoptotic BCL-2 family for cancer therapy. Nat Commun 8:16078

Kaefer A et al (2014) Mechanism-based pharmacokinetic/pharmacodynamic meta-analysis of navitoclax (ABT-263) induced thrombocytopenia. Cancer Chemother Pharmacol 74:593–602

Khaw SL et al (2014) Both leukaemic and normal peripheral B lymphoid cells are highly sensitive to the selective pharmacological inhibition of prosurvival Bcl-2 with ABT-199. Leukemia 28:1207–1215

Khaw SL et al (2016) Venetoclax responses of pediatric ALL xenografts reveal sensitivity of MLL-rearranged leukemia. Blood 128:1382–1395

Kipps TJ et al (2015) A phase 2 study of the BH3 mimetic BCL2 inhibitor navitoclax (ABT-263) with or without rituximab, in previously untreated B-cell chronic lymphocytic leukemia. Leuk Lymphoma 56:2826–2833

Konopleva M et al (2016) Efficacy and biological correlates of response in a phase II study of venetoclax monotherapy in patients with acute myelogenous leukemia. Cancer Discov 6:1106–1117

Korsmeyer SJ et al (2000) Pro-apoptotic cascade activates BID, which oligomerizes BAK or BAX into pores that result in the release of cytochrome c. Cell Death Differ 7:1166–1173

Kotschy A et al (2016) The MCL1 inhibitor S63845 is tolerable and effective in diverse cancer models. Nature 538:477–482

Kumar SK et al (2015) Safety and efficacy of venetoclax (ABT-199/GDC-0199) monotherapy for relapsed/refractory multiple myeloma: phase 1 preliminary results. Blood 126

Lam LT et al (2017) Vulnerability of small-cell lung cancer to apoptosis induced by the combination of BET bromodomain proteins and BCL2 inhibitors. Mol Cancer Ther 16:1511–1520

Lee JH et al (2004) Inactivating mutation of the pro-apoptotic geneBID in gastric cancer. J Pathol 202:439–445

Leonard JT et al (2016) Targeting BCL-2 and ABL/LYN in Philadelphia chromosome-positive acute lymphoblastic leukemia. Sci Transl Med 8, 354ra114-354ra114

Lessene G et al (2013) Structure-guided design of a selective BCL-XL inhibitor. Nat Chem Biol 9:390–397

Li CJ et al (2016) Novel Bruton's tyrosine kinase inhibitor Bgb-3111 demonstrates potent activity in mantle cell lymphoma. Blood 128

Liu-Dumlao T, Kantarjian H, Thomas DA, O'Brien S, Ravandi F (2012) Philadelphia-positive acute lymphoblastic leukemia: current treatment options. Curr Oncol Rep 14:387–394

Meijerink JP et al (1998) Hematopoietic malignancies demonstrate loss-of-function mutations of BAX. Blood 91:2991–2997

Merino R, Ding L, Veis DJ, Korsmeyer SJ, Nuñez G (1994) Developmental regulation of the Bcl-2 protein and susceptibility to cell death in B lymphocytes. EMBO J 13:683–691

Miyashita T, Reed JC (1995) Tumor suppressor p53 is a direct transcriptional activator of the human bax gene. Cell 80:293–299

Monni O et al (1997) BCL2 overexpression associated with chromosomal amplification in diffuse large B-cell lymphoma. Blood 90

Moreau P et al (2017) Promising efficacy and acceptable safety of venetoclax plus bortezomib and dexamethasone in relapsed/refractory MM. Blood blood-2017-06-788323. https://doi.org/10.1182/blood-2017-06-788323

Motoyama N et al (1995) Massive cell death of immature hematopoietic cells and neurons in Bcl-x-deficient mice. Science 267:1506–1510

NCT01794507. A study evaluating ABT-199 in multiple myeloma subjects who are receiving bortezomib and dexamethasone as standard therapy—full text view—ClinicalTrials.gov

NCT02391480. A study evaluating the safety and pharmacokinetics of ABBV-075 in subjects with cancer—full text view—ClinicalTrials.gov

NCT02755597. A study evaluating venetoclax (ABT-199) in multiple myeloma subjects who are receiving bortezomib and dexamethasone as standard therapy—full text view—ClinicalTrials.gov

NCT02758665. Trial of ibrutinib plus venetoclax plus obinutuzumab in patients with CLL (CLL2-GiVe)-full text view-ClinicalTrials.gov

NCT02987400. Combination of obinutuzumab and venetoclax in relapsed or refractory DLBCL—full text view—ClinicalTrials.gov

NCT03112174. Study of ibrutinib combined with venetoclax in subjects with mantle cell lymphoma (SYMPATICO)—full text view—ClinicalTrials.gov

NCT03181126 & AbbVie. A study of venetoclax in combination with navitoclax and chemotherapy in subjects with relapsed acute lymphoblastic leukemia—full text view—ClinicalTrials.gov

NCT03236857. A study of the safety and pharmacokinetics of venetoclax in pediatric and young adult patients with relapsed or refractory malignancies—full text view—ClinicalTrials.gov

NCT03314181. A study of combination therapy with venetoclax, daratumumab and dexamethasone (with and without bortezomib) in subjects with relapsed or refractory multiple myeloma—full text view—ClinicalTrials.gov

Nguyen M et al (2007) Small molecule obatoclax (GX15-070) antagonizes MCL-1 and overcomes MCL-1-mediated resistance to apoptosis. Proc Natl Acad Sci 104:19512–19517

Niederst MJ, Engelman JA (2013) Bypass mechanisms of resistance to receptor tyrosine kinase inhibition in lung cancer. Sci Signal 6, re6

O'Brien SM et al (2005) Phase I to II multicenter study of oblimersen sodium, a Bcl-2 antisense oligonucleotide, in patients with advanced chronic lymphocytic leukemia. J Clin Oncol 23:7697–7702

O'Brien S et al (2009) 5-year survival in patients with relapsed or refractory chronic lymphocytic leukemia in a randomized, phase III trial of fludarabine plus cyclophosphamide with or without oblimersen. J Clin Oncol 27:5208–5212

O'Connor L et al (1998) Bim: a novel member of the Bcl-2 family that promotes apoptosis. EMBO J 17:384–395

Oda E et al (2000) Noxa, a BH3-only member of the Bcl-2 family and candidate mediator of p53-induced apoptosis. Science 288:1053–1058

Oltersdorf T et al (2005) An inhibitor of Bcl-2 family proteins induces regression of solid tumours. Nature 435:677–681

Opferman JT et al (2003) Development and maintenance of B and T lymphocytes requires antiapoptotic MCL-1. Nature 426:671–676

Opferman JT et al (2005) Obligate role of anti-apoptotic MCL-1 in the survival of hematopoietic stem cells. Science 307:1101–1104

Pan R et al (2014) Selective BCL-2 inhibition by ABT-199 causes on-target cell death in acute myeloid leukemia. Cancer Discov 4:362–375

Park D et al (2013) Novel small-molecule inhibitors of Bcl-XL to treat lung cancer. Cancer Res 73:5485–5496

Perillo B, Sasso A, Abbondanza C, Palumbo G (2000) 17beta-estradiol inhibits apoptosis in MCF-7 cells, inducing bcl-2 expression via two estrogen-responsive elements present in the coding sequence. Mol Cell Biol 20:2890–2901

Pui C-H et al (2015) Clinical utility of sequential minimal residual disease measurements in the context of risk-based therapy in childhood acute lymphoblastic leukaemia: a prospective study. Lancet Oncol 16:465–474

Punnoose EA et al (2016) Expression profile of BCL-2, BCL-XL, and MCL-1 predicts pharmacological response to the BCL-2 selective antagonist venetoclax in multiple myeloma models. Mol Cancer Ther 15:1132–1144

Reed JC, Stein C, Subasinghe C, Haldar S, Croce CM, Yum S, Cohen J (1990) Antisense-mediated inhibition of BCL2 protooncogene expression and leukemic cell growth and survival: comparisons of phosphodiester and phosphorothioate oligodeoxynucleotides. Cancer Res 50:6565–6570

Rinkenberger JL, Horning S, Klocke B, Roth K, Korsmeyer SJ (2000) Mcl-1 deficiency results in peri-implantation embryonic lethality. Genes Dev 14:23–27

Roberts AW et al (2012) Substantial susceptibility of chronic lymphocytic leukemia to BCL2 inhibition: results of a phase I study of navitoclax in patients with relapsed or refractory disease. J Clin Oncol 30:488–496

Roberts AW et al (2016) Targeting BCL2 with venetoclax in relapsed chronic lymphocytic leukemia. N Engl J Med 374:311–322

Roberts AW, Stilgenbauer S, Seymour JF, Huang DCS (2017) Venetoclax in patients with previously treated chronic lymphocytic leukemia. Clin Cancer Res 23:4527–4533

Robertson LE, Plunkett W, McConnell K, Keating MJ, McDonnell TJ (1996) Bcl-2 expression in chronic lymphocytic leukemia and its correlation with the induction of apoptosis and clinical outcome. Leukemia 10:456–459

Rudin CM et al (2012) Phase II study of single-agent navitoclax (ABT-263) and biomarker correlates in patients with relapsed small cell lung cancer. Clin Cancer Res 18:3163–3169

Seymour JF, Kipps TJ, Eichhorst BF, Hillmen P, D'Rozario JM, Assouline S, Owen CJ, Gerecitano J, Robak T, De la Serna J, Jaeger U, Cartron G, Montillo M, Humerickhouse R, Elizabet APK. Venetoclax plus rituximab is superior to bendamustine plus rituximab in patients with relapsed/refractory chronic lymphocytic leukemia—results from pre-planned interim analysis of the randomized phase 3 murano study. ASH Abstract 2017 (2017)

Seymour JF et al (2017) Venetoclax plus rituximab in relapsed or refractory chronic lymphocytic leukaemia: a phase 1b study. Lancet Oncol 18:230–240

Souers AJ et al (2013) ABT-199, a potent and selective BCL-2 inhibitor, achieves antitumor activity while sparing platelets. Nat Med 19:202–208

Stilgenbauer S et al (2016) Venetoclax in relapsed or refractory chronic lymphocytic leukaemia with 17p deletion: a multicentre, open-label, phase 2 study. Lancet Oncol 17:768–778

Sturm I et al (2000) Impaired BAX protein expression in breast cancer: mutational analysis of the BAX and the p53 gene. Int J Cancer 87:517–521

Tahir SK et al (2017) Potential mechanisms of resistance to venetoclax and strategies to circumvent it. BMC Cancer 17:399

Teh T-C et al (2017) Enhancing venetoclax activity in acute myeloid leukemia by co-targeting MCL1. Leukemia. https://doi.org/10.1038/leu.2017.243

Tolcher AW et al (2015) Safety, efficacy, and pharmacokinetics of navitoclax (ABT-263) in combination with erlotinib in patients with advanced solid tumors. Cancer Chemother Pharmacol 76:1025–1032

Tse C et al (2008) ABT-263: a potent and orally bioavailable Bcl-2 family inhibitor. Cancer Res 68:3421–3428

Tsujimoto Y, Cossman J, Jaffe E, Croce CM (1985) Involvement of the bcl-2 gene in human follicular lymphoma. Science 228:1440–1443

Vaillant F et al (2013) Targeting BCL-2 with the BH3 mimetic ABT-199 in estrogen receptor-positive breast cancer. Cancer Cell 24:120–129 van Delft MF et al (2006) The BH3 mimetic ABT-737 targets selective Bcl-2 proteins and efficiently induces apoptosis via Bak/Bax if Mcl-1 is neutralized. Cancer Cell 10:389–399

Varadarajan S et al (2013a) Evaluation and critical assessment of putative MCL-1 inhibitors. Cell Death Differ 20:1475–1484

Varadarajan S et al (2013b) Sabutoclax (BI97C1) and BI112D1, putative inhibitors of MCL-1, induce mitochondrial fragmentation either upstream of or independent of apoptosis. Neoplasia 15:568–578

Veis DJ, Sentman CL, Bach EA, Korsmeyer SJ (1993) Expression of the Bcl-2 protein in murine and human thymocytes and in peripheral T lymphocytes. J. Immunol. 151:2546–2554

Vogler M, Dinsdale D, Dyer MJS, Cohen GM (2013) ABT-199 selectively inhibits BCL2 but not BCL2L1 and efficiently induces apoptosis of chronic lymphocytic leukaemic cells but not platelets. Br J Haematol 163:139–142

Wei MC et al (2000) tBID, a membrane-targeted death ligand, oligomerizes BAK to release cytochrome c. Genes Dev 14:2060–2071

Weiss J, Gajek T, Köhler B, Haefeli W (2016) Venetoclax (ABT-199) might act as a perpetrator in pharmacokinetic drug-drug interactions. Pharmaceutics 8:5

Wilson WH et al (2010) Navitoclax, a targeted high-affinity inhibitor of BCL-2, in lymphoid malignancies: a phase 1 dose-escalation study of safety, pharmacokinetics, pharmacodynamics, and antitumour activity. Lancet Oncol 11:1149–1159

Woyach JA, Johnson AJ (2015) Targeted therapies in CLL: mechanisms of resistance and strategies for management. Blood 126

Idelalisib

Katja Zirlik and Hendrik Veelken

Contents

K. Zirlik
Department of Medicine I: Hematology, Oncology, and Stem Cell Transplantation,
University Medical Center Freiburg, Hugstetterstr. 55, 79106 Freiburg, Germany
e-mail: Katja.Zirlik@zetup.ch

K. Zirlik
Tumor and Breast Center ZeTuP, St. Gallen, Switzerland

H. Veelken (✉)
Department of Hematology, Leiden University Medical Center, Leiden, The Netherlands
e-mail: J.H.Veelken@lumc.nl

© Springer International Publishing AG, part of Springer Nature 2018
U. M. Martens (ed.), *Small Molecules in Hematology*, Recent Results
in Cancer Research 211, https://doi.org/10.1007/978-3-319-91439-8_12

Abstract

Idelalisib (GS-1101, CAL-101, Zydelig®) is an orally bioavailable, small-molecule inhibitor of the delta isoform (p110δ) of the enzyme phospho-inositide 3-kinase (PI3K). In contrast to the other PI3K isoforms, PI3Kδ is expressed selectively in hematopoietic cells. PI3Kδ signaling is active in many B-cell leukemias and lymphomas. By inhibiting the PI3Kδ protein, idelalisib blocks several cellular signaling pathways that maintain B-cell viability. Idelalisib is the first PI3K inhibitor approved by the US Food and Drug Administration (FDA). Treatment with idelalisib is indicated in relapsed/refractory chronic lymphocytic leukemia (CLL), follicular lymphoma (FL), and small lymphocytic lymphoma (SLL). This review presents the preclinical and clinical activity of idelalisib with a focus on clinical studies in CLL.

Keywords

Idelalisib · Kinase inhibitor · Chronic lymphocytic leukemia (CLL) ·
PI 3 Kinase

1 Introduction

The management of lymphoid malignancies has greatly evolved during the last decade with the advent of biological, more targeted therapies (Awan and Byrd 2014; Byrd et al. 2014a; Danilov 2013; Jahangiri et al. 2014; Jain and O'Brien 2016; Marini et al. 2017; Molica 2017; Morabito et al. 2015; Niemann et al. 2013; Sanford et al. 2015; Vitale et al. 2017). Since its initial description, the PI3K pathway has been an attractive target for anticancer therapy. The PI3K pathway seems to play an important role in the development of various solid malignancies, such as melanoma, lung, colorectal, and breast cancers (Janku 2017). More recently, the role of the PI3K pathway in the pathophysiology of hematological malignancies has been appreciated (Akinleye et al. 2013; Alinari et al. 2012; Brown 2016; Burger and Okkenhaug 2014; Fruman and Rommel 2011; Gilbert 2014; Gockeritz et al. 2015; Hewett et al. 2016; Macias-Perez and Flinn 2013; Okoli et al. 2015; Pongas and Cheson 2016; Seiler et al. 2016; Vanhaesebroeck and Khwaja 2014; Yap et al. 2015). CLL, a malignancy of mature B lymphocytes, remains the most prevalent leukemia in Western adult patients. Though the clinical outcome has improved considerably through the introduction of immunochemotherapy and presumably better supportive care, CLL treatment may be challenging, particularly as the incidence of CLL increases with age (Rai 2015; Ysebaert et al. 2015). Therefore, new treatment strategies to improve efficacy, survival rate, and safety profile are needed.

The B-cell receptor (BCR) signaling pathway plays a key role in the pathogenesis of CLL (Chiorazzi et al. 2005; Herishanu et al. 2011; ten Hacken and Burger 2016; Duhren-von Minden et al. 2012). BCR signaling is mediated in part by the activation of the delta isoform of phosphatidylinositol 3-kinase (PI3Kδ). The delta isoform is one of four catalytic isoforms (p110 α, β, γ, and δ) that differ in their tissue expression, with PI3Kδ being highly expressed in lymphoid cells (Okkenhaug and Vanhaesebroeck 2003) and acting as the most critical isoform for the malignant phenotype in CLL (Herman et al. 2010). It activates the serine–threonine kinases (AKT) and mammalian target of rapamycin (mTOR) and exerts multiple effects on cell metabolism, migration, survival, proliferation, and differentiation (Fig. 1) (Bodo et al. 2013; Hoellenriegel et al. 2011; Lannutti et al. 2011; Maffei et al. 2015; Puri and Gold 2012). Given the functional significance of the BCR, strategies to target BCR signaling have appeared as emerging therapeutic options (Arnason and Brown 2017; Choi and Kipps 2012; Fruman and Cantley 2014; Jerkeman et al. 2017; Jeyakumar and O'Brien 2016; Niemann and Wiestner 2013; Pula et al. 2017; ten Hacken and Burger 2014; Wiestner 2012; Wiestner

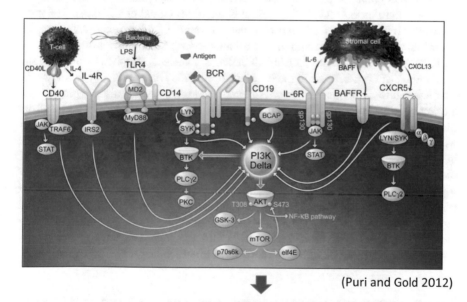

(Puri and Gold 2012)

Survival, Proliferation, Homing, Chemokine secretion, Adhesion

Fig. 1 Pathways utilizing PI3Kδ signaling. PI3Kδ is a central signaling enzyme that mediates the effects of multiple receptors on B cells. PI3Kδ signaling is important for B-cell survival, migration, and activation, functioning downstream of the B-cell antigen receptor (BCR) and its co-receptor CD19, chemokine receptors (CXCR5), and activation/co-stimulatory receptors such as CD40 and Toll-like receptors (TLRs). Cytokines derived from lymphoid stromal cells (BAFF, IL-6) and T cells (IL-4) that are essential for the expansion and survival of B-cells also require PI3Kδ for their actions and bind receptors that activate PI3Kδ. Akt is the major downstream target of PI3Kδ. Once phosphorylated, Akt is activated and in turn phosphorylates other downstream substrates, including mTOR (Puri and Gold 2012)

2014; Wiestner 2015). In fact, inhibitors of BCR signaling, especially those targeting the BCR-associated kinases SYK, BTK, and PI3Ks have shown promising clinical results (Sharman and Di Paolo 2016). Idelalisib (formerly called GS-1101 and CAL-101) is a potent, oral, selective small-molecule inhibitor of PI3Kδ. Idelalisib was approved by the US Food and Drug Administration in July 2014 for the treatment of relapsed CLL, in combination with rituximab, in patients who do not qualify for other chemotherapeutic agents, except rituximab monotherapy due to the presence of comorbidities. Idelalisib also received an accelerated approval for relapsed follicular lymphoma and small lymphocytic lymphoma after failing at least two systemic therapies (Markham 2014; Miller et al. 2015; Traynor 2014; Yang et al. 2015). The European Commission has also granted marketing authorization for idelalisib: (1) in combination with rituximab for the treatment of adult patients with CLL who received ≥ 1 prior therapy or as first-line treatment in the presence of a 17p deletion or TP53 mutation in patients unsuitable for chemo-immuno-therapy and (2) as monotherapy in the treatment of adult patients with follicular lymphoma refractory to two prior lines of treatment. The safety profile of idelalisib appeared acceptable in patients with recurrent B-cell lymphomas treated for up to 4 years in the Phase I and II trials (Flinn et al. 2014; Gopal et al. 2014). The most frequent adverse events were diarrhea, nausea, fatigue, and pyrexia. As seen with other inhibitors of BCR signaling, in particular the BTK inhibitor ibrutinib and the SYK inhibitor fostamatinib, idelalisib induces transient lymphocytosis resulting from egress of CLL cells from the microenvironment. This peculiar lymphocytosis, also referred to as "leukemic flare," is not considered to signify disease progression any more (Cheson et al. 2012; Fiorcari et al. 2013). However, a series of upfront trials were terminated early because of an increased risk of fatal infections for patients randomized to combinations containing idelalisib. Idelalisib prescribing information includes now a black box warning for fatal and severe hepatotoxicity, diarrhea or colitis, pneumonitis, fatal and/or serious infections, and intestinal perforation. An understanding of these unusual toxicities, as well as good institutional policies for their management, will gain important as more PI3K inhibitors are approved and become incorporated into routine practice. Many clinical studies with idelalisib in hematological malignancies in different treatment lines and combinations are ongoing. Results are summarized in this review.

2 Structure and Mechanisms of Action

The chemical name for idelalisib is 5-fluoro-3-phenyl-2-[(1S)-1-(9H-purin-6-ylamino)-propyl]quinazolin-4(3H)-one (Fig. 2) (Somoza et al. 2015). It has a molecular formula of $C_{22}H_{18}FN_7O$ and a molecular weight of 415.42.

Idelalisib was initially developed by ICOS as a potential treatment of inflammatory diseases. Later on, Calistoga Pharmaceuticals and now Gilead Sciences (following its acquisition of Calistoga) performed preclinical testing and phase I clinical trials with a focus on the treatment of hematological cancers.

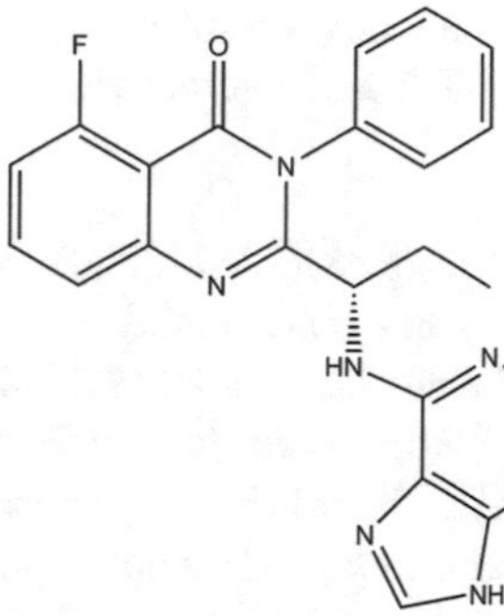

Fig. 2 Chemical structure of idelalisib (5-fluoro-3-phenyl-2-[(1S)-1-(9H-purin-6-ylamino)propyl] quinazolin-4(3H)-one) (Somoza et al. 2015)

In vitro, Idelalisib showed high potency against PI3Kδ with an IC_{50} value of 2.5 nM (Lannutti et al. 2011). In contrast, the IC_{50} values for PI3Kα, PI3Kβ, and PI3Kγ were 820, 565, and 89 nM, respectively (Lannutti et al. 2011). In cell-based assays, idelalisib blocked FcεRI p110δ-mediated CD63 expression in basophils with an EC_{50} of 8 nM, which was 240- to 2500-fold selective for PI3Kδ over the other class I PI3K isoforms. Idelalisib has a favorable pharmacokinetic profile with a plasma half-life of 8 h, and oral bioavailability of 39 and 79% in rats and dogs, respectively. Using tumor cell lines and primary patient samples representing multiple B-cell malignancies, idelalisib blocks the constitutive activation of the p110δ-dependent PI3K pathway, resulting in decreased phosphorylation of AKT and other downstream effectors.

3   Preclinical Data

3.1   Idelalisib in CLL

Ex vivo treatment of primary CLL cells with idelalisib in various concentrations established that

1. CLL cells express PI3Kδ in abundance at both gene and protein level;
2. idelalisib can induce apoptosis in CLL cells, although responses varied;
3. the induction of apoptosis was selective for CLL cells as compared with normal B cells or other hematopoietic cells;
4. the induction of apoptosis occurred independently of prognostic markers such as cytogenetic abnormality or immunoglobulin heavy chain variable region heavy chain *(IGHV)* mutational status;
5. the mechanism of action seemed to be associated with induction of apoptosis through caspase activation; and

6. CAL-101 antagonized CLL cell survival mechanisms by blocking the protective effect of CD40-ligand (CD40L) and microenvironment stimuli (Herman et al. 2010).

Further experimental studies suggested that idelalisib could overcome both bone marrow stromal cell- (BMSC-) and endothelial cell- (EC-) mediated CLL cell protection, indicating that idelalisib inhibits BMCS- and EC-derived pro-survival signals (Fiorcari et al. 2013). Furthermore, idelalisib can inhibit both the chemotaxis toward CXCL12 and CXCL13 and the migration beneath stroma cell layers, suggesting a potential mobilization effect (Hoellenriegel et al. 2011). Furthermore, idelalisib inhibits chemokine (such as CCL3 and CCL4) and cytokine (such as TNF and interleukin-6) secretion mediated by BCR stimulation or nurse-like cells. Concurrent with these findings, the sensitivity of CLL cells to other cytotoxic drugs (such as fludarabine and bendamustine) was increased (Hoellenriegel et al. 2011; Modi et al. 2017). Similarly, ex vivo data suggested that idelalisib could sensitize stroma-exposed CLL cells to other agents by inhibition of stroma-CLL contact, leading to an increase in mitochondrial apoptotic priming of CLL cells (Davids et al. 2012). In summary, these ex vivo data suggest that idelalisib may be beneficial in the treatment of CLL by directly inducing apoptosis and inhibiting microenvironmental interactions.

Combined inhibition of PI3Kδ by idelalisib and Syk by GS-9973 in primary peripheral blood and bone marrow CLL samples reduced CLL survival, synergistically induced growth inhibition, and further disrupted chemokine signaling at nanomolar concentrations, including in bone marrow derived and poor risk samples (Burke et al. 2014). These data suggest increased clinical activity by simultaneous targeting of these kinases.

3.2 Idelalisib in other Hematological Malignancies

Idelalisib yielded no activity against non-neoplastic mononuclear cells, but 26% of CLL and 23% of B-cell acute lymphoblastic leukemia samples were sensitive to idelalisib (Lannutti et al. 2011). In contrast, only 3% of acute myeloid leukemia and 0% of myeloproliferative neoplasm samples showed sensitivity to idelalisib, indicating that idelalisib has a greater therapeutic potential for lymphoid malignancies. In addition, idelalisib downregulated p-Akt expression in diffuse large B-cell lymphoma (DLBCL), mantle cell lymphoma (MCL), and follicular lymphoma (FL) cell lines, and induced a several-fold increase in the levels of apoptotic markers, such as caspase 3 and poly(ADP-ribose) polymerase cleavage (Lannutti et al. 2011).

High levels of p110δ and p-Akt were also found in five out of five investigated Hodgkin lymphoma (HL) cell lines. Exposure to CAL-101 not only decreased levels of p110δ and p-Akt but also disrupted tumor microenvironment-mediated survival signals mediated by CCL5, CCL17, and CCL22 in co-cultures of HL cells and BMSCs (Meadows et al. 2012).

In plasma cell myeloma (PCM), in vitro experiments demonstrated that

1. All PCM cell lines were shown to express PI3Kδ;
2. Idelalisib was highly selective against p110δ-positive PCM cells by inducing caspase-dependent apoptosis in dose-dependent fashion but with minimal cytotoxicity in p110δ-negative cells;
3. Idelalisib inhibited the Akt phosphorylation in p110δ-positive PCM cells;
4. Idelalisib decreased PCM viability in the presence of BMSCs, and
5. Idelalisib had a synergistic effect with bortezomib, a proteasome inhibitor approved by the FDA for the treatment of PCM and MCL (Ikeda et al. 2010).

The PI3K pathway is known to be closely involved in BCR-ABL transformation and the tumorigenesis of chronic myeloid leukemia (CML), suggesting that PI3K may be a potential target for CML therapy. Idelalisib inhibited proliferation of K562 chronic myeloid leukemia cells and induced apoptosis with increased expression of pro-apoptotic molecules such as Bad and Bax, cleavage of caspase-9, -8, and -3, and PARP, in contrast to downregulation of anti-apoptotic protein Bcl-2 (Chen et al. 2016). In addition, combination of idelalisib with imatinib led to a synergistic anti-proliferative effect on K562 cells, together with enhanced activity of G1 arrest and apoptosis induction, suggesting potential application in CML therapy.

4 Clinical Data

4.1 Clinical Trials with Idelalisib

More than 50 clinical trials have been registered with idelalisib so far (http://www.clinicaltrials.gov). Currently, 20 trials are listed as active, the greater part of which are phase II and III trials in hematological malignancies (Table 1). Idelalisib has shown clinical activity and a tolerable safety profile in phase II and III trials.

4.2 Idelalisib in CLL

The initial efficacy of idelalisib in CLL was demonstrated in a phase I trial treating patients with relapsed or refractory CLL (Brown et al. 2014). Fifty-four patients with adverse characteristics, including bulky lymphadenopathy, extensive prior therapy, refractory disease, unmutated *IGVH*, and deletion of 17p or *TP53* mutations, were included. 81% of patients had a nodal response. Median progression-free survival (PFS) was 15.8 months, but at the recommended phase II dose of 150 mg twice a day or higher, it was 32 months. The most common grade 3 adverse events included pneumonia in 20% of patients and neutropenic fever in 11% of patients (Brown et al. 2014).

Table 1 Registered active interventional clinical trials (phase I–III) with idelalisib

Indication	Phase I	Phase I/II	Phase II	Phase III
B-cell hematological malignancies	3		1	
Indolent B-cell lymphoma (FL, SLL, LPL, MZL)			1	
FL, MCL	1			1
CLL, SLL			1	
CLL	2		2	4
FL				1
Waldenström's macroglobinaemia			1	
MCL		1		
NSCLC		1		

Reference: www.clinicaltrials.gov
FL follicular lymphoma, *MCL* mantle cell lymphoma, *SLL* small lymphocytic lymphoma, *LPL* lymphoplasmacytic lymphoma, *MZL* marginal zone lymphoma, *CLL* chronic lymphocytic leukemia, *NSCLC* non-small cell lung cancer

The approval of idelalisib in combination with rituximab for the treatment of patients with relapsed CLL was based on a randomized, double-blind, placebo-controlled phase III clinical trial (Furman et al. 2014). This clinical trial enrolled 220 patients with relapsed CLL who required treatment and were unable to tolerate standard chemo-immunotherapy due to coexisting medical conditions, reduced renal function or neutropenia or thrombocytopenia resulting from myelo-toxic effects of prior therapy with cytotoxic agents. Patients received idelalisib plus rituximab or placebo plus rituximab until disease progression or unacceptable toxicity. The primary endpoint was PFS. As recommended by the data and safety monitoring board, the trial was stopped early at the pre-specified first interim analysis because of the positive results seen with idelalisib. At 24 weeks, the PFS rate was 93% in patients receiving idelalisib plus rituximab compared with 46% in patients receiving placebo plus rituximab. At 12 months, the overall survival (OS) rate in the idelalisib plus rituximab group (92%) was significantly higher than the OS rate in the placebo plus rituximab group (80%; HR for death, 0.28; 95% CI, 0.09–0.86; $p = 0.02$). In the idelalisib plus rituximab group, the overall response rate (ORR) was 81% compared with 13% in the placebo plus rituximab group ($p < 0.001$). All responses were partial responses (Furman et al. 2014).

Idelalisib treatment has been associated with a dramatic lymph node response, but eradication of disease and relapse in high-risk disease remain challenges. Idelalisib in combination with rituximab and bendamustine (idelalisib BR) as compared to rituximab and bendamustine (BR) was investigated in a randomized, phase III, placebo-controlled, double-blind trial, treating patients with relapsed or refractory CLL (Zelenetz et al. 2017). At a median follow-up of 14 months, the median PFS was 20.8 months in the idelalisib-containing arm and 11.1 months in the placebo arm ($p < 0.0001$). An increased risk of grade 3 or higher infections was seen in the idelalisib-containing arm (39 vs. 25%). Updated efficacy data recently demonstrated that the combination of idelalisib BR had improved overall survival relative to BR (not reached vs. 41 months, $p = 0.036$) (Zelenetz et al. 2016).

The efficacy and safety of idelalisib in combination with the second-generation anti-CD20 antibody, ofatumumab, was investigated in a randomized phase 3 trial for previously treated CLL patients. The idelalisib plus ofatumumab combination resulted in better PFS compared with ofatumumab alone in patients with relapsed CLL (16.3 months vs. 8 months, adjusted hazard ratio (HR) 0.27, 95% CI 0.19–0.39, $p < 0.0001$), including in those with high-risk disease. Idelalisib in combination with ofatumumab might represent a new treatment alternative for this patient population (Jones et al. 2017).

Given the efficacy seen with idelalisib in patients with relapsed/refractory CLL, and the activity of rituximab in treatment-naive patients, a phase II open-label study of idelalisib in combination with rituximab in older patients with previously untreated CLL or small lymphocytic lymphoma was performed (O'Brien et al. 2015). The ORR was 97%, including 19% complete responses. The ORR was 100% in patients with del(17p)/*TP53* mutations and 97% in those with unmated *IGVH*. PFS was 83% at 36 months. The most frequent adverse events (any grade) were diarrhea (including colitis) (64%), rash (58%), pyrexia (42%), and nausea (38%). Elevated alanine transaminase/aspartate transaminase was seen in 67% of patients (23% grade >3). These data suggest that toxicity rates may be higher in the front-line setting. Concurrent with this, results from a phase II clinical trial of front-line idelalisib used in combination with the anti-CD20 monoclonal antibody ofatumumab indicated frequent occurrence of often severe immune-mediated transaminitis, potentially through inhibition of regulatory T cells (Lampson et al. 2016). In March 2016, Gilead closed seven randomized trials of idelalisib in B-cell malignancies (5 in treatment-naive patients) due to an excess of infectious deaths.

Several studies are actively evaluating idelalisib in CLL in combination with, e.g., Bcl-2 inhibitors, Btk inhibitors, CD19 or CD20 antibodies, or PD-1 inhibitors. These include a phase II investigation of idelalisib with the Bcl-2 inhibitor venetoclax for patients with CLL that have relapsed or are refractory to prior therapy with a BCR pathway inhibitor (NCT02141282). A phase II study to evaluate safety and preliminary efficacy of the Fc-enhanced CD19 antibody MOR00208 combined with idelalisib or venetoclax in adult patients with relapsed or refractory CLL or SLL pretreated with a BTK inhibitor (e.g., ibrutinib) as single agent or as part of combination therapy is also currently underway (NCT02639910). In addition, the combination of the BTK inhibitor tirabrutinib and idelalisib with or without obinutuzumab in adults with relapsed or refractory CLL is currently tested in a phase II study (NCT02968563).

Otlertuzumab (TRU-016) is a novel humanized anti-CD37 protein therapeutic. The safety and efficacy of otlertuzumab is currently evaluated in a Phase Ib trial when administered in combination with rituximab or obinutuzumab, in combination with idelalisib and rituximab, or in combination with ibrutinib in patients with CLL (NCT01644253). The PD-1 inhibitor pembrolizumab it currently explored alone or with idelalisib or ibrutinib in patients with relapsed or refractory CLL or other low-grade B-cell lymphomas (NCT02332980).

4.3 Idelalisib in Relapsed Small Lymphocytic Lymphoma

Idelalisib is indicated for the treatment of patients with relapsed small lymphocytic lymphoma (SLL), the nodal form of CLL, who have received at least two prior systemic therapies. Accelerated approval was granted for this indication based on ORR. The safety and efficacy of idelalisib in patients with relapsed SLL were explicitly evaluated in the DELTA clinical trial (Gopal et al. 2014). Overall, 26 patients with relapsed SLL received 150 mg of idelalisib orally twice daily until evidence of disease progression or unacceptable toxicity. The study's primary end point was Independent Review Committee-assessed ORR. Among these 26 patients with relapsed SLL, the ORR was 58% (95% CI, 37–77%), and all responses were partial responses (Gopal et al. 2014). An improvement in survival or disease-related symptoms has not yet been established for idelalisib in relapsed SLL.

4.4 Idelalisib in Relapsed Follicular Lymphoma

In relapsed follicular lymphoma (FL), idelalisib was approved under the accelerated approval program based on ORR data. Idelalisib is indicated for the treatment of patients with relapsed FL who received at least two prior systemic therapies.

The safety and efficacy of idelalisib in patients with relapsed FL were evaluated in the DELTA clinical trial, a single-arm, multicenter clinical trial that included 72 patients with relapsed FL who had received at least two prior treatments (Gopal et al. 2014). The primary endpoint was Independent Review Committee-assessed ORR. Among the 72 patients with relapsed FL who received idelalisib, the ORR was 54% (95% CI, 42–66%), including 6 complete responses (8%) and 33 partial responses (46%).

To better characterize the efficacy and safety of idelalisib treatment for patients with refractory FL, a subsequent subgroup analysis of patients enrolled in this study was performed (Salles et al. 2017). The ORR was 55.6% ($n = 40/72$; 95% CI 43.4–67.3; $p < 0.001$ for testing against the null hypothesis) in patients with FL overall and did not differ when stratified by FL grade. Idelalisib was effective across evaluated patient categories, regardless of the number of prior therapies, refractoriness to previous regimens, bulky disease, and age. Median PFS with idelalisib was 11.0 months (95% CI, 8.0–14.0) overall. At the time of data cutoff, median OS had not been reached. At 24 months, OS was estimated to be 69.8%, and all patients achieving a CR had survived. In these heavily pretreated patients with relapsed/refractory FL, idelalisib monotherapy demonstrated an acceptable and manageable safety profile. Diarrhea, colitis, and transaminase elevations were generally manageable with dose interruption/reduction or drug discontinuation. In conclusion, these data suggest that patients with high-risk FL may benefit from a targeted therapy such as idelalisib (Salles et al. 2017).

Similarly, a multicenter UK-wide compassionate use program evaluating the efficacy of idelalisib monotherapy in relapsed, refractory FL ($n = 79$), showed an ORR of 57% (CR/unconfirmed CR 15%; PR 42%) in 65 assessable cases. The median PFS was 7.1 months (95% CI 5.0–9.1 months) and median OS was not reached. This is the only real-world series outlining the efficacy and survival of idelalisib-treated relapsed and refractory FL (Eyre et al. 2017).

Idelalisib treatment in patients with high-risk follicular lymphoma and early relapse after initial chemo-immunotherapy induced an ORR of 56.8% (21 out of 37) with 5 complete responses (13.5%) and 16 partial responses (43.2%). These results are the first to describe the efficacy and safety of idelalisib in patients with FL relapsing early following first-line chemo-immunotherapy and suggest that idelalisib may provide a viable therapeutic option for patients with double-refractory FL with early relapse after initial therapy (Gopal et al. 2017b).

4.5 Idelalisib in Other Indolent and Aggressive B-Cell Lymphomas

The efficacy of idelalisib monotherapy was first reported in a phase I dose-ranging study of 64 patients with previously treated indolent B-cell lymphomas (FL $n = 38$; SLL $n = 11$; marginal zone lymphoma (MZL) $n = 6$; lymphoplasmacytic lymphoma (LPL) $n = 9$) (Flinn et al. 2014). Patients had received a median of 4 prior therapies, and 58% were refractory to the last prior therapy. The ORR was 47% ($n = 30$) in the total study population and 59% in patients treated with continuous higher doses. Responding patients had a rapid reduction in lymphadenopathy with a median time to response of 1.3 months. Because the median PFS was longer in patients treated with higher dose continuous therapy (16.8 months; range: 1–37 months) than in patients receiving lower doses or intermittent therapy (3.7 months; range: 0.5–33 months), idelalisib doses of >150 mg twice daily were identified for further study.

In a phase I study of idelalisib in patients with relapsed and refractory MCL, the ORR was 16 of 40 patients (40%), with CR in 2 of 40 patients (5%). Median DOR was 2.7 months, and 1-year PFS was 22%, providing proof of concept that targeting PI3Kd is a viable strategy in MCL (Kahl et al. 2014).

To evaluate the safety and activity of idelalisib in combination with immunotherapy, chemotherapy, or both, 79 patients with relapsed/refractory indolent B-cell lymphoma were enrolled in a phase I study in three treatment groups based on investigators preference: (1) idelalisib + rituximab, (2) idelalisib + bendamustine, or (3) idelalisib + rituximab + bendamustine (de Vos et al. 2016). Lymphoma subtypes included FL (59 patients, 74.7%), SLL (15 patients, 19.0%), and MZL (5 patients, 6.3%). The ORR for the idelalisib + rituximab, idelalisib + bendamustine, and idelalisib + rituximab + bendamustine groups were 75, 88, and 79%, respectively. The median PFS was 37.1 months overall:

29.7 months for idelalisib + rituximab, 32.8 for idelalisib and bendamustine, and 37.1 months for idelalisib + rituximab + bendamustine. The most common grade ≥ 3 adverse events and laboratory abnormalities were neutropenia (41%), pneumonia (19%), transaminase elevations (16%), diarrhea/colitis (15%), and rash (9%). The safety and efficacy reflected in these early data, however, stand in contrast with later observations of significant toxicity in subsequent phase 3 trials in frontline CLL and less heavily pretreated indolent B-cell lymphoma patients. These findings highlight the limitations of phase I trial data in the assessment of new regimens. Therefore, the safety of novel combinations should be proven in phase III trials before adoption in clinical practice.

Similarly, a phase II study evaluating the safety and effectivity of the combination of idelalisib and the Syk inhibitor entospletinib in patients with relapsed or refractory CLL or non-Hodgkin lymphoma including MCL and DLBCL was terminated early due to an unexpectedly high rate of pneumonitis in 18% of patients (severe in 11 of 12 cases) (Barr et al. 2016), whereas the combination of idelalisib and the selective Syk inhibitor GS-9973 has shown promising synergistic preclinical activity (Burke et al. 2014).

The safety and tolerability of idelalisib, lenalidomide, and rituximab was investigated in phase I trials in patients with relapsed and refractory MCL and FL (Smith et al. 2017). The primary endpoint of safety and tolerability was not met due to unexpected dose-limiting toxicities coinciding with rituximab. Both studies were amended to remove rituximab, but two of three additional patients developed grade 3 rashes and one had grade 3 AST elevation. Both trials were then permanently closed.

Recently, results of a phase II study of idelalisib for relapsed and refractory classical Hodgkin's lymphoma (HL) were presented (Gopal et al. 2017a). Twenty-five patients who had previously received a median of five therapies, including 18 (72%) with failed autologous stem cell transplant and 23 (92%) with failed brentuximab vedotin, were enrolled in the study. Idelalisib was tolerable and had modest single-agent activity in these heavily pretreated patients with an ORR of 20% and a median PFS of 2.3 months. Rational combinations with other novel agents may improve response rate and duration of response.

4.6   Idelalisib in Merkel-Cell Carcinoma

Aberrant activation of the PI3K pathway may be a potential therapeutic target in Merkel-cell carcinoma. Indeed, activation of the PI3K pathway was detected both in Merkel-cell polyomavirus-negative tumor tissues and in tumor cells (Nardi et al. 2012; Shao et al. 2013). In a recent case report, a patient with metastatic Merkel-cell carcinoma showing high expression of PI3Kδ in the tumor cells was treated with idelalisib, resulting in a rapid and complete response. Unfortunately, the patient died from other causes before long-term response could be measured (Shiver et al. 2015). Although the cause of high expression of PI3Kδ in Merkel-cell carcinoma is unclear, the efficacy of idelalisib provides evidence that targeting of PI3Kδ in Merkel-cell carcinoma is warranted.

5 Toxicity

Selective inhibition of the PI3Kδ isoform be idelalisib minimizes adverse events (AEs) from inhibition of other PI3K signaling pathways involved in normal function of the healthy cells. Overall, idelalisib was fairly well tolerated (Falchi et al. 2016) with the most common AEs in patients receiving idelalisib and rituximab being pyrexia, fatigue, nausea, and diarrhea (Keating 2015). Therapy interruption occurred in 3.6% of patients across all studies with 1.3% requiring a dose reduction (Coutre et al. 2015). In the pivotal phase III study, AEs led to treatment discontinuation in 8% of the patients; majority of which were due to gastrointestinal and skin toxicities (Furman et al. 2014).

However, following the initial trials investigating the use of idelalisib in relapsed and refractory CLL, a series of upfront trials were terminated secondary to the observation of increased risk of death related to infection for patients randomized to combinations containing idelalisib. This experience was communicated to healthcare professionals via an FDA alert, and a black box warning for fatal hepatotoxicity, severe diarrhea or colitis, pneumonitis, serious infections and intestinal perforation is now included in the idelalisib product insert (http://www.fda.gov/Drugs/DrugSafety/ucm490618.htm). The majority of deaths was due to bacterial sepsis sometimes associated with neutropenia, but pneumocystis jiroveci pneumonia (PJP) and cytomegalovirus (CMV) infections were also seen, leading to the recommendation that patients receiving idelalisib should be on PJP prophylaxis and should be monitored regularly for the development of CMV infection.

In addition to the increased rate of death related to infection, increased likely autoimmune toxicity related to lymphocytic infiltrates was observed in the upfront setting. In a phase II study investigating the combination of idelalisib and ofatumumab as upfront therapy for CLL, 19 out of 24 patients (79%) experienced a grade 1 or higher elevation in transaminases and 13 patients (54%) experienced grade 3 or higher transaminitis (Lampson et al. 2016). The development of transaminitis occurred before the initiation of ofatumumab, at a median time of 28 days. A lymphocytic infiltrate was seen on liver biopsy specimens taken from 2 patients with transaminitis. A decrease in peripheral blood regulatory T cells was seen in patients experiencing toxicity on therapy, which is consistent with an immune-mediated mechanism. All cases of transaminitis resolved either with drug hold or the initiation of immunosuppression, or both. Significant risk factors for the development of hepatotoxicity were younger age and mutated *IGHV* (Lampson et al. 2016). Histopathological examination during idelalisib-associated diarrhea or colitis in relapsed patients revealed similar findings with a mixed appearance with both apoptotic and ischemic and inflammatory features (Louie et al. 2015; Weidner et al. 2015).

One potential mechanism for the development of the hepatic lymphocytic infiltrate is the effects of PI3K inhibition on regulatory T cells (Tregs). PI3K activity has been shown to be critical to Treg development and function. Initial studies with PI3K-deficient mice demonstrated decreased numbers of Tregs and decreased Treg function (Oak et al. 2006; Patton et al. 2006). Furthermore, Tregs from mice with a kinase-dead mutant p110δ PI3K have inferior suppressive capacity relative to wild-type Tregs (Patton et al. 2011). Given the increased risk of infection and risk of death related to infection coupled with significant idelalisib-mediated liver, colonic (Hammami et al. 2017), and pulmonary injury (Barr et al. 2016; Gupta and Li 2016; Haustraete et al. 2016), the use of idelalisib continues to be adapted to these risks (Greenwell et al. 2017).

An expert panel of hematologists and one gastroenterologist has provided further guidance for the management of idelalisib treatment-emergent diarrhea/colitis (Coutre et al. 2015). Based on anecdotal effectiveness, the panel recommended that once infectious source has been ruled out, budesonide or steroid (oral or intravenous) therapy should be initiated and continued until diarrhea resolves. Any patient presenting with pulmonary symptoms should be evaluated for pneumonitis. Additional warnings and precautions from the US prescribing information include severe cutaneous reactions (Gabriel et al. 2017; Huilaja et al. 2017), anaphylaxis, neutropenia, and embryo-fetal toxicity.

6 Drug Interactions

Idelalisib and its major inactive metabolite GS-563117 are implicated in the inhibition or induction of various CYP isoenzymes or transporters (Jin et al. 2015; Liewer and Huddleston 2015).

Midazolam (CYP3A substrate) exposure was significantly increased by the co-administration of idelalisib, reflecting inhibition of CYP3A by GS-563117 (Jin et al. 2015). A drug interaction between idelalisib and diazepam, also a CYP3A4 substrate, resulted in altered mental status and respiratory failure resulting in hospitalization. After discontinuation of both agents, the patient recovered quickly (Bossaer and Chakraborty 2017). Therefore, co-administration of idelalisib with CYP3A substrates should be avoided.

Both idelalisib and GS-563117 exposure were significantly reduced by co-administration of the potent CYP3A inducer rifampicin (Jin et al. 2015). The US prescribing information states that co-administration of idelalisib with strong CYP3A inducers such as rifampicin, phenytoin, hypericum (St John's wort), or carbamazepine should be avoided.

In contrast, idelalisib exposure was increased by co-administration of the strong CYP3A inhibitor ketoconazole. Monitoring for signs of idelalisib toxicity is recommended in patients receiving concomitant therapy with strong CYP3A inhibitors. The EU summary of product characteristics recommends caution when co-administering idelalisib and CYP2C8 substrates with a narrow therapeutic index (e.g., paclitaxel) or substrates of CYP2C9, CYP2C19, CYP2B6 or UGT with a narrow therapeutic index (e.g., warfarin, phenytoin).

7 Biomarkers

With changing treatment paradigms, particularly the use of oral targeted therapies, the value of predictive and prognostic factors to determine treatment choice are shifting. Traditional risk factors, including disease stage and lymphocyte doubling time, are becoming less relevant for treatment selection, and the predictive value of cytogenetic and molecular markers on response to treatment with novel agents is being redefined based on the outcomes of recent trials.

A number of biomarkers have been developed in CLL that fulfill the definition of prognostic factors, while conversely, few biomarkers meet the definition of predictive biomarkers. The presence of a deletion of chromosome 17p (del17p) and mutated *TP53* represents the most relevant disease characteristics that guide the choice of therapy in patients with CLL. Both del17p and mutated *TP53* are associated with poor response to chemotherapy-based regimens, short PFS, and poor OS, independently of *IGHV* mutation status (Hallek et al. 2010). Recent trials have demonstrated activity of novel targeted agents in patients with del17p/*TP53*-mutant CLL (Furman et al. 2014; Byrd et al. 2014b). These results have significantly changed outcomes for this subgroup for whom previous options to increase the duration of response were largely limited to stem cell transplant in eligible patients. Because leukemic clones may evolve, del17p and *TP53* mutations analyses should be repeated at each disease progression requiring treatment. BCR inhibitors ibrutinib and idelalisib are considered the preferred first-line therapy for patients with del17p/*TP53*-mutant CLL and are a category 1 recommendation for patients with CLL without del17p/*TP53* mutation who are frail, or are ≥ 65 years of age, or younger with significant comorbidities, according to the National Comprehensive Cancer Network (NCCN) guidelines on CLL.

Patients with mutated *IGHV* genes receiving chemo-immunotherapy often maintain disease remission in the long term and almost all *IGHV* unmutated CLL patients are projected to progress after chemo-immunotherapy (Fischer et al. 2016). In contrast, upon treatment with ibrutinib or idelalisib, the PFS of *IGHV* unmutated patients is similar to that of *IGHV* mutated cases (Furman et al. 2014; Burger et al. 2015). Accordingly, the most recent guidelines support *IGHV* mutations analysis as desirable at the time of treatment requirements.

Ibrutinib and idelalisib overcome the relevance of biomarkers reflecting patients' frailty. In the relapsed–refractory setting, patient's age does not affect ibrutinib or idelalisib safety and efficacy (Furman et al. 2014; Byrd et al. 2014b). Though guideline recommendations are lacking and the level of evidence is low, comorbidities support the choice of one novel agents among the others when multiple options are available. Most of the recent trials stratify patient inclusion criteria according to the cumulative illness rating scale (CIRS) with a cutoff of 6 to define fit and less fit patients (Eichhorst et al. 2016).

Regarding prognostic factors, identified to be significantly associated with CLL outcome, more recently, an international collaboration developed a comprehensive CLL-International Prognostic Index (IPI) (2016). The CLL-IPI score is based on five robust and widely used prognostic biomarkers (age, clinical stage, 17p13 deletion and/or TP53 mutation, *IGHV* mutations status, and β2-microglobulin levels) and incorporates both clinical and biological CLL aspects. Based on these biomarkers, a prognostic index was derived that identified four risk groups with significantly different survival at 5 years. The CLL-IPI score was developed in patients diagnosed in the chemo+/− immunotherapy era. The significant impact of novel targeted agents on patients' survival and the mitigation of historical prognostic factors when these drugs are used prompt the reevaluation and validation of the clinical usefulness of CLL prognostic scores in cohort of patients treated with the new drugs.

8 Summary and Perspectives

Idelalisib, the first FDA-approved PI3Kδ inhibitor, is an important addition to treatment options for patients with B-cell lymphomas. Its use is approved as single agent for patients with FL or SLL relapsed after 2 prior regimens and in combination with rituximab for patients with relapsed CLL for whom single-agent rituximab would be an appropriate therapy. Idelalisib has shown impressive clinical activity both as a single agent and in combination therapy, even in high-risk subtypes of indolent B-cell lymphoma, and is usually well tolerated. PI3Kδ inhibition appears to antagonize both intrinsic and extrinsic cell survival signals, decreases the survival of CLL cells directly, and abrogates cellular interactions between CLL cells and components of the tissue microenvironment that normally sustain leukemia and lymphoma cells in a protective niche.

Recent clinical trial data have demonstrated increased risk of death secondary to infections when idelalisib is used frontline. In addition, idelalisib has been shown to promote the development of immune-mediated colitis, hepatitis, and pneumonitis. Additional research is needed to better understand the mechanisms underlying the off-target toxicities, whether they can be predicted by features of the disease or the patient's genetics, and how they can be minimized. Ongoing clinical studies are evaluating idelalisib in combination studies to potentially expand its utility in B-cell malignancies and solid tumors.

In addition, PI3Kδ also plays a critical role in the activation, proliferation, and tissue homing of self-reactive B cells that contribute to autoimmune diseases, in particular innate-like B-cell populations such as marginal zone (MZ) B cells and B-1 cells that have been strongly linked to autoimmunity. Inhibitors of PI3Kδ, either alone or in combination with B-cell depletion, showed activity in treating autoimmune diseases such as lupus, rheumatoid arthritis, and type 1 diabetes (Puri and Gold 2012). Further research is needed to determine if PI3K inhibitors specific for other isoforms are effective against autoimmune diseases; however, PI3Kδ inhibitors may represent also a promising therapeutic approach for treating these diseases (Foster et al. 2012; Vyas and Vohora 2017).

References

Akinleye A, Avvaru P, Furqan M, Song Y, Liu D (2013) Phosphatidylinositol 3-kinase (PI3K) inhibitors as cancer therapeutics. J Hematol Oncol 6(1):88

Alinari L, Christian B, Baiocchi RA (2012) Novel targeted therapies for mantle cell lymphoma. Oncotarget 3(2):203–211

An international prognostic index for patients with chronic lymphocytic leukaemia (CLL-IPI) (2016) A meta-analysis of individual patient data. Lancet Oncol 17(6):779–790

Arnason JE, Brown JR (2017) Targeting B cell signaling in chronic lymphocytic leukemia. Curr Oncol Rep 19(9):61

Awan FT, Byrd JC (2014) New strategies in chronic lymphocytic leukemia: shifting treatment paradigms. Clin Cancer Res 20(23):5869–5874

Barr PM, Saylors GB, Spurgeon SE et al (2016) Phase 2 study of idelalisib and entospletinib: pneumonitis limits combination therapy in relapsed refractory CLL and NHL. Blood 127 (20):2411–2415

Bodo J, Zhao X, Sharma A et al (2013) The phosphatidylinositol 3-kinases (PI3K) inhibitor GS-1101 synergistically potentiates histone deacetylase inhibitor-induced proliferation inhibition and apoptosis through the inactivation of PI3K and extracellular signal-regulated kinase pathways. Br J Haematol 163(1):72–80

Bossaer JB, Chakraborty K (2017) Drug interaction between idelalisib and diazepam resulting in altered mental status and respiratory failure. J Oncol Pharm Pract 23(6):470–472

Brown JR (2016) The PI3K pathway: clinical inhibition in chronic lymphocytic leukemia. Semin Oncol 43(2):260–264

Brown JR, Byrd JC, Coutre SE et al (2014) Idelalisib, an inhibitor of phosphatidylinositol 3-kinase p110δ, for relapsed/refractory chronic lymphocytic leukemia. Blood 123(22):3390–3397

Burger JA, Okkenhaug K (2014) Haematological cancer: idelalisib-targeting PI3Kδ in patients with B cell malignancies. Nat Rev Clin Oncol 11(4):184–186

Burger JA, Tedeschi A, Barr PM et al (2015) Ibrutinib as initial therapy for patients with chronic lymphocytic leukemia. N Engl J Med 373(25):2425–2437

Burke RT, Meadows S, Loriaux MM et al (2014) A potential therapeutic strategy for chronic lymphocytic leukemia by combining Idelalisib and GS-9973, a novel spleen tyrosine kinase (Syk) inhibitor. Oncotarget 5(4):908–915

Byrd JC, Jones JJ, Woyach JA, Johnson AJ, Flynn JM (2014a) Entering the era of targeted therapy for chronic lymphocytic leukemia: impact on the practicing clinician. J Clin Oncol 32 (27):3039–3047

Byrd JC, Brown JR, O'Brien S et al (2014b) Ibrutinib versus ofatumumab in previously treated chronic lymphoid leukemia. N Engl J Med 371(3):213–223

Chen Y, Zhou Q, Zhang L et al (2016) Idelalisib induces G1 arrest and apoptosis in chronic myeloid leukemia K562 cells. Oncol Rep 36(6):3643–3650

Cheson BD, Byrd JC, Rai KR et al (2012) Novel targeted agents and the need to refine clinical end points in chronic lymphocytic leukemia. J Clin Oncol 30(23):2820–2822

Chiorazzi N, Rai KR, Ferrarini M (2005) Chronic lymphocytic leukemia. N Engl J Med 352 (8):804–815

Choi MY, Kipps TJ (2012) Inhibitors of B-cell receptor signaling for patients with B-cell malignancies. Cancer J 18(5):404–410

Coutre SE, Barrientos JC, Brown JR et al (2015) Management of adverse events associated with idelalisib treatment: expert panel opinion. Leuk Lymphoma 56(10):2779–2786

Danilov AV (2013) Targeted therapy in chronic lymphocytic leukemia: past, present, and future. Clin Ther 35(9):1258–1270

Davids MS, Deng J, Wiestner A et al (2012) Decreased mitochondrial apoptotic priming underlies stroma-mediated treatment resistance in chronic lymphocytic leukemia. Blood 120(17):3501–3509

de Vos S, Wagner-Johnston N, Coutre S et al (2016) Combinations of idelalisib with rituximab and/or bendamustine in patients with recurrent indolent non-Hodgkin lymphoma. Blood Adv 1 (2):122–131

Duhren-von Minden M, Ubelhart R, Schneider D et al (2012) Chronic lymphocytic leukaemia is driven by antigen-independent cell-autonomous signalling. Nature 489(7415):309–312

Eichhorst B, Fink AM, Bahlo J et al (2016) First-line chemoimmunotherapy with bendamustine and rituximab versus fludarabine, cyclophosphamide, and rituximab in patients with advanced chronic lymphocytic leukaemia (CLL10): an international, open-label, randomised, phase 3, non-inferiority trial. Lancet Oncol 17(7):928–942

Eyre TA, Osborne WL, Gallop-Evans E et al (2017) Results of a multicentre UK-wide compassionate use programme evaluating the efficacy of idelalisib monotherapy in relapsed, refractory follicular lymphoma. Br J Haematol

Falchi L, Baron JM, Orlikowski CA, Ferrajoli A (2016) BCR signaling inhibitors: an overview of toxicities associated with ibrutinib and idelalisib in patients with chronic lymphocytic leukemia. Mediterr J Hematol Infect Dis 8(1):e2016011

Fiorcari S, Brown WS, McIntyre BW et al (2013) The PI3-kinase delta inhibitor idelalisib (GS-1101) targets integrin-mediated adhesion of chronic lymphocytic leukemia (CLL) cell to endothelial and marrow stromal cells. PLoS One 8(12):e83830

Fischer K, Bahlo J, Fink AM et al (2016) Long-term remissions after FCR chemoimmunotherapy in previously untreated patients with CLL: updated results of the CLL8 trial. Blood 127 (2):208–215

Flinn IW, Kahl BS, Leonard JP et al (2014) Idelalisib, a selective inhibitor of phosphatidylinositol 3-kinase-δ, as therapy for previously treated indolent non-Hodgkin lymphoma. Blood 123 (22):3406–3413

Foster JG, Blunt MD, Carter E, Ward SG (2012) Inhibition of PI3K signaling spurs new therapeutic opportunities in inflammatory/autoimmune diseases and hematological malignancies. Pharmacol Rev 64(4):1027–1054

Fruman DA, Cantley LC (2014) Idelalisib—a PI3Kδ inhibitor for B-cell cancers. N Engl J Med 370(11):1061–1062

Fruman DA, Rommel C (2011) PI3Kδ inhibitors in cancer: rationale and serendipity merge in the clinic. Cancer Discov 1(7):562–572

Furman RR, Sharman JP, Coutre SE et al (2014) Idelalisib and rituximab in relapsed chronic lymphocytic leukemia. N Engl J Med 370(11):997–1007

Gabriel JG, Kapila A, Gonzalez-Estrada A (2017) A severe case of cutaneous adverse drug reaction secondary to a novice drug: idelalisib. J Investig Med High Impact Case Rep 5 (2):2324709617711463

Gilbert JA (2014) Idelalisib: targeting PI3Kδ in B-cell malignancies. Lancet Oncol 15(3):e108

Gockeritz E, Kerwien S, Baumann M et al (2015) Efficacy of phosphatidylinositol-3 kinase inhibitors with diverse isoform selectivity profiles for inhibiting the survival of chronic lymphocytic leukemia cells. Int J Cancer 137(9):2234–2242

Gopal AK, Fanale MA, Moskowitz CH et al (2017a) Phase II study of idelalisib, a selective inhibitor of PI3Kδ, for relapsed/refractory classical Hodgkin lymphoma. Ann Oncol 28 (5):1057–1063

Gopal AK, Kahl BS, de Vos S et al (2014) PI3Kδ inhibition by idelalisib in patients with relapsed indolent lymphoma. N Engl J Med 370(11):1008–1018

Gopal AK, Kahl BS, Flowers CR et al (2017b) Idelalisib is effective in patients with high-risk follicular lymphoma and early relapse after initial chemoimmunotherapy. Blood 129 (22):3037–3039

Greenwell IB, Ip A, Cohen JB (2017) PI3K inhibitors: understanding toxicity mechanisms and management. Oncology (Williston Park) 31(11):821–828

Gupta A, Li HC (2016) Idelalisib-induced pneumonitis. BMJ Case Rep 2016

Hallek M, Fischer K, Fingerle-Rowson G et al (2010) Addition of rituximab to fludarabine and cyclophosphamide in patients with chronic lymphocytic leukaemia: a randomised, open-label, phase 3 trial. Lancet 376(9747):1164–1174

Hammami MB, Al-Taee A, Meeks M et al (2017) Idelalisib-induced colitis and skin eruption mimicking graft-versus-host disease. Clin J Gastroenterol 10(2):142–146

Haustraete E, Obert J, Diab S et al (2016) Idelalisib-related pneumonitis. Eur Respir J 47(4):1280–1283

Herishanu Y, Perez-Galan P, Liu D et al (2011) The lymph node microenvironment promotes B-cell receptor signaling, NF-κB activation, and tumor proliferation in chronic lymphocytic leukemia. Blood 117(2):563–574

Herman SE, Gordon AL, Wagner AJ et al (2010) Phosphatidylinositol 3-kinase-δ inhibitor CAL-101 shows promising preclinical activity in chronic lymphocytic leukemia by antagonizing intrinsic and extrinsic cellular survival signals. Blood 116(12):2078–2088

Hewett YG, Uprety D, Shah BK (2016) Idelalisib—a PI3Kδ targeting agent for B-cell malignancies. J Oncol Pharm Pract 22(2):284–288

Hoellenriegel J, Meadows SA, Sivina M et al (2011) The phosphoinositide 3'-kinase delta inhibitor, CAL-101, inhibits B-cell receptor signaling and chemokine networks in chronic lymphocytic leukemia. Blood 118(13):3603–3612

Huilaja L, Lindgren O, Soronen M, Siitonen T, Tasanen K (2017) A slowly developed severe cutaneous adverse reaction to idelalisib. J Eur Acad Dermatol Venereol

Ikeda H, Hideshima T, Fulciniti M et al (2010) PI3K/p110δ is a novel therapeutic target in multiple myeloma. Blood 116(9):1460–1468

Jahangiri S, Friedberg J, Barr P (2014) Emerging protein kinase inhibitors for the treatment of non-Hodgkin's lymphoma. Expert Opin Emerg Drugs 19(3):367–383

Jain N, O'Brien S (2016) Targeted therapies for CLL: practical issues with the changing treatment paradigm. Blood Rev 30(3):233–244

Janku F (2017) Phosphoinositide 3-kinase (PI3K) pathway inhibitors in solid tumors: from laboratory to patients. Cancer Treat Rev 59:93–101

Jerkeman M, Hallek M, Dreyling M, Thieblemont C, Kimby E, Staudt L (2017) Targeting of B-cell receptor signalling in B-cell malignancies. J Intern Med 282(5):415–428

Jeyakumar D, O'Brien S (2016) B cell receptor inhibition as a target for CLL therapy. Best Pract Res Clin Haematol 29(1):2–14

Jin F, Robeson M, Zhou H et al (2015) Clinical drug interaction profile of idelalisib in healthy subjects. J Clin Pharmacol 55(8):909–919

Jones JA, Robak T, Brown JR et al (2017) Efficacy and safety of idelalisib in combination with ofatumumab for previously treated chronic lymphocytic leukaemia: an open-label, randomised phase 3 trial. Lancet Haematol 4(3):e114–e126

Kahl BS, Spurgeon SE, Furman RR et al (2014) A phase 1 study of the PI3Kδ inhibitor idelalisib in patients with relapsed/refractory mantle cell lymphoma (MCL). Blood 123(22):3398–3405

Keating GM (2015) Idelalisib: a review of its use in chronic lymphocytic leukaemia and indolent non-Hodgkin's lymphoma. Target Oncol 10(1):141–151

Lampson BL, Kasar SN, Matos TR et al (2016) Idelalisib given front-line for treatment of chronic lymphocytic leukemia causes frequent immune-mediated hepatotoxicity. Blood 128(2):195–203

Lannutti BJ, Meadows SA, Herman SE et al (2011) CAL-101, a p110δ selective phosphatidylinositol-3-kinase inhibitor for the treatment of B-cell malignancies, inhibits PI3K signaling and cellular viability. Blood 117(2):591–594

Liewer S, Huddleston AN (2015) Oral targeted therapies: managing drug interactions, enhancing adherence and optimizing medication safety in lymphoma patients. Expert Rev Anticancer Ther 15(4):453–464

Louie CY, DiMaio MA, Matsukuma KE, Coutre SE, Berry GJ, Longacre TA (2015) Idelalisib-associated enterocolitis: clinicopathologic features and distinction from other enterocolitides. Am J Surg Pathol 39(12):1653–1660

Macias-Perez IM, Flinn IW (2013) GS-1101: a delta-specific PI3K inhibitor in chronic lymphocytic leukemia. Curr Hematol Malig Rep 8(1):22–27

Maffei R, Fiorcari S, Martinelli S, Potenza L, Luppi M, Marasca R (2015) Targeting neoplastic B cells and harnessing microenvironment: the "double face" of ibrutinib and idelalisib. J Hematol Oncol 8:60

Marini BL, Samanas L, Perissinotti AJ (2017) Expanding the armamentarium for chronic lymphocytic leukemia: a review of novel agents in the management of chronic lymphocytic leukemia. J Oncol Pharm Pract 23(7):502–517

Markham A (2014) Idelalisib: first global approval. Drugs 74(14):1701–1707

Meadows SA, Vega F, Kashishian A et al (2012) PI3Kδ inhibitor, GS-1101 (CAL-101), attenuates pathway signaling, induces apoptosis, and overcomes signals from the microenvironment in cellular models of Hodgkin lymphoma. Blood 119(8):1897–1900

Miller BW, Przepiorka D, de Claro RA et al (2015) FDA approval: idelalisib monotherapy for the treatment of patients with follicular lymphoma and small lymphocytic lymphoma. Clin Cancer Res 21(7):1525–1529

Modi P, Balakrishnan K, Yang Q, Wierda WG, Keating MJ, Gandhi V (2017) Idelalisib and bendamustine combination is synergistic and increases DNA damage response in chronic lymphocytic leukemia cells. Oncotarget 8(10):16259–16274

Molica S (2017) Targeted therapy in the treatment of chronic lymphocytic leukemia: facts, shortcomings and hopes for the future. Expert Rev Hematol 10(5):425–432

Morabito F, Gentile M, Seymour JF, Polliack A (2015) Ibrutinib, idelalisib and obinutuzumab for the treatment of patients with chronic lymphocytic leukemia: three new arrows aiming at the target. Leuk Lymphoma 56(12):3250–3256

Nardi V, Song Y, Santamaria-Barria JA et al (2012) Activation of PI3K signaling in Merkel cell carcinoma. Clin Cancer Res 18(5):1227–1236

Niemann CU, Jones J, Wiestner A (2013) Towards targeted therapy of chronic lymphocytic leukemia. Adv Exp Med Biol 792:259–291

Niemann CU, Wiestner A (2013) B-cell receptor signaling as a driver of lymphoma development and evolution. Semin Cancer Biol 23(6):410–421

O'Brien SM, Lamanna N, Kipps TJ et al (2015) A phase 2 study of idelalisib plus rituximab in treatment-naive older patients with chronic lymphocytic leukemia. Blood 126(25):2686–2694

Oak JS, Deane JA, Kharas MG et al (2006) Sjogren's syndrome-like disease in mice with T cells lacking class 1A phosphoinositide-3-kinase. Proc Natl Acad Sci U S A 103(45):16882–16887

Okkenhaug K, Vanhaesebroeck B (2003) PI3K in lymphocyte development, differentiation and activation. Nat Rev Immunol 3(4):317–330

Okoli TC, Peer CJ, Dunleavy K, Figg WD (2015) Targeted PI3Kδ inhibition by the small molecule idelalisib as a novel therapy in indolent non-Hodgkin lymphoma. Cancer Biol Ther 16(2):204–206

Patton DT, Garden OA, Pearce WP et al (2006) Cutting edge: the phosphoinositide 3-kinase p110δ is critical for the function of CD4+CD25+Foxp3+ regulatory T cells. J Immunol 177 (10):6598–6602

Patton DT, Wilson MD, Rowan WC, Soond DR, Okkenhaug K (2011) The PI3K p110δ regulates expression of CD38 on regulatory T cells. PLoS One 6(3):e17359

Pongas G, Cheson BD (2016) PI3K signaling pathway in normal B cells and indolent B-cell malignancies. Semin Oncol 43(6):647–654

Pula A, Stawiski K, Braun M, Iskierka-Jazdzewska E, Robak T (2017) Efficacy and safety of B-cell receptor signaling pathway inhibitors in relapsed/refractory chronic lymphocytic leukemia: a systematic review and meta-analysis of randomized clinical trials. Leuk Lymphoma 1–11

Puri KD, Gold MR (2012) Selective inhibitors of phosphoinositide 3-kinase delta: modulators of B-cell function with potential for treating autoimmune inflammatory diseases and B-cell malignancies. Front Immunol 3:256

Rai KR (2015) Therapeutic potential of new B cell-targeted agents in the treatment of elderly and unfit patients with chronic lymphocytic leukemia. J Hematol Oncol 8:85

Salles G, Schuster SJ, de Vos S et al (2017) Efficacy and safety of idelalisib in patients with relapsed, rituximab- and alkylating agent-refractory follicular lymphoma: a subgroup analysis of a phase 2 study. Haematologica 102(4):e156–e159

Sanford DS, Wierda WG, Burger JA, Keating MJ, O'Brien SM (2015) Three newly approved drugs for chronic lymphocytic leukemia: incorporating ibrutinib, idelalisib, and obinutuzumab into clinical practice. Clin Lymphoma Myeloma Leuk 15(7):385–391

Seiler T, Hutter G, Dreyling M (2016) The emerging role of PI3K inhibitors in the treatment of hematological malignancies: preclinical data and clinical progress to date. Drugs 76(6):639–646

Shao Q, Byrum SD, Moreland LE et al (2013) A proteomic study of human Merkel cell carcinoma. J Proteomics Bioinform 6:275–282

Sharman J, Di Paolo J (2016) Targeting B-cell receptor signaling kinases in chronic lymphocytic leukemia: the promise of entospletinib. Ther Adv Hematol 7(3):157–170

Shiver MB, Mahmoud F, Gao L (2015) Response to idelalisib in a patient with stage IV Merkel-cell carcinoma. N Engl J Med 373(16):1580–1582

Smith SM, Pitcher BN, Jung SH et al (2017) Safety and tolerability of idelalisib, lenalidomide, and rituximab in relapsed and refractory lymphoma: the alliance for clinical trials in oncology A051201 and A051202 phase 1 trials. Lancet Haematol 4(4):e176–e182

Somoza JR, Koditek D, Villasenor AG et al (2015) Structural, biochemical, and biophysical characterization of idelalisib binding to phosphoinositide 3-kinase δ. J Biol Chem 290 (13):8439–8446

ten Hacken E, Burger JA (2014) Molecular pathways: targeting the microenvironment in chronic lymphocytic leukemia—focus on the B-cell receptor. Clin Cancer Res 20(3):548–556

ten Hacken E, Burger JA (2016) Microenvironment interactions and B-cell receptor signaling in chronic lymphocytic leukemia: implications for disease pathogenesis and treatment. Biochim Biophys Acta 1863(3):401–413

Traynor K (2014) Idelalisib approved for three blood cancers. Am J Health Syst Pharm 71 (17):1430

Vanhaesebroeck B, Khwaja A (2014) PI3Kδ inhibition hits a sensitive spot in B cell malignancies. Cancer Cell 25(3):269–271

Vitale C, Griggio V, Todaro M, Salvetti C, Boccadoro M, Coscia M (2017) Magic pills: new oral drugs to treat chronic lymphocytic leukemia. Expert Opin Pharmacother 18(4):411–425

Vyas P, Vohora D (2017) Phosphoinositide-3-kinases as the novel therapeutic targets for the inflammatory diseases: current and future perspectives. Curr Drug Targets 18(14):1622–1640

Weidner AS, Panarelli NC, Geyer JT et al (2015) Idelalisib-associated colitis: histologic findings in 14 patients. Am J Surg Pathol 39(12):1661–1667

Wiestner A (2012) Emerging role of kinase-targeted strategies in chronic lymphocytic leukemia. Hematology Am Soc Hematol Educ Program 2012:88–96

Wiestner A (2014) BCR pathway inhibition as therapy for chronic lymphocytic leukemia and lymphoplasmacytic lymphoma. Hematology Am Soc Hematol Educ Program 2014(1):125–134

Wiestner A (2015) The role of B-cell receptor inhibitors in the treatment of patients with chronic lymphocytic leukemia. Haematologica 100(12):1495–1507

Yang Q, Modi P, Newcomb T, Queva C, Gandhi V (2015) Idelalisib: first-in-class PI3K delta inhibitor for the treatment of chronic lymphocytic leukemia, small lymphocytic leukemia, and follicular lymphoma. Clin Cancer Res 21(7):1537–1542

Yap TA, Bjerke L, Clarke PA, Workman P (2015) Drugging PI3K in cancer: refining targets and therapeutic strategies. Curr Opin Pharmacol 23:98–107

Ysebaert L, Feugier P, Michallet AS (2015) Management of elderly patients with chronic lymphocytic leukemia in the era of targeted therapies. Curr Opin Oncol 27(5):365–370

Zelenetz AD, Barrientos JC, Brown JR et al (2017) Idelalisib or placebo in combination with bendamustine and rituximab in patients with relapsed or refractory chronic lymphocytic leukaemia: interim results from a phase 3, randomised, double-blind, placebo-controlled trial. Lancet Oncol 18(3):297–311

Zelenetz AD, Brown JR, Delgado J, Eradat H, Ghia P, Jacob A (2016) Updated analysis of overall survival in randomized phase III study of idelalisib in combination with bendamustine and rituximab in patients with relapsed/refractory CLL. Blood 128(22):a231

Carfilzomib

Monika Engelhardt, Magdalena Szymaniak-Vits, Stefanie Ajayi,
Sandra Maria Dold, Stefan Jürgen Müller, Sophia Scheubeck
and Ralph Wäsch

Contents

M. Engelhardt (✉) · M. Szymaniak-Vits · S. Ajayi · S. M. Dold · S. J. Müller
S. Scheubeck · R. Wäsch
Hematology and Oncology, Faculty of Medicine,
University of Freiburg, Hugstetter Str. 55, 79106 Freiburg, Germany
e-mail: monika.engelhardt@uniklinik-freiburg.de

M. Engelhardt · S. Ajayi
Comprehensive Cancer Center Freiburg (CCCF), Hugstetter Str. 55, 79106 Freiburg,
Germany

© Springer International Publishing AG, part of Springer Nature 2018
U. M. Martens (ed.), *Small Molecules in Hematology*, Recent Results
in Cancer Research 211, https://doi.org/10.1007/978-3-319-91439-8_13

Abstract

Carfilzomib (CFZ) is a potent, second-generation proteasome inhibitor (PI), with significant activity as a single agent and in combination with other antimyeloma agents in patients with relapsed or refractory multiple myeloma (RRMM). CFZ binds selectively and irreversibly to its target and leads to antiproliferative and proapoptotic effects on cancer cells. This irreversible inhibition is dose- and time-dependent in vitro and in vivo. CFZ as monotherapy and in combination with other antimyeloma agents (e.g., as CFZ and dexamethasone [Kd]) achieved very good responses, progression-free survival (PFS) and overall survival (OS). In several ongoing studies, CFZ is being investigated in triplet and quadruplet schedules of CFZ, lenalidomide and dexamethasone (KRd), CFZ, cyclophosphamide, dexamethasone (KCd) and with antibodies, like elotuzumab or daratumumab. The multitude of completed and ongoing studies confirmed a tolerable safety profile of CFZ, a significantly lower incidence of neuropathy compared to bortezomib (BTZ) and a slightly higher incidence of cardiotoxicity, which is closely observed and precautions taken to avoid them as best as possible. In July 2012, the US Food and Drug Administration (FDA) approved CFZ as a single agent for RRMM patients with disease progression after two prior therapies, including BTZ and immunomodulatory drugs (IMiDs). The combination of KRd and Kd followed, being approved by both FDA and European Medicines Agency (EMA) in 2015 and 2016, respectively. Moreover, CFZ is being evaluated in patients with newly diagnosed MM (NDMM), in high-risk smoldering MM and for maintenance approaches.

Keywords

Novel proteasome inhibitor · Irreversible · Carfilzomib · Relapsed/refractory disease · Multiple myeloma

1 Introduction

Multiple myeloma (MM) is characterized by proliferation of monoclonal plasma cells (PCs) in the bone marrow (BM) and accounts for approximately 10% of hematological malignancies (Rajkumar and Kumar 2016). The treatment of MM has substantially changed in the last decade due to the introduction of novel agents (NA) with new specific target structures against malignant cells. Among immunomodulatory drugs (IMiD), novel immunotherapies, including antibodies and various others (such as histone deacetylase inhibitors [HDACi]), proteasome inhibitors (PIs) play a pivotal role in the treatment of MM today.

Proteasomes are present in all eukaryotic cells. They degrade proteins and influence multiple cellular processes, including proliferation and DNA repair, so that their inhibition leads to cell cycle arrest and apoptosis. Unique immunoproteasomes exist in cells of immune or hematopoietic origin, where the catalytic sites differ from the constitutive proteasomes. Both constitutive and immunoproteasomes are expressed in MM cells and are targeted by PIs (Kortuem and Stewart 2013).

After the introduction of the first PI bortezomib (BTZ/V), second- and third-generation PIs have been developed, aiming to be potentially more efficacious and less toxic, including an improved polyneuropathy (PNP) side effect profile. Carfilzomib (CFZ/K) is a potent, selective, and irreversible second-generation PI, which granted approval for the treatment of relapsed/refractory MM (RRMM). The US Food and Drug Administration (FDA) approved CFZ monotherapy in RRMM patients in 2012. Moreover, the combination of CFZ, lenalidomide and dexamethasone (KRd) and CFZ and dexamethasone (Kd) followed, being approved by both FDA and European Medicines Agency (EMA) in 2015 and 2016, respectively.

In several clinical studies, CFZ has shown substantial antitumor activity in hematological malignancies, while exhibiting a well-tolerated side effect profile: The ENDEAVOR study compared Kd versus BTZ plus dexamethasone (Vd) and determined a longer progression-free survival (PFS) and lower risk of painful PNP with Kd (Dimopoulos et al. 2016). In the ASPIRE study, superiority of KRd vs. Rd, with unprecedented PFS differences in RRMM, was shown, and study results have recently been updated (Stewart et al. 2017). However, cardiac toxicity has been observed in a small proportion of patients, leading to the determination of potential risks and precautions that have been defined as relevant to observe to prudently use CFZ (Rajkumar and Kumar 2016). CFZ guideline papers are under way to guide these decisions and to conduct best surveillance and co-medication in different CFZ regimens (S. Bringhen, personal communication, 2018).

2 Structure and Mechanism of Action

CFZ, formerly known as PR-171 (Khan and Stewart 2011; Stewart 2012), is a PI that irreversibly interacts with the proteasome (Khan and Stewart 2011). Since it belongs to the epoxyketone-based PIs, CFZ is structurally and functionally distinct from BTZ (Khan and Stewart 2011; Demo et al. 2007). Due to the irreversible binding of CFZ, the response is more sustained than with the reversible BTZ (Demo et al. 2007) and the proteasome activity is decreased to less than 20%. Only by a new synthesis of the proteasome subunits and a new compilation it is possible to restore this irreversible binding (Kuhn et al. 2007). This CFZ property leads to minimal off-target inhibition to other proteases (Khan and Stewart 2011).

The proteasome itself is a multicatalytic protease complex (Fig. 1), that is responsible for the ubiquitin-dependent turnover of cellular proteins (Ciechanover 2005; Dalton 2004; Kisselev and Goldberg 2001). The inhibition of the proteasome leads to an accumulation of proteins in the cell guiding the cell into apoptosis (Adams 2004). Two units form the 26S proteasome, the 19S and the 20S units. This 20S unit consists of four stacked rings, two α-rings and two β-rings, of each seven subunits (α_1–α_7; β_1–β_7). The inner two β-subunit rings encode for three major catalytic activities, the caspase-like (C-L) proteolytic activity (β_1), the trypsin-like (T-L) (β_2), and the chymotrypsin-like (CT-L) proteolytic activity (β_7) (Kisselev and

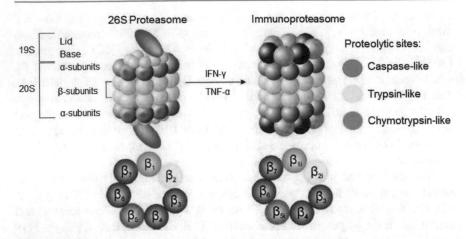

Fig. 1 Structure of the 26S proteasome and immunoproteasome with the three different catalytic sites. In cells from hematopoietic origin different factors like interferon (IFN)-γ and tumor necrosis factor (TNF)-α lead to the synthesis of the immunoproteasome. The arrangement of the three different catalytic sites is displayed between the proteasome and the immunoproteasome. Adapted from Kubiczkova et al. (2014), Kisselev and Goldberg (2001), Ciechanover (2005)

Goldberg 2005; Kuhn et al. 2009). Hematologically derived tumor cells express a variant 20S core, the i20S, making it an ideal target for PIs in the treatment of hematological cancers (Parlati et al. 2009). Since the CT-L activity is the rate limiting step of the proteolysis, it is the primary target for this drug class (Rock et al. 1994). The approval of BTZ led to the validation of the ubiquitin–proteasome pathway as a target for cancer therapy (Demo et al. 2007).

The epoxyketone-based CFZ is a potent and highly selective inhibitor of the CT-L catalytic subunit of the i20S proteasome or so-called immunoproteasome (Kuhn et al. 2007; O'Connor et al. 2009). The inhibition has an antiproliferative and proapoptotic effect on the cancer cell. The high selectivity of CFZ eliminates the potential off-target activity with other cellular proteases (Demo et al. 2007; Kuhn et al. 2007; Parlati et al. 2009). The epoxyketone structure (Fig. 2) leads to this

Fig. 2 Chemical structure of carfilzomib, an epoxyketone-based irreversible proteasome inhibitor (Kubiczkova et al. 2014)

Table 1 Characteristics and key features of carfilzomib

Pharmacodynamics

Active moiety	Proteasome target	Key cellular effects	Binding
Tetrapeptide epoxyketone	CT-L subunit	Caspase-3, 7, 8, 9; JNK, eIF2, NOXA	Irreversible (N-terminal to threonine)

Application notes

Dosage	Half-life (min)	Application
20–56 mg/m^2	<30	Intravenous

CT-L—chymotrypsin-like, eIF2—eukaryotic Initiation Factor 2, JNK—c-Jun N-terminal *kinase*, NOXA PMAIP1—phorbol-12-myristate-13-acetate-induced protein 1, mg—milligram; m—meter
Adapted from Kuhn et al. (2007), Tsakiri et al. (2013), Kubiczkova et al. (2014)

special characteristic of CFZ, due to the specificity of the NH_2-terminal threonine residue of the kinase ending in the inhibition of the enzyme activity (Kuhn et al. 2007).

By binding to the proteasome, CFZ forms a unique six-atom ring structure with the β_5-subunit that leads to an intramolecular cyclization and morpholino adduction (Kisselev and Goldberg 2001; Ruschak et al. 2011). This process is a two-step mechanism composed of the nucleophilic attack of the oxygen from the hydroxyl group of threonine 1 (Thr1) to carbon of the epoxyketone leading to the formation of a hemiacetal. In the second steps, the α-amino nitrogen of Thr1 nucleophilically attacks the C_2 carbon–epoxide ring, as a result this forms the morpholine adduct (Kisselev and Goldberg 2001; Ruschak et al. 2011).

The blockage of the proteasome induces several external and internal apoptotic cascades in the cell, like the elevation of the Caspases-3, 7, 8, 9. Additionally, the activation of c-Jun N-terminal kinase (JNK), the mitochondrial membrane depolarization, and a cytochrome c release is associated with programmed cell death. Furthermore, the accumulation of non-functional proteins and an increased level of NOXA induce ER stress connected with a decreased level of phosphorylated eukaryotic initiation factor 2 (eIF2) (Kuhn et al. 2007; Parlati et al. 2009). CFZ also promotes mesenchymal stem cell (MSC) differentiation into osteoclasts, similar to BTZ (Hu et al. 2013).

With no increased toxicity, CFZ can induce apoptosis in BTZ-naïve and pre-treated MM cells (Demo et al. 2007; Kuhn et al. 2007). Other mechanisms are also important for the toxicity of PIs, like dissociation half-life, pharmacokinetic, and pharmacodynamics (Table 1). Since CFZ as an epoxyketone PI has a significantly milder impact on the neuromusculatory system, this has been postulated as one reason for CFZ's lower neurotoxicity (Tsakiri et al. 2013).

3 Preclinical Data

The most exclusively expressed mammalian cytosolic 26S proteasome consists of two regulatory 19S cap subunits and one 20S core particle including two outer α-rings and two inner β-rings with three catalytically active sites (chymotrypsin-, trypsin-, and caspase-like proteolytic sites). Hence, the proteasomal ubiquitin-dependent proteolysis plays a crucial role in cellular homeostasis, particularly in excessively paraprotein-expressing MM cells (Kisselev et al. 2012). The epoxyketone class PI CFZ is a potent and highly selective, covalent inhibitor of the chymotrypsin-like (CT-L) activity within the 20S core subunit (Khan and Stewart 2011), leads to cellular protein accumulation and finally induces apoptosis. Moreover, CFZ demonstrated to overcome BTZ resistance in MM patient-derived cell culture models and worked synergistically in combination with dexamethasone in vitro (Kuhn et al. 2007). Additionally, CFZ, different to BTZ, can overcome BM stroma protection by inhibiting phosphorylated C-X-C chemokine receptor type 4 (pCXCR-4) and can cause downregulation of the cell surface marker CD138 in myeloma cells in vitro (Waldschmidt et al. 2017). In mice and monkeys, two consecutive intravenous (IV) boluses within 24 h (e.g., 1, 2; 8, 9; 15, 16; of a 28-day cycle) could demonstrate reduction of tumor growth and did cumulatively inhibit proteasomal activity, while a once-weekly schedule allowed proteasome recovery (Demo et al. 2007).

4 Clinical Data

CFZ is a second-generation PI that received approval for the treatment of RRMM patients, who have received at least two prior therapies, including BTZ and one IMiD. CFZ is active as a single agent and in combination with others antimyeloma agents.

4.1 Relapsed and Refractory MM (RRMM)

4.1.1 Single-Agent CFZ—Phase I/II Studies
The efficacy of CFZ in heavily pretreated, RRMM has been evaluated in a number of phase II trials. PX-171-003 was a multicenter, open-label, single-arm, phase II study. This registration trial led to FDA approval of CFZ in RRMM: 266 patients with prior exposure to BTZ and IMiDs were enrolled in this study. The median number of prior therapy lines was 5. CFZ was administered IV two consecutive days each week for three weeks in the 28-day treatment cycle. Patient received 20 mg/m^2 at a daily dose in cycle 1, and 27 mg/m^2 in subsequent cycles, until disease progression, unacceptable toxicity, or for a maximum of 12 cycles. The overall response rate (ORR) was 23.7%, with a median duration of response of

7.8 months. PFS and OS in response evaluable patients ($n = 257$) were 3.7 and 15.6 months, respectively. The therapy was generally well tolerated; 190 patients discontinued treatment due to progressive disease (59%) or AEs (12%). Dose reduction due to adverse events (AEs) was required in 17.7%. Drug-related AEs of all grades were most frequently fatigue (37%), nausea (3%), and thrombocytopenia (Jagannath et al. 2012; Siegel et al. 2012).

Vij et al. performed other clinical CFZ trials: The PX-171-004 trial enrolled 129 BTZ-naïve patients and 35 patients with prior BTZ treatment. In the first phase of the trial, CFZ was administrated in cohort 1 (94 patients) with 20 mg/m^2 IV on days 1, 2, 8, 9, 15, 16, every 28 days for up to 12 cycles. In the second phase of the study, 67 patients who tolerated 20 mg/m^2 CFZ during cycle 1 received an escalated dose of 27 mg/m^2 beginning in cycle 2. ORR in the BTZ-naïve cohort was 47.6%, while in the BTZ-pretreated cohort was 17.1%. In the BTZ-naïve cohort, the clinical benefit rate (CBR) was 61.9% after 6 CFZ-cycles (Vij et al. 2012b); whereas in BTZ-pretreated patients 31.4%. The median duration of response (DOR) was >10.6 months (Vij et al. 2012a). No differences in tolerability between both cohorts were observed. The most common reported AEs were non-hematological and included fatigue, nausea, dyspnea, which were primarily $\leq$ grade 2. Grade 3/4 events were less common and included thrombocytopenia, neutropenia, and lymphopenia, while PNP was rarely observed. No dose modification was required in patients with baseline renal function impairment. Both PX-171-003 and PX-171-004 studies demonstrated that CFZ was tolerable and active in RRMM, suggested a more rewarding activity in patients with lesser pretreatment (as has been univocally shown for other antimyeloma agents) and the PX-171-004 trial confirmed a dose–response relationship with single-agent CFZ (20 vs. 27 mg/m^2) (Jakubowiak 2014).

The open-label, multicenter phase II study PX-171-005 was designed to assess the influence of renal impairment (RI) on CFZ's pharmacokinetics (PK) in RRMM. Badros et al. (2013) enrolled 50 patients with varying degrees of renal function, ranging from normal to long-term dialysis patients. Patients received CFZ via IV infusion over 2–10 min on days 1, 2, 8, 9, 15, 16 of 28-day cycles for up to 12 cycles. The starting dose was 15 mg/m^2 in cycle 1. If tolerated, the CFZ dose was increased to 20 mg/m^2 in cycle 2 and to 27 mg/m^2 in cycle 3 and subsequent cycles. The results demonstrated a similar duration of drug exposure and clearance regardless of renal function with a similar rate of proteasomal ChT-L activity inhibition. Toxicities were similar between groups, and the incidence of AEs was independent of renal status. No dose modification was required. Therefore, CFZ was proposed as an appropriate treatment also in patients with severe RI, albeit admittedly, this phase II trial was small, which limits the general applicability of this subgroup analysis.

4.1.2 CFZ in Combination with Dexamethasone (Kd)—Phase I/II Study

In 2016, Berenson et al. presented results of the phase I/II, multicenter, single-arm, dose-escalation CHAMPION-1 study. This was the first clinical trial, which evaluated the safety and efficacy of once-weekly Kd in RRMM. CFZ was administered as a 30-min IV infusion on days 1, 8, and 15 of a 28-day cycle: 27 patients were enrolled in the phase I, dose-escalation study and received CFZ at 20 mg/m^2 on cycle 1 day 1. Subsequent doses were escalated in a standard 3 + 3 dose-escalation schema to 45, 56, 70, or 88 mg/m^2, to determine the maximum tolerated dose (MTD). In the phase 2 portion, 89 patients received CFZ at the MTD of the same schedule as in the phase 1 portion. All patients received additional dexamethasone with 40 mg (IV or orally) on days 1, 8, 15, and 22 for the first 8 cycles, whereas this was omitted on day 22 from cycle 9 and onward. Investigators observed no dose-limiting toxicities (DLT) across the 45, 56, and 70 mg/m^2 cohorts. The MTD of CFZ was therefore determined as 70 mg/m^2. The median PFS in 104 patients treated with the MTD was 12.6 months, the ORR was 77%, and 48 patients achieved $\geq$ VGPR. The frequency of any grade and $\geq$ grade 3 AEs was similar or lower than those reported in the Kd group of the phase III ENDEAVOR study (Berenson et al. 2016). This regime is evaluated in the phase III ARROW study, which compares the efficacy and safety of once-weekly 20/70 mg/m^2 Kd versus twice-weekly 20/27 mg/m^2 Kd in RRMM.

4.1.3 CFZ in Combination with Immunomodulatory Drugs (IMiDs)—Phase Ib/II Study

In June 2008, Wang et al. started the phase Ib/II study PX-171-006 to evaluate CFZ in combination with standard-dose lenalidomide (25 mg/d, days 1–21) and low-dose dexamethasone (40 mg once weekly) (KRd) in RRMM. CFZ was initiated at 15 mg/m^2 and was escalated to a maximal dose of 27 mg/m^2: 84 patients were treated in 28-day cycles; of those 62% within the maximum planned dose (MPD) cohort. The ORR was 69% and median PFS was 11.8 months. ORR, duration of response (DOR), and PFS in the MPD cohort were even better with 76.9%, 22.1, and 15.4 months, respectively. The AEs led to dose reduction in 7.7% and to treatment discontinuation in 19.2% of patients. Frequent hematological AEs of any grade were lymphopenia, neutropenia, and anemia, and common non-hematological AEs like fatigue and diarrhea. Grade 3/4 events were generally hematological and included lymphopenia (48.1%), neutropenia (32.7%), thrombocytopenia (19.2%), and anemia (19.2%) (Wang et al. 2013a). Results of this trial demonstrated that KRd was well tolerated and highly active in RRMM.

Therefore, Shah et al. (2015) designed an open-label, multicenter, phase I study of CFZ, pomalidomide, and dexamethasone. All 32 patients had been refractory to prior lenalidomide, and almost all were also BTZ-refractory. They received CFZ 20/27 mg/m^2 over 30 min on days 1, 2, 8, 9, 15, 16, pomalidomide 4 mg once daily on days 1–21 and dexamethasone 40 mg on days 1, 8, 15, and 22, every 28 days for the first 6 cycles. After termination of 6 cycles, maintenance therapy with CFZ on days 1, 2, 15, and 16 and pomalidomide on days 1–21 was continued. Patients received a median of 7 cycles. The ORR was 50% and the median PFS 7.2 months. Maintenance in cycle 7 was performed in 17 patients. Of the 32 enrolled patients, 8 required dose reduction and 7 treatment discontinuation due to AEs.

4.1.4 CFZ in Combination with Cyclophosphamide and Dexamethasone (KCd)—Phase II Study

Yong et al. (2017) presented at the American Society of Hematology Meeting 2017 results of the phase II MUK *five* study. The aim of this study was to compare the activity and safety of 6 cycles of CFZ versus 8 cycle of BTZ in triplet combination with cyclophosphamide and dexamethasone (KCd vs. VCd). A total of 300 patients at first relapse, or refractory to no more than 1 previous line of therapy, were randomized, 201 to KCd and 99 to VCd group. Participants in the KCd arm received CFZ 20/36 mg/m^2 biweekly (weeks 1–3) as IV infusion in the 28-day cycle, in the VCd arm BTZ 1.3 mg/m^2 was administered biweekly (weeks 1 and 2) subcutaneously in 21-day cycles. Both groups received cyclophosphamide 500 mg and dexamethasone 40 mg orally weekly. Patients in the KCd group with at least stable disease after 6 cycles of therapy were randomized to receive maintenance CFZ or no further treatment, patients in the VCd group did not receive maintenance. In the KCd arm, 81.6% of patients received all 6 treatment cycles, versus 53.5% with 8 completed cycles in the VCd arm. KCd group achieved significant higher major response ($\geq$ VGPR) at 24 weeks (40.2 vs. 31.9% for VCd). The OS for KCd and VCd was 84 and 68.1%, respectively. Treatment emergent neuropathy occurred more often in the VCd arm (56.3 vs. 21.4% with KCd). The incidence of $\geq$ grade 3 neuropathy or $\geq$ grade 2 neuropathy with pain was lower in the KCd group (1.5 vs. 19.8% with VCd). Cardiac SAEs were reported in 4.2% of patients in the KCd arm (vs. 1.4% VCd arm), neurological SAEs occurred more frequently in the VCd arm (8.1 vs. 0.7%). The results of this study showed that patients in the KCd arm achieved better OS, the regimen was generally well tolerated, and the incidence of neuropathy was significant lower than in the VCd arm.

4.1.5 Phase III CFZ Combination Trials: KRd (ASPIRE), KD (ENDEAVOR), and CFZ Alone (FOCUS)

Due to the promising results of KRd in phase I and II trials, Stewart et al. started a randomized, open-label, multicenter, phase III study in July 2010, which led to FDA approval of KRd in RRMM. This ASPIRE study was designed to compare the combination of KRd versus Rd. The investigators enrolled 792 RRMM patients who had previously received 1–3 prior lines, the median being 2 in both groups, with 66% having received prior BTZ- and 20% R-regimens. CFZ was administrated as a 10-min infusion on days 1, 2, 8, 9, 15, and 16 of cycles 1–12 (starting dose 20 mg/m^2 on days 1 and 2 of cycle 1 and 27 mg/m^2 thereafter) and on days 1, 2, 15, and 16 during cycles 13 through 18. Patients in both groups received 25 mg lenalidomide on days 1–21 and 40 mg dexamethasone on days 1, 8, 15, and 22 of a 28-days cycle until disease progression. The primary study endpoint was PFS in the intent-to-treat population. Secondary endpoints included OS, ORR, DOR, quality of life, and safety. The KRd group demonstrated significantly longer PFS (median 26.3 months) compared to Rd (17.6 months). The median OS was also shown to be improved (Stewart et al. 2017). The ORR was 87.1% with KRd versus 66.7% with Rd, including CRs or better in 31.8 versus 9.3%, respectively. The median DOR with KRd versus Rd was 28.6 versus 21.2 months, respectively. KRd-patient in the <70-year age subgroup reported improved health-related quality of life (HRQOL) in comparison to the Rd control group. No significant differences were observed between the KRd and Rd groups in the >70-year age subgroup (Stewart et al. 2016). Over 18 months, the global health status/quality of life (GHS-QoL) was greater in patients in the KRd than those in the Rd arm. Patients in the KRd group experienced a longer time to GHS/QoL deterioration than the Rd group, with the median time to deterioration (≥ 5 points) of 10.3 versus 4.8 months, respectively. Dyspnea (2.8 vs. 1.8%), cardiac failure (3.8 vs. 1.8%), ischemic heart disease (3.3 vs. 2.1%), hypertension (4.3 vs. 1.8%), and acute renal failure (3.3 vs. 3.1%) occurred more often with KRd. There was no difference between KRd und Rd groups in the incidence of PNP (17.1 vs. 17%, respectively). Treatment discontinuation due to AEs appeared in 15% with KRd versus 17.7% with Rd. The findings of the ASPIRE study demonstrated that KRd resulted in significantly improved ORR, PFS, and OS in RRMM patients. KRd also showed a favorable benefit-risk profile compared with Rd, irrespective of previous treatment (Stewart et al. 2015; Dimopoulos et al. 2017b, c).

In January 2016, Dimopoulos et al. presented results of the randomized, open-label, multicenter ENDEAVOR study, which compared Kd versus Vd in RRMM patients, who had received 1–3 previous therapies. Prior treatments could include BTZ, if patients achieved at least a partial response (PR) upon PI-treatment before relapse or progression. A total of 929 patients were enrolled and stratified by previous PIs, prior lines of therapy, ISS stage, and route of BTZ delivery, if randomized to Vd. CFZ was given as a 30-min infusion on days 1, 2, 8, 9, 15, and 16 of 28-day cycles (20 mg/m^2 d1 and 2 of cycle 1; 56 mg/m^2 thereafter). BTZ was administrated as IV bolus or subcutaneously, with a dose of 1.3 mg/m^2 on days 1, 4, 8, and 11 of 21-days cycle. Patients received 20 mg dexamethasone on days 1, 2, 8, 9, 15, 16, 22, 23 in the Kd group and on days 1, 2, 4, 5, 8, 9, 11, 12 in the VD group. Patients were treated until progression, withdrawal of consent or unacceptable toxicity. In the first interim analysis, the ORR was significantly higher with Kd versus Vd (77 vs. 63%, respectively), including VGPR or better in 54% with Kd and 29% with Vd. The PFS also favored Kd versus Vd (median 18.7 vs. 9.4 months, respectively). The median DOR was 21.3 months for Kd and 10.4 months for Vd. These results translated into prolonged OS (Kd: 47.6 vs. Vd: 40 months) and suggested that therapy with the selective, irreversible PI CFZ may induce higher responses, PFS and OS in RRMM than with BTZ. Of note, significantly higher GHS-QoL was reported in the CFZ group, albeit 99% of patients in both groups had any grade AEs. The incidence of grade 2 or worsened PNP was significantly higher in the Vd than Kd group (35 vs. 7%, respectively). The most frequent $\geq$ grade 3 AEs, which led to treatment discontinuation in the Kd group were cardiac failure, decrease in ejection fraction, asthenia, and acute renal failure and with Vd PNP, fatigue, dyspnea, and diarrhea. The median time to discontinuation in the Kd group was 6.8 and 4.3 months in the Vd group. Dose reduction due to AEs was necessary in 32% of patients in the Kd group and in 50% in the Vd group. The results of the study demonstrated that Kd versus Vd led to significantly and clinically meaningful improvements in OS, PFS, and objective response in RRMM (Dimopoulos et al. 2016, 2017a).

Hajek et al. (2012) presented results of the randomized, phase III, open-label, multicenter study FOCUS (PX-171-011), which investigated CFZ monotherapy versus low-dose corticosteroids with optional cyclophosphamide. A total of 315 patients were enrolled into this study and comprised the intent-to-treat population. The median number of 5 prior regimens was extensive. The median treatment duration was higher in the CFZ than in the control group (16.3 vs. 10.7 weeks, respectively). Median PFS in the CFZ group was 3.7 months compared with 3.3 months in the control group. Patients in the control group started next anti-myeloma therapy earlier than in the CFZ group. The median ORR in the CFZ group was 19.1 versus 11.4% in the control group. Moreover, the number of patients achieving minimal response or better was higher with CFZ than in the control population (31.2 vs. 20.8%, respectively). Incidence of treatment-related AEs was similar in both groups. Findings of this FOCUS study confirmed the safety profile of CFZ and suggested that CFZ in advanced and highly pretreated MM patients needs combination partners.

4.2 Newly Diagnosed Multiple Myeloma (NDMM)

CFZ as monotherapy and in combination with other antimyeloma agents has been investigated in newly diagnosed MM (NDMM) patients in several ongoing and completed studies:

CYKLONE is a phase Ib/II study designed to investigate CFZ in 64 transplant-eligible NDMM patients. Patients were treated with the 4-agent combination of CFZ (days 1, 2, 8, 9, 15, 16), 300 mg/m^2 cyclophosphamide (days 1, 8, 15), 100 mg thalidomide (days 1–28), and 40 mg dexamethasone (days 1, 8, 15, 22) in 28-day cycles. CFZ was dose-escalated at 4 dose levels to determine the MTD, which was 20/36 mg/m^2. Those 59% of patients treated at the MTD in the phase II part achieved a VGPR or better. In the overall population, the ORR was 91% and 44 patients achieved ≥ VGPR. Mikhael et al. demonstrated that the CYKLONE combination led to rapid and deep responses with limited neuropathy, cardiac or pulmonary toxicity in NDMM patients (Mikhael et al. 2015).

Bringhen et al. (2014) assessed the safety and efficacy of CFZ in combination with cyclophosphamide and dexamethasone (KCd) in NDMM patients ≥ 65 years of age and ineligible for autologous stem cell transplantation (ASCT) in a multi-center, open-label phase II trial. Investigators enrolled 58 patients, who received KCd for up to 9 cycles, followed by maintenance with CFZ until progression or intolerance. Patients received oral cyclophosphamide 300 mg/m^2 and dexamethasone 40 mg on days 1, 8, and 15; CFZ (20/36 mg/m^2) was administrated as 30-min infusions on days 1, 2, 8, 9, 15, 16. In the maintenance phase, patients were treated with 36 mg/m^2 CFZ on days 1, 2, 15, 16 every 28 days. Response was prompt and showed improvement over time. After a median of 9 cycles of KCd, 71% of patients achieved ≥ VGPR. After a median follow-up of 18 months, the 2-year

PFS and OS were 76 and 87%, respectively. The rate of $\geq$ grade 3 AEs was low, and the most common toxicities were neutropenia (20%), anemia (11%), and cardiopulmonary events (7%). This KCd regime showed a good safety profile and high efficacy with prominent CR rates, also in elderly patients.

Bringhen and colleague also presented results of weekly CFZ, combined with cyclophosphamide and dexamethasone. Patients were treated with CFZ on days 1, 8, and 15 of a 28-day cycle. A total of 63 patients were enrolled in the phase I and phase II of the study, 54 of them received recommended phase 2 dose 70 mg/m^2. At least very good PR was achieved in 36 (66%) of these 54 patients. The frequency of hematological and non-hematological AEs was similar to, or lower, than reported in previous study with twice-weekly CFZ (Bringhen et al. 2017).

Currently, a comparative trial of KRd versus KCD in younger patients, eligible for ASCT, is being performed by the GIMEMA (Italian) study group, preliminary results suggesting similar efficacy and toxicity for both induction schedules (Gay et al. 2017).

Several triplet and quadruplet schedules of KRD, KCD, e.g., with both antibodies elotuzumab and daratumumab, are being assessed in phase II/III clinical trials (e.g., DSMM; GMMG). The results of these studies are eagerly expected.

5 Toxicity

Most common side effects of CFZ reported in trials have been anemia, dyspnea, diarrhea, nausea, and fatigue. In the comparative analysis of 4 sequential phase II trials (PX-171-003-A0, PX-171-003-A1, PX-171-004, and PX-171-005) in 526 patients receiving single-agent CFZ at doses ranging from 15 to 27 mg/m^2, most common hematological toxicities (grade $\geq$ 3) were thrombocytopenia (23.4%), anemia (22.4%), lymphopenia (18.1%), and neutropenia (10.3%). Non-hematological toxicities were generally grade 1/2, although grade 3/4 grade toxicities did include pneumonia (10.5%), cardiac failure (9.5%), fatigue (7.6%), and RI (7.2%) (Harvey 2014; Muchtar et al. 2016). CFZ may bear the risk of cardiac toxicity, predominantly in patients with pre-existing cardiac impairment. Probably it is a direct result of reduced proteasome activity in the cardiac myocytes (Li and Wang 2011). Cardiovascular events were likewise reported in BTZ patients. Thus, this effect was particularly compared in the ENDEAVOR study, which demonstrated a higher frequency of any cardiac events of any grade in the Kd versus Vd group (12 vs. 4%). The most commonly reported cardiovascular events were new onset or worsening congestive heart failure, arrhythmia (mostly of low grade), myocardial infarction, pulmonary hypertension, sudden cardiac death, and an asymptomatic decrease in left ventricular ejection fraction (LVEF). Echocardiography, cardiac magnetic resonance imaging (MRI), or longer term blood pressure monitoring are recommended in patients with risk factors for cardiac events. Patients who developed cardiac toxicity should be regularly monitored regarding blood pressure, LVEF, heart rate, cardiac ischemia, dyspnea, and volume overload.

Infusion-related reactions (IRR) occurred following CFZ administration in >10% of patients. Within the first 24–48 h of CFZ application, IRR were reported and characterized by a constellation of symptoms, including fever, rigor, chills, arthralgia, myalgia, facial flushing, facial edema, vomiting, weakness, dyspnea, hypotension, syncope, chest tightness, and angina. IRR under CFZ may be prevented or allayed with dexamethasone prophylaxis. The toxicity profile of CFZ is intensively investigated in many phase I, II, and III studies. CFZ is generally considered well-tolerated, with a manageable toxicity profile for most patients (Table 2).

Table 2 Management of adverse events (AEs) in MM patients receiving CFZ

Toxicity	Recommended action

Hematological toxicity
Neutropenia (grade 3/4)
Thrombocytopenia (grade 4)
	• Withhold dose
	• If fully recovered before next scheduled dose, continue at same dose level
	  • Thrombocytopenia: If the patient recovers to grade 3 thrombocytopenia, reduce dose by one dose level
	  • Neutropenia: If the patient recovers to grade 2 neutropenia, reduce dose by one dose level
	• If tolerated, the reduced dose may be escalated to the previous dose at the discretion of the physician

Cardiac toxicity Grade 3 or 4, new onset or worsening of • congestive heart failure • decreased left ventricular function • or myocardial ischemia	• Withhold until resolved or returned to baseline, stop fluid administration • After resolution, consider restarting CFZ at 1 dose level reduction (KRd: $27 \text{ mg/m}^2 \rightarrow 20 \text{ mg/m}^2 \rightarrow 15 \text{ mg/m}^2$, Kd: $56 \text{ mg/m}^2 \rightarrow 45 \text{ mg/m}^2\ 36 \text{ mg/m}^2 \rightarrow 27 \text{ mg/m}^2$) based on a benefit/risk assessment • Resuming therapy: Follow-up EKG and biomarker monitoring (BNP or NT-pro-BNP) are recommended • If tolerated, the reduced dose may be escalated to the previous dose at the discretion of the physician
Pulmonary hypertension or *Peripheral neuropathy (grad 3/4)*	• Withhold until resolved or returned to baseline • Restart at the dose used prior to the event or reduced dose at the discretion of the physicians • If tolerated, the reduced dose may be escalated to the previous dose at the discretion of the physician
Pulmonary complications *(grade 3/4) or* *Other grade 3/4 non-hematological* *toxicities*	• Withhold until resolved or returned to baseline • Consider restarting at the next scheduled treatment with one dose level reduction • If tolerated, the reduced dose may be escalated to the previous dose at the discretion of the physician

(continued)

Table 2 (continued)

Toxicity	Recommended action
Hepatic toxicity *Grade 3/4 elevation of transaminases,* *bilirubin or other liver abnormalities*	• Withhold until resolved or returned to baseline • After resolution, consider if restarting CFZ is appropriate • If appropriate, reinitiate at the reduced dose with frequent monitoring of liver function • If tolerated, the reduced dose may be escalated to the previous dose at the discretion of the physician
Renal toxicity *Serum creatinine ≥ 2x baseline*	• Withhold until renal function has recovered to Grade 1 or to baseline and monitor renal function • If attributable to CFZ, restart at the next scheduled treatment at a reduced dose • If not attributable to CFZ, restart at the dose used prior to the event • If tolerated, the reduced dose may be escalated to the previous dose at the discretion of the physician

Adapted from Harvey (2014), Ludwig et al. (2017)

6 Drug Interactions

CFZ is characterized by a high systemic clearance and a short half-life period in patients with solid tumors ($t_{1/2}$). It is mainly metabolized via peptidase cleavage and epoxide hydrolysis (Yang et al. 2011). In vitro studies demonstrated that CFZ did not induce effects on human CYP 1A2 and CYP 3A4 in cultured fresh human hepatocytes. Cytochrome P450-mediated metabolism plays a marginal role in elimination of CFZ. The open-label, phase I, non-randomized, clinical drug interaction study enrolled 18 patients with solid tumors: 17 of them received at least 1 dose of CFZ and 67% ($n = 12$) completed a full cycle of administration. Repeated administration of CFZ (on day 1 + 16) did not result in significant interactions with midazolam via pharmacokinetics. The results of this study demonstrate that CFZ can be administered with other medications that are substrates of CYP3A4 (Wang et al. 2013b). It is unknown if CFZ is an inducer of CYP1A2, 2C8, 2C9, 2C19, and 2B6. Caution should be observed when combined with products which are substrates of these enzymes, including oral contraceptives (Onyx Pharmaceuticals 2012).

7 Biomarkers

Valid biomarkers that are predictive of response to therapy, survival and AEs are clinically relevant. Bhutani et al. showed that CXCR4 modulation after one day of CFZ monotherapy was predictive of early clinical response to KRd. Patients who responded to CFZ at 24 h with a decrease or no change in CXCR4 expression in PCs showed early clinical response in cycles 1–3 compared to those who had an increase in CXCR4 expression (Bhutani et al. 2014). Moreover, an increased expression of tight junction protein (TJP1) could be observed during the adaptive response mediating CFZ resistance in the LP-1/CFZ cell line (Riz and Hawley 2017). A strong association between higher immunoglobulin expression and sensitivity of CFZ was noted. Combined IGH and Fc gamma receptor 2B (FCGR2B) expression constitutes a retrospective validated biomarker that classifies CFZ response with 70% sensitivity and 94% specificity (Tuch et al. 2014). Also the difference between involved and uninvolved serum heavy-light chains (HLC) after 2 cycles of KRd was suggested as an independent predictor of early CR, as well as minimal residual disease (MRD) among high-risk smoldering myeloma (SMM) and NDMM patients treated with KRd. Normalization of the HLC ratio after 2 cycles of KRd appeared significantly associated with obtained nCR/CR/sCR (Bhutani et al. 2013). The 19S proteasome levels were predictive of response and survival. In patients receiving combination therapy with KRd, higher pretreatment 19S proteasome levels correlated with deeper clinical response to treatment. Additionally, higher pretreatment proteasome levels were predictive of improved duration of response and PFS (Korde et al. 2014). Furthermore, Jonsson et al. (2015) suggested early change in tumor size based on M-protein modeling as an early biomarker for survival in MM following exposure to single-agent CFZ. Four circulating micro-RNAs (miRNAs) were identified to be related to different PFS in patients treated with KRd. MiR-103a and miR-199 were associated with deceased risk of PFS, whereas miR-278 and miR-99 were associated with increased risk for progression. Cardiovascular events are known complications to CFZ and eagerly explored to be predicted in MM patients. Matrix metalloproteinase-1 (MMP-1) has been suggested as a potential biomarker for patients at risk for cardiovascular events when treated with CFZ. MM patients who developed cardiovascular events had 37% lower MMP-1 compared to those without (Lendvai et al. 2015). Albeit these biomarkers are further explored, their routine clinical use is inapt (Table 3).

Table 3 Biomarkers for response, PFS/OS, and cardiovascular events

Response	PFS/OS	CV events
19S proteasome levels	ECTS	MMP-1
CXCR4 modulation	miRNAs (miR-99, -199, -103a, and -378)	
TJP-1		
IGH & FCGR2B-expression		
HLC		

PFS—progression-free survival, *OS*—overall survival, *CV*—cardiovascular, *CXCR4*—CXC-chemokine receptor type 4, *TJP-1*—tight junction protein-1, *IGH*—immunoglobulin heavy chain, *FCGR2B*—low-affinity immunoglobulin gamma Fc region receptor II-b, *HLC*—serum heavy-light chain, *ECTS*—early change in tumor size, *miRNA*—microRNA, *RNA*—ribonucleic acid, *MMP-1*—matrix metalloproteinase-1

8 Summary and Perspective

CFZ is a potent PI and important component of antimyeloma treatment in a variety of regimens, including Kd, KRd, and KCd. CFZ has also been investigated with other IMiDs, such as pomalidomide and thalidomide, with different alkylators (e.g., CFZ-Bendamustine-Dex) and antibodies like daratumumab or elotuzumab in clinical trials. Due to its substantial efficacy and good tolerability, it is used in doublet, triplet, and quadruplet combinations, both in younger and older, ASCT-eligible and -ineligible patients. CFZ is considered a potent relapse option in MM patients who have relapsed after and/or are refractory to both BTZ and IMiD. The findings from ongoing phase II and multiple phase III studies will help to determine optional dosing regimens and to establish the position of CFZ in relapse, first- and subsequent-line therapy and maintenance approaches in even more depth in the near future.

References

Adams J (2004) The proteasome: a suitable antineoplastic target. Nat Rev Cancer 4:349. https://doi.org/10.1038/nrc1361

Badros AZ, Vij R, Martin T et al (2013) Carfilzomib in multiple myeloma patients with renal impairment: pharmacokinetics and safety. Leukemia 27:1707–1714. https://doi.org/10.1038/leu.2013.29

Berenson JR, Cartmell A, Bessudo A et al (2016) CHAMPION-1: a phase 1/2 study of once-weekly carfilzomib and dexamethasone for relapsed or refractory multiple myeloma. Blood 127:3360–3368. https://doi.org/10.1182/blood-2015-11-683854

Bhutani M, Costello R, Korde N et al (2013) Serum heavy-light chains (HLC) and free light chains (FLC) As predictors for early CR In newly diagnosed myeloma patients treated with carfilzomib, lenalidomide, and dexamethasone (CRd). Blood 122:762

Bhutani M, Lee M-J, Tomita Y et al (2014) Early biomarkers of response to carfilzomib in multiple myeloma (MM): modulation of CXCR4 and induction of autophagy. J Clin Oncol 32:e19572–e19572. https://doi.org/10.1200/jco.2014.32.15_suppl.e19572

Bringhen S, Petrucci MT, Larocca A et al (2014) Carfilzomib, cyclophosphamide, and dexamethasone in patients with newly diagnosed multiple myeloma: a multicenter, phase 2 study. Blood 124:63–69. https://doi.org/10.1182/blood-2014-03-563759

Bringhen S, D'Agostino M, Paoli LD et al (2017) Phase 1/2 study of weekly carfilzomib, cyclophosphamide, dexamethasone in newly diagnosed transplant-ineligible myeloma. Leukemia. https://doi.org/10.1038/leu.2017.327

Ciechanover A (2005) Proteolysis: from the lysosome to ubiquitin and the proteasome. Nat Rev Mol Cell Biol 6:79. https://doi.org/10.1038/nrm1552

Dalton WS (2004) The proteasome. Semin Oncol 31:3–9. https://doi.org/10.1053/j.seminoncol.2004.10.012

Demo SD, Kirk CJ, Aujay MA et al (2007) Antitumor activity of PR-171, a novel irreversible inhibitor of the proteasome. Cancer Res 67:6383–6391. https://doi.org/10.1158/0008-5472.CAN-06-4086

Dimopoulos MA, Moreau P, Palumbo A et al (2016) Carfilzomib and dexamethasone versus bortezomib and dexamethasone for patients with relapsed or refractory multiple myeloma (ENDEAVOR): a randomised, phase 3, open-label, multicentre study. Lancet Oncol 17:27–38. https://doi.org/10.1016/S1470-2045(15)00464-7

Dimopoulos MA, Goldschmidt H, Niesvizky R et al (2017a) Carfilzomib or bortezomib in relapsed or refractory multiple myeloma (ENDEAVOR): an interim overall survival analysis of an open-label, randomised, phase 3 trial. Lancet Oncol 18:1327–1337. https://doi.org/10.1016/S1470-2045(17)30578-8

Dimopoulos MA, Stewart AK, Masszi T et al (2017b) Carfilzomib–lenalidomide–dexamethasone vs lenalidomide–dexamethasone in relapsed multiple myeloma by previous treatment. Blood Cancer J 7:e554. https://doi.org/10.1038/bcj.2017.31

Dimopoulos MA, Stewart AK, Masszi T et al (2017c) Carfilzomib, lenalidomide, and dexamethasone in patients with relapsed multiple myeloma categorised by age: secondary analysis from the phase 3 ASPIRE study. Br J Haematol 177:404–413. https://doi.org/10.1111/bjh.14549

Gay FM, Scalabrini DR, Belotti A et al (2017) Paper: A randomized study of carfilzomib-lenalidomide-dexamethasone vs carfilzomib-cyclophosphamide-dexamethasone induction in newly diagnosed myeloma patients eligible for transplant: high efficacy in high- and standard-risk patients

Hájek R, Bryce R, Ro S et al (2012) Design and rationale of FOCUS (PX-171-011): a randomized, open-label, phase 3 study of carfilzomib versus best supportive care regimen in patients with relapsed and refractory multiple myeloma (R/R MM). BMC Cancer 12:415. https://doi.org/10.1186/1471-2407-12-415

Harvey RD (2014) Incidence and management of adverse events in patients with relapsed and/or refractory multiple myeloma receiving single-agent carfilzomib. Clin Pharmacol Adv Appl 6:87–96. https://doi.org/10.2147/CPAA.S62512

Hu B, Chen Y, Usmani SZ et al (2013) Characterization of the molecular mechanism of the bone-anabolic activity of carfilzomib in multiple myeloma. PLoS ONE 8:e74191. https://doi.org/10.1371/journal.pone.0074191

Jagannath S, Vij R, Stewart AK et al (2012) An open-label single-arm pilot phase II study (PX-171-003-A0) of low-dose, single-agent carfilzomib in patients with relapsed and refractory multiple myeloma. Clin Lymphoma Myeloma Leuk 12:310–318. https://doi.org/10.1016/j.clml.2012.08.003

Jakubowiak AJ (2014) Evolution of carfilzomib dose and schedule in patients with multiple myeloma: a historical overview. Cancer Treat Rev 40:781–790. https://doi.org/10.1016/j.ctrv.2014.02.005

Jonsson F, Ou Y, Claret L et al (2015) A tumor growth inhibition model based on M-protein levels in subjects with relapsed/refractory multiple myeloma following single-agent carfilzomib use. CPT Pharmacomet Syst Pharmacol 4:711–719. https://doi.org/10.1002/psp4.12044

Khan ML, Stewart AK (2011) Carfilzomib: a novel second-generation proteasome inhibitor. Future Oncol 7:607–612. https://doi.org/10.2217/fon.11.42

Kisselev AF, Goldberg AL (2001) Proteasome inhibitors: from research tools to drug candidates. Chem Biol 8:739–758. https://doi.org/10.1016/S1074-5521(01)00056-4

Kisselev AF, Goldberg AL (2005) Monitoring activity and inhibition of 26S proteasomes with fluorogenic peptide substrates. In: Methods in enzymology. Academic Press, pp 364–378

Kisselev AF, van der Linden WA, Overkleeft HS (2012) Proteasome inhibitors: an expanding army attacking a unique target. Chem Biol 19:99–115. https://doi.org/10.1016/j.chembiol.2012.01.003

Korde N, Dosani T, Simakova O et al (2014) Biomarker proteasome levels predict response to combination therapy with carfilzomib, lenalidomide, and dexamethasone in newly diagnosed multiple myeloma patients. Blood 124:2080

Kortuem KM, Stewart AK (2013) Carfilzomib. Blood 121:893–897. https://doi.org/10.1182/blood-2012-10-459883

Kubiczkova L, Pour L, Sedlarikova L et al (2014) Proteasome inhibitors—molecular basis and current perspectives in multiple myeloma. J Cell Mol Med 18:947–961. https://doi.org/10.1111/jcmm.12279

Kuhn DJ, Chen Q, Voorhees PM et al (2007) Potent activity of carfilzomib, a novel, irreversible inhibitor of the ubiquitin-proteasome pathway, against preclinical models of multiple myeloma. Blood 110:3281–3290. https://doi.org/10.1182/blood-2007-01-065888

Kuhn DJ, Hunsucker SA, Chen Q et al (2009) Targeted inhibition of the immunoproteasome is a potent strategy against models of multiple myeloma that overcomes resistance to conventional drugs and nonspecific proteasome inhibitors. Blood 113:4667–4676. https://doi.org/10.1182/blood-2008-07-171637

Lendvai N, Devlin S, Patel M, Knapp KM (2015) Paper: Biomarkers of cardiotoxicity among multiple myeloma patients subsequently treated with proteasome inhibitor therapy

Li Y-F, Wang X (2011) The role of the proteasome in heart disease. Biochim Biophys Acta 1809:141–149. https://doi.org/10.1016/j.bbagrm.2010.09.001

Ludwig H, Delforge M, Facon T et al (2017) Prevention and management of adverse events of novel agents in multiple myeloma: a consensus of the european myeloma network. Leukemia. https://doi.org/10.1038/leu.2017.353

Mikhael JR, Reeder CB, Libby EN et al (2015) Phase Ib/II trial of CYKLONE (cyclophosphamide, carfilzomib, thalidomide and dexamethasone) for newly diagnosed myeloma. Br J Haematol 169:219–227. https://doi.org/10.1111/bjh.13296

Muchtar E, Gertz MA, Magen H (2016) A practical review on carfilzomib in multiple myeloma. Eur J Haematol 96:564–577. https://doi.org/10.1111/ejh.12749

O'Connor OA, Stewart AK, Vallone M et al (2009) A phase 1 dose escalation study of the safety and pharmacokinetics of the novel proteasome inhibitor carfilzomib (PR-171) in patients with hematologic malignancies. Clin Cancer Res Off J Am Assoc Cancer Res 15:7085–7091. https://doi.org/10.1158/1078-0432.CCR-09-0822

Onyx Pharmaceuticals (2012) Kyprolis® (carfilzomib) prescribing information

Parlati F, Lee SJ, Aujay M et al (2009) Carfilzomib can induce tumor cell death through selective inhibition of the chymotrypsin-like activity of the proteasome. Blood 114:3439–3447. https://doi.org/10.1182/blood-2009-05-223677

Rajkumar SV, Kumar S (2016) Multiple myeloma: diagnosis and treatment. Mayo Clin Proc 91:101–119. https://doi.org/10.1016/j.mayocp.2015.11.007

Riz I, Hawley RG (2017) Increased expression of the tight junction protein TJP1/ZO-1 is associated with upregulation of TAZ-TEAD activity and an adult tissue stem cell signature in carfilzomib-resistant multiple myeloma cells and high-risk multiple myeloma patients. Oncoscience 4:79–94. https://doi.org/10.18632/oncoscience.356

Rock KL, Gramm C, Rothstein L et al (1994) Inhibitors of the proteasome block the degradation of most cell proteins and the generation of peptides presented on MHC class I molecules. Cell 78:761–771

Ruschak AM, Slassi M, Kay LE, Schimmer AD (2011) Novel proteasome inhibitors to overcome bortezomib resistance. J Natl Cancer Inst 103:1007–1017. https://doi.org/10.1093/jnci/djr160

Shah JJ, Stadtmauer EA, Abonour R et al (2015) Carfilzomib, pomalidomide, and dexamethasone for relapsed or refractory myeloma. Blood 126:2284–2290. https://doi.org/10.1182/blood-2015-05-643320

Siegel DS, Martin T, Wang M et al (2012) A phase 2 study of single-agent carfilzomib (PX-171-003-A1) in patients with relapsed and refractory multiple myeloma. Blood 120:2817–2825. https://doi.org/10.1182/blood-2012-05-425934

Stewart AK (2012) Novel therapeutics in multiple myeloma. Hematol Amst Neth 17:S105–S108. https://doi.org/10.1179/102453312X13336169156131

Stewart AK, Rajkumar SV, Dimopoulos MA et al (2015) Carfilzomib, lenalidomide, and dexamethasone for relapsed multiple myeloma. N Engl J Med 372:142–152. https://doi.org/10.1056/NEJMoa1411321

Stewart AK, Dimopoulos MA, Masszi T et al (2016) Health-Related quality-of-life results from the open-label, randomized, phase III ASPIRE trial evaluating carfilzomib, lenalidomide, and dexamethasone versus lenalidomide and dexamethasone in patients with relapsed multiple myeloma. J Clin Oncol Off J Am Soc Clin Oncol 34:3921–3930. https://doi.org/10.1200/JCO. 2016.66.9648

Stewart AK, Siegel D, Ludwig H et al (2017) Overall survival (OS) of patients with relapsed/refractory multiple myeloma (RRMM) treated with carfilzomib, lenalidomide, and dexamethasone (KRd) versus lenalidomide and dexamethasone (Rd): final analysis from the randomized phase 3 aspire trial. Blood 130:743

Tsakiri EN, Kastritis E, Bagratuni T et al (2013) The novel proteasome inhibitors carfilzomib and oprozomib induce milder degenerative effects compared to bortezomib when administered via oral feeding in an in vivo drosophila experimental model: a biological platform to evaluate safety/efficacy of proteasome inhibitors. Blood 122:1930

Tuch BB, Loehr A, Degenhardt JD et al (2014) Abstract 898: Expression of immunoglobulin and its receptor are major determinants of multiple myeloma patient sensitivity to proteasome inhibitors. Cancer Res 74:898. https://doi.org/10.1158/1538-7445.AM2014-898

Vij R, Siegel DS, Jagannath S et al (2012a) An open-label, single-arm, phase 2 study of single-agent carfilzomib in patients with relapsed and/or refractory multiple myeloma who have been previously treated with bortezomib. Br J Haematol 158:739–748. https://doi.org/10. 1111/j.1365-2141.2012.09232.x

Vij R, Wang M, Kaufman JL et al (2012b) An open-label, single-arm, phase 2 (PX-171-004) study of single-agent carfilzomib in bortezomib-naive patients with relapsed and/or refractory multiple myeloma. Blood 119:5661–5670. https://doi.org/10.1182/blood-2012-03-414359

Waldschmidt JM, Simon A, Wider D et al (2017) CXCL12 and CXCR7 are relevant targets to reverse cell adhesion-mediated drug resistance in multiple myeloma. Br J Haematol 179:36–49. https://doi.org/10.1111/bjh.14807

Wang M, Martin T, Bensinger W et al (2013a) Phase 2 dose-expansion study (PX-171-006) of carfilzomib, lenalidomide, and low-dose dexamethasone in relapsed or progressive multiple myeloma. Blood 122:3122–3128. https://doi.org/10.1182/blood-2013-07-511170

Wang Z, Yang J, Kirk C et al (2013b) Clinical pharmacokinetics, metabolism, and drug-drug interaction of carfilzomib. Drug Metab Dispos Biol Fate Chem 41:230–237. https://doi.org/10. 1124/dmd.112.047662

Yang J, Wang Z, Fang Y et al (2011) Pharmacokinetics, pharmacodynamics, metabolism, distribution, and excretion of carfilzomib in rats. Drug Metab Dispos 39:1873–1882. https:// doi.org/10.1124/dmd.111.039164

Yong K, Hinsley S, Auner HW et al (2017) Carfilzomib, cyclophosphamide and dexamethasone (KCD) versus bortezomib, cyclophosphamide and dexamethasone (VCD) for treatment of first relapse or primary refractory multiple myeloma (MM): first final analysis of the phase 2 Muk five study. Blood 130:835

Acalabrutinib, A Second-Generation Bruton's Tyrosine Kinase Inhibitor

Katharina Kriegsmann, Mark Kriegsmann
and Mathias Witzens-Harig

Contents

K. Kriegsmann (✉) · M. Witzens-Harig
Department of Hematology, Oncology and Rheumatology, Heidelberg University, Heidelberg,
Germany
e-mail: katharina.kriegsmann@med.uni-heidelberg.de

M. Kriegsmann
Institute of Pathology, Heidelberg University, Heidelberg, Germany

© Springer International Publishing AG, part of Springer Nature 2018
U. M. Martens (ed.), *Small Molecules in Hematology*, Recent Results
in Cancer Research 211, https://doi.org/10.1007/978-3-319-91439-8_14

Abstract

The Bruton's tyrosine kinase (BTK) is an essential in the B-cell receptor (BCR) signaling pathway which was identified as crucial in the pathogenesis of B-cell malignancies. Ibrutinib, a first-in-class BTK inhibitor, has been approved for the treatment of distinct B-cell malignancies. To overcome off-target side effects of and emerging resistances to ibrutinib, more selective second-generation BTK inhibitors were developed. Acalabrutinib is a novel second-generation BTK inhibitor and has shown promising safety and efficacy profiles in phase 1/2 clinical trials in patients with relapsed CLL and pretreated MCL. Recently, acalabrutinib was approved by the FDA for treatment of adult patients with MCL who received at least one prior therapy. However, clinical trials on a direct comparison between ibrutinib and acalabrutinib and on combination treatment options with other agents as CD20 antibodies are warranted.

Keywords

Acalabrutinib · Bruton's tyrosine kinase · Hematologic malignancies

1 Introduction

B-cell receptor (BCR) signaling pathway has been identified to play an important role in the pathogenesis and progression of B-cell malignancies (Bojarczuk et al. 2015). As Bruton's tyrosine kinase (BTK) is an essential kinase in the BCR signaling pathway, ibrutinib, a first-in-class BTK inhibitor, has been approved for the treatment of chronic lymphocytic leukemia (CLL), mantle cell lymphoma (MCL), marginal zone lymphoma and Waldenstrom's macroglobulinemia (WM) (Thompson and Burger 2017; Agency EM 2017; Martin et al. 2016; Kapoor et al. 2017; Noy et al. 2017). More specific second-generation BTK inhibitors were developed to overcome off-target side effects of and emerging resistances to ibrutinib (Wu et al. 2016). Herein, the mechanism of action, preclinical and clinical data, including toxicity profile and drug interactions of the novel second-generation BTK inhibitor, acalabrutinib (also known as ACP-196), are summarized.

2 Structure and Mechanism of Action

The molecular formula of acalabrutinib is $C_{26}H_{23}N_7O_2$, the chemical name 4-{8-Amino-3-[(2S)-1-(2-butynoyl)-2-pyrrolidinyl]imidazo[1,5-a]pyrazin-1-yl}-N-(2-pyridinyl)benzamide, and the molar mass 465.507 g/mol (AstraZeneca 2017). The chemical structure is shown in Fig. 1.

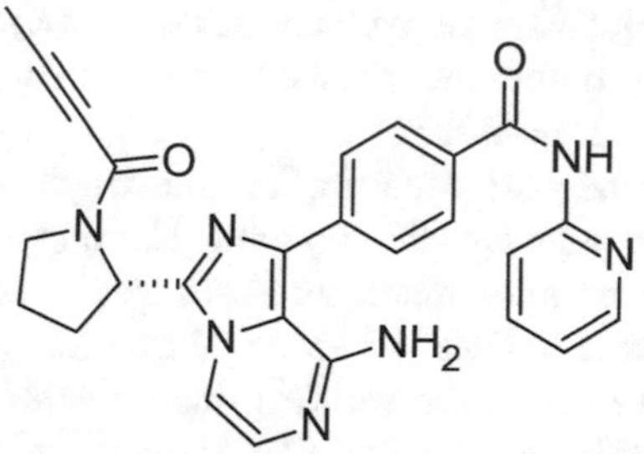

Fig. 1 Chemical structure of acalabrutinib. The figure was used in agreement with the Wikimedia Commons License

Acalabrutinib and its active metabolite, ACP-5862, bind covalently to a cysteine residue (Cys481) in the adenosine triphosphate- (ATP-) binding pocket of BTK via a reactive butynamide group thereby acting as an irreversible small-molecule inhibitor of BTK (Barf et al. 2017; Wu et al. 2016). Acalabrutinib was demonstrated to inhibit BTK with a half maximal inhibitory concentration (IC$_{50}$) of 5.1 ± 1.0 nM in the immobilized metal ion affinity-based fluorescence polarization (IMAP) assay (Barf et al. 2017; Byrd et al. 2016). In vitro, increasing concentrations of acalabrutinib led to a dose-dependent inhibition of the BCR signaling pathway in primary human CLL cells (Byrd et al. 2016).

In order to determine the selectivity of acalabrutinib, inhibitory assays on kinases with a cysteine residue in the same position as BTK were performed. Herein, acalabrutinib showed almost no inhibitory activity on epidermal growth factor receptor (EGFR), IL2-inducible T-cell kinase (ITK) and tyrosine-protein kinase Tec (TEC) (Barf et al. 2017; Byrd et al. 2016; Patel et al. 2017). These findings indicated a higher selectivity of acalabrutinib over ibrutinib with reduced off-target side effects. In this regard, ibrutinib but not acalabrutinib treatment resulted in a reduced platelet–vessel wall interaction compared to healthy controls in a humanized mouse model of thrombosis. These results demonstrated that acalabrutinib did not inhibit platelet activity, probably due to its improved selectively (Byrd et al. 2016).

3 Preclinical Data

Preclinical in vivo data on single-agent activity of acalabrutinib were obtained from mouse and canine animal models.

Herman et al. demonstrated acalabrutinib to be a potent inhibitor of BTK in two murine models of human CLL: the human NSG (NOD-Scid-IL2Rgc^{null}) primary CLL xenograft model and the Eµ-TCL-1 adoptive transfer model. In both mouse models, acalabrutinib treatment had on-target effects including decreased activation of key signaling molecules such as BTK, phospholipase C-γ2 (PLCγ2), ribosomal protein S6, and extracellular signal regulated kinase (ERK). Moreover, a significant inhibition of CLL cell proliferation, reduced tumor burden, and increased survival were observed (Herman et al. 2017).

In a model of spontaneously occurring canine lymphoma, a B-cell malignancy similar to human diffuse large B-cell lymphoma, Harrington et al. proved activity of acalabrutinib. In particular, upon treatment at dosages of 2.5–20 mg/kg every 12 or 24 h an overall response rate (ORR) of 25% and a median progression-free survival (PFS) of 22.5 days have been observed (Harrington et al. 2016).

These preclinical studies provided detailed insights into the mechanism of action of acalabrutinib and paved the way for subsequent clinical trials.

4 Clinical Data

The safety and efficacy of single-agent acalabrutinib was evaluated in phase 1/2 clinical trials in relapsed CLL and previously pretreated MCL.

In an uncontrolled multicenter study (NCT02029443) acalabrutinib was administered orally at a dose of 100–400 mg once daily (phase 1 dose escalation) and 100 mg twice daily (phase 2) to 61 patients with relapsed CLL (median of three previous therapies). Among the recruited patients, 75% had an unmutated immunoglobulin variable-region heavy-chain gene, 31% a chromosome 17p13.1 deletion, and 29% a chromosome 11q22.3 deletion. The median age was 62 (range 44–84) years. Compared to once-daily dosing, the twice-daily application improved the kinase occupancy allowing continues BTK inhibition without increasing toxic effects. The ORR was 95%, including 10% of patients with partial response (PR) with lymphocytosis and 85% with a PR, after a median follow-up of 14.3 months. Stable disease (SD) was observed in the remaining 5% of patients. In patients with a chromosome 17p13.1 deletion, the ORR was 100%. Only one patient, with a chromosome 17p13.1 deletion, experienced disease progression during therapy. Interestingly, at progression a C481S mutation in BTK (major clone) and a L845F mutation in PLCγ2 (minor clone) was found in this patient. Overall, acalabrutinib showed promising efficacy in relapsed CLL (Byrd et al. 2016). Based on these data, a subsequent phase 3 clinical trial comparing acalabrutinib versus ibrutinib in pretreated patients with high-risk CLL has been initiated (NCT02477696). Further clinical trials evaluating acalabrutinib in combination with other agents in CLL are ongoing (Table 1).

In another phase 2 open-label, single-arm clinical trial (ACE-LY-004, NCT02213926) acalabrutinib was administered at a dosage of 100 mg twice daily until progression. 124 patients with relapsed/refractory MCL (median of two previous treatments, including 18% of patients with prior stem cell transplant) were included. Previous BTK treatment was defined as an exclusion criterion. The median age was 68 (range 42–90) years. 44 and 17% of patients had intermediate or high risk with regard to MCL International Prognostic Index (MIPI), respectively. At a median follow-up of 15.2 months, the ORR was 80%, with a 40% complete

Table 1 Acalabrutinib trials in hematologic malignancies[a]

Phase	Agents	Diseases	NCT No	Status
1	Acalabrutinib + ACP-319	CLL	NCT02157324	Active, not recruiting
1	Acalabrutinib	B-cell malignancies	NCT03198650	Recruiting
1b	Acalabrutinib + Dexamethasone vs. Acalabrutinib	MM	NCT02211014	Active, not recruiting
1b	Acalabrutinib + Bendamustine + Rituximab	MCL	NCT02717624	Active, not recruiting
1b	Acalabrutinib + Obinutuzumab + Venetoclax and Acalabrutinib + Rituximab + Venetoclax	CLL, SLL, PLL	NCT02296918	Active, not recruiting
1b	Acalabrutinib	DLBCL	NCT02112526	Unknown
1/2	Acalabrutinib + Vistusertib	B-cell malignancies	NCT03205046	Recruiting
1/2	Acalabrutinib	CLL, Richters syndrome, SLL, PLL	NCT02029443	Active, not recruiting
1/2	Acalabrutinib + AZD6738 vs. AZD6738	CLL	NCT03328273	Not yet recruiting
1/2	Acalabrutinib + ACP-319	B-cell malignancies	NCT02328014	Recruiting
1b/2	Acalabrutinib + Pembrolizumab	Hematologic malignancies	NCT02362035	Active, not recruiting
1b/2	Acalabrutinib + Rituximab vs. Acalabrutinib	FL	NCT02180711	Active, not recruiting
2	Acalabrutinib	WM	NCT02180724	Active, not recruiting
2	Acalabrutinib	MCL	NCT02213926	Active, not recruiting
2	Acalabrutinib	CLL	NCT02717611	Active, not recruiting

(continued)

Table 1 (continued)

Phase	Agents	Diseases	NCT No	Status
2	Acalabrutinib	CLL, SLL	NCT02337829	Recruiting
3	Acalabrutinib + Bendamustine + Rituximab vs. Placebo + Bendamustine + Rituximab	MCL	NCT02972840	Recruiting
3	Acalabrutinib vs. Rituximab + Idelalisib or Rituximab + Bendamustine	CLL	NCT02970318	Recruiting
3	Acalabrutinib vs. Ibrutinib	CLL	NCT02477696	Recruiting
3	Acalabrutinib + Obinutuzumab vs. Acalabrutinib vs. Obinutuzumab + Chlorambucil	CLL	NCT02475681	Active, not recruiting

[a]As registered at ClinicalTrials.gov (2017)

CLL chronic lymphocytic leukemia, *DLBCL* diffuse large B-cell lymphoma, *FL* follicular lymphoma, *MCL* mantel cell lymphoma, *MM* multiple myeloma, *PLL* prolymphocytic leukemia, *SLL* small lymphocytic leukemia, *vs.* versus, *WM* Waldenstrom's macroglobulinemia response (CR) and 40% PR rate (AstraZeneca 2017b). These data demonstrated the potential impact of acalabrutinib in treatment of relapsed/refractory MCL and led to an accelerated Food and Drug Administration (FDA) approval of Calquence® (acalabrutinib) for treatment of adult patients with MCL who received at least one prior therapy (FDA 2017).

5 Toxicity

Side effects of acalabrutinib were reported in the two previously described phase 1/2 clinical trials.

The most common non-hematological side effects described in the acalabrutinib/relapsed CLL trial (NCT02029443) were headache (43%), diarrhea (39%), weight gain (26%), pyrexia (23%), upper respiratory tract infection (23%), hypertension (20%) and nausea (20%). Severe (grade $\geq$ 3) diarrhea, weight gain, pyrexia, fatigue, hypertension, and arthralgia were rare (2–7%). Grade 1–2 petechiae were reported in 16% of patients, grade $\geq$ 3 anemia and neutropenia in 2% of patients, respectively. Overall, no dose-limiting toxicities in the phase 1 part of the trial and no cases of atrial fibrillation (common during ibrutinib treatment) were observed (Byrd et al. 2016).

In the acalabrutinib/pretreated MCL study (ACE-LY-004, NCT02213926) anemia (46%), thrombocytopenia (44%), headache (39%), neutropenia (36%), diarrhea (31%), fatigue (28%), myalgia (21%), bruising (21%), nausea (19%), and rash (18%) were common side effects. Grade $\geq$ 3 non-hematological events included diarrhea, headache, abdominal pain as well as vomiting and were also rare (2–3%). Grade $\geq$ 3 anemia, thrombocytopenia and neutropenia were observed in 10, 12, and 15% of patients, respectively. Dose-adjustment and treatment discontinuation was reported in 2 and 7% of patients (AstraZeneca 2017a, b).

6 Drug Interactions

Acalabrutinib is predominantly metabolized by CYP3A enzymes in the liver. Therefore, plasma concentrations and side effects were elevated when administered in combination with moderate and strong CYP3A inhibitors such as itraconazole, erythromycin, fluconazole, or diltiazem. On the other hand, co-administration of CYP3A inducers, like rifampicin, resulted in reduced plasma concentration. Furthermore, solubility of acalabrutinib was affected by the pH. Thus, co-administration with antacids and proton pump inhibitors decreased absorption. In combination with CYP3A inhibitors, CYP3A inducers or gastric acid-reducing agents dose adjustments and/or separate dosing are recommended (AstraZeneca 2017).

7　Biomarkers

So far, no predictive or prognostic biomarkers were reported for acalabrutinib.

8　Summary and Perspective

Acalabrutinib is a novel second-generation BTK inhibitor with improved selectivity compared to the first-in-class BTK inhibitor ibrutinib. Acalabrutinib showed promising safety and efficacy profiles in phase 1/2 clinical trials in patients with relapsed CLL and pretreated MCL. In contrast to ibrutinib, so far no cases of atrial fibrillation have been reported during treatment with acalabrutinib. Recently, acalabrutinib was approved by the FDA for treatment of adult patients with MCL who received at least one prior therapy. However, clinical trials and a direct comparison between ibrutinib and acalabrutinib are warranted to reveal the superiority and possible resistance mechanisms of acalabrutinib. Currently, several phase 1, 2, and 3 clinical trials on acalabrutinib single-agent activity and combinations with other agents in hematologic malignancies (Table 1) and solid tumors (Table 2) are ongoing. As indicated in preclinical studies, combinations of acalabrutinib with other agents as CD20 antibodies, phosphoinositide 3 (PI3) kinase and BCL-2 inhibitors will likely increase rates and duration of response (Patel et al. 2017; Niemann et al. 2017; Golay et al. 2017; Deng et al. 2017) Finally, additional selective BTK inhibitors, as ONO/GS-4059, CC-292, BGB-3111, are currently

Table 2　Acalabrutinib trials in solid tumors[a]

Phase	Agents	Diseases	NCT No	Status
1b/2	Acalabrutinib	Glioblastoma multiforme	NCT02586857	Recruiting
2	Acalabrutinib + Pembrolizumab versus Acalabrutinib	Ovarian cancer	NCT02537444	Active, not recruiting
2	Acalabrutinib + Pembrolizumab versus Pembrolizumab	Non-small lung cancer	NCT02448303	Active, not recruiting
2	Acalabrutinib + Pembrolizumab	Head and neck squamous cell carcinoma	NCT02454179	Active, not recruiting
2	Acalabrutinib + Pembrolizumab	Metastatic urothelial carcinoma	NCT02351739	Active, not recruiting
2	Acalabrutinib + Pembrolizumab versus Acalabrutinib	Metastatic pancreatic cancer	NCT02362048	Active, not recruiting
2	Acalabrutinib + Nab-paclitaxel	Metastatic pancreatic cancer	NCT02570711	Terminated
2	Acalabrutinib + Methotrexate versus Methotrexate + Placebo	Rheumatoid arthritis	NCT02387762	Completed

[a]As registered at ClinicalTrials.gov. (2017)

tested in B-cell malignancy models and early phase clinical trials (Thompson and Burger 2017; Robak and Robak 2017; Vidal-Crespo et al. 2017; Wu et al. 2017; Walter et al. 2016).

References

Agency EM (2017) Ibrutinib [monograph on the internet]. Available from: http://www.ema.europa.eu/ema/index.jsp?curl=pages/medicines/human/medicines/003791/human_med_001801.jsp&mid=WC0b01ac058001d124

AstraZeneca (2017a) Prescribing information of CALQUENCE (acalabrutinib) [monograph on the internet]. Available from: https://www.accessdata.fda.gov/drugsatfda_docs/label/2017/210259s000lbl.pdf

AstraZeneca (2017b) S FDA approves AstraZeneca's Calquence (acalabrutinib) for adult patients with previously-treated mantle cell lymphoma [monograph on the internet]. Available from: https://www.astrazeneca.com/media-centre/press-releases/2017/us-fda-approves-astrazenecas-calquence-acalabrutinib-for-adult-patients-with-previously-treated-mantle-cell-lymphoma-24102017.html

Barf T, Covey T, Izumi R, van de Kar B, Gulrajani M, van Lith B, van Hoek M, de Zwart E, Mittag D, Demont D, Verkaik S, Krantz F, Pearson PG, Ulrich R, Kaptein A (2017) Acalabrutinib (ACP-196): a covalent bruton tyrosine kinase inhibitor with a differentiated selectivity and in vivo potency profile. J Pharmacol Exp Ther 363:240–252

Bojarczuk K, Bobrowicz M, Dwojak M, Miazek N, Zapala P, Bunes A, Siernicka M, Rozanska M, Winiarska M (2015) B-cell receptor signaling in the pathogenesis of lymphoid malignancies. Blood Cells Mol Dis 55:255–265

Byrd JC, Harrington B, O'Brien S, Jones JA, Schuh A, Devereux S, Chaves J, Wierda WG, Awan FT, Brown JR, Hillmen P, Stephens DM, Ghia P, Barrientos JC, Pagel JM, Woyach J, Johnson D, Huang J, Wang X, Kaptein A, Lannutti BJ, Covey T, Fardis M, McGreivy J, Hamdy A, Rothbaum W, Izumi R, Diacovo TG, Johnson AJ, Furman RR (2016) Acalabrutinib (ACP-196) in relapsed chronic lymphocytic leukemia. N Engl J Med 374:323–332

ClinicalTrials.gov (2017) Acalabrutinib (ACP-196) clinical trials [monograph on the internet]. Available from: https://clinicaltrials.gov/ct2/results?cond=&term=acalabrutinib&cntry1=&state1=&Search=Search

Deng J, Isik E, Fernandes SM, Brown JR, Letai A, Davids MS (2017) Bruton's tyrosine kinase inhibition increases BCL-2 dependence and enhances sensitivity to venetoclax in chronic lymphocytic leukemia. Leukemia 31:2075–2084

FDA (2017) FDA grants accelerated approval to acalabrutinib for mantle cell lymphoma [monograph on the internet]. Available from: https://www.fda.gov/Drugs/InformationOnDrugs/ApprovedDrugs/ucm583106.htm

Golay J, Ubiali G, Introna M (2017) The specific Bruton tyrosine kinase inhibitor acalabrutinib (ACP-196) shows favorable in vitro activity against chronic lymphocytic leukemia B cells with CD20 antibodies. Haematologica 102:e400–e403

Harrington BK, Gardner HL, Izumi R, Hamdy A, Rothbaum W, Coombes KR, Covey T, Kaptein A, Gulrajani M, Van Lith B, Krejsa C, Coss CC, Russell DS, Zhang X, Urie BK, London CA, Byrd JC, Johnson AJ, Kisseberth WC (2016) Preclinical evaluation of the novel BTK inhibitor acalabrutinib in canine models of B-cell non-hodgkin lymphoma. PLoS ONE 11:e0159607

Herman SEM, Montraveta A, Niemann CU, Mora-Jensen H, Gulrajani M, Krantz F, Mantel R, Smith LL, McClanahan F, Harrington BK, Colomer D, Covey T, Byrd JC, Izumi R, Kaptein A, Ulrich R, Johnson AJ, Lannutti BJ, Wiestner A, Woyach JA (2017) The Bruton tyrosine kinase (BTK) inhibitor acalabrutinib demonstrates potent on-target effects and efficacy in two mouse models of chronic lymphocytic Leukemia. Clin Cancer Res 23:2831–2841

Kapoor P, Ansell SM, Fonseca R, Chanan-Khan A, Kyle RA, Kumar SK, Mikhael JR, Witzig TE, Mauermann M, Dispenzieri A, Ailawadhi S, Stewart AK, Lacy MQ, Thompson CA, Buadi FK, Dingli D, Morice WG, Go RS, Jevremovic D, Sher T, King RL, Braggio E, Novak A, Roy V, Ketterling RP, Greipp PT, Grogan M, Micallef IN, Bergsagel PL, Colgan JP, Leung N, Gonsalves WI, Lin Y, Inwards DJ, Hayman SR, Nowakowski GS, Johnston PB, Russell SJ, Markovic SN, Zeldenrust SR, Hwa YL, Lust JA, Porrata LF, Habermann TM, Rajkumar SV, Gertz MA, Reeder CB (2017) Diagnosis and Management of Waldenstrom Macroglobuline- mia: mayo stratification of macroglobulinemia and risk-adapted therapy (mSMART) guidelines 2016. JAMA Oncol 3:1257–1265

Martin P, Maddocks K, Leonard JP, Ruan J, Goy A, Wagner-Johnston N, Rule S, Advani R, Iberri D, Phillips T, Spurgeon S, Kozin E, Noto K, Chen Z, Jurczak W, Auer R, Chmielowska E, Stilgenbauer S, Bloehdorn J, Portell C, Williams ME, Dreyling M, Barr PM, Chen-Kiang S, DiLiberto M, Furman RR, Blum KA (2016) Postibrutinib outcomes in patients with mantle cell lymphoma. Blood 127:1559–1663

Niemann CU, Mora-Jensen HI, Dadashian EL, Krantz F, Covey T, Chen SS, Chiorazzi N, Izumi R, Ulrich R, Lannutti BJ, Wiestner A, Herman SEM (2017) Combined BTK and PI3Kdelta inhibition with acalabrutinib and ACP-319 improves survival and tumor control in CLL mouse model. Clin Cancer Res 23:5814–5823

Noy A, de Vos S, Thieblemont C, Martin P, Flowers CR, Morschhauser F, Collins GP, Ma S, Coleman M, Peles S, Smith S, Barrientos JC, Smith A, Munneke B, Dimery I, Beaupre DM, Chen R (2017) Targeting Bruton tyrosine kinase with ibrutinib in relapsed/refractory marginal zone lymphoma. Blood 129:2224–2232

Patel VK, Lamothe B, Ayres ML, Gay J, Cheung J, Balakrishnan K, Ivan C, Morse J, Nelson M, Keating MJ, Wierda WG, Marszalek JR, Gandhi V (2017) Pharmacodynamics and proteomic analysis of acalabrutinib therapy: Similarity of on-target effects to ibrutinib and rationale for combination therapy. Leukemia

Robak P, Robak T (2017) Novel synthetic drugs currently in clinical development for chronic lymphocytic leukemia. Expert Opin Investig Drugs 26:1249–1265

Thompson PA, Burger JA (2017) Bruton's tyrosine kinase inhibitors: first and second generation agents for patients with Chronic Lymphocytic Leukemia (CLL). Expert Opin Investig Drugs 1–12

Vidal-Crespo A, Rodriguez V, Matas-Cespedes A, Lee E, Rivas-Delgado A, Gine E, Navarro A, Bea S, Campo E, Lopez-Guillermo A, Lopez-Guerra M, Roue G, Colomer D, Perez-Galan P (2017) The Bruton tyrosine kinase inhibitor CC-292 shows activity in mantle cell lymphoma and synergizes with lenalidomide and NIK inhibitors depending on nuclear factor-kappaB mutational status. Haematologica 102:e447–e451

Walter HS, Rule SA, Dyer MJ, Karlin L, Jones C, Cazin B, Quittet P, Shah N, Hutchinson CV, Honda H, Duffy K, Birkett J, Jamieson V, Courtenay-Luck N, Yoshizawa T, Sharpe J, Ohno T, Abe S, Nishimura A, Cartron G, Morschhauser F, Fegan C, Salles G (2016) A phase 1 clinical trial of the selective BTK inhibitor ONO/GS-4059 in relapsed and refractory mature B-cell malignancies. Blood 127:411–419

Wu J, Liu C, Tsui ST, Liu D (2016a) Second-generation inhibitors of Bruton tyrosine kinase. J Hematol Oncol 9:80

Wu J, Zhang M, Liu D (2016b) Acalabrutinib (ACP-196): a selective second-generation BTK inhibitor. J Hematol Oncol 9:21

Wu J, Zhang M, Liu D (2017) Bruton tyrosine kinase inhibitor ONO/GS-4059: from bench to bedside. Oncotarget 8:7201–7207